AF904801

ANTIBODY ENGINEERING

Edited by **Thomas Böldicke**

Antibody Engineering
http://dx.doi.org/10.5772/65238
Edited by Thomas Böldicke

Contributors

Theam Soon Lim, Chia Chiu Lim, Teiji Sawa, Taizo Uda, Oliver Backhaus, Yoshiro Hanyu, Mieko Kato, Adalbert Krawczyk, Philipp Diebolder, Chiuan Herng Leow, Qin Cheng, Katja Fischer, James McCarthy, Jan Gettemans, Anneleen Steels, Laurence Bertier, Atis Chakrabarti, Lavanya Suneetha, Sujai Suneetha, Prasanna Marsakatla, Supriya Suneetha, Ana Maria Moro, Lilian Rumi Tsuruta, Mariana Lopes Dos Santos, Karolina Vorcakova, Juraj Pec, Tatiana Pecova, Klara Martinaskova

Published by InTech
Janeza Trdine 9, 51000 Rijeka, Croatia

© The Editor(s) and the Author(s) 2018
The moral rights of the editor(s) and the author(s) have been asserted.
All rights to the book as a whole are reserved by InTech. The book as a whole (compilation) cannot be reproduced, distributed or used for commercial or non-commercial purposes without InTech's written permission. Enquiries concerning the use of the book should be directed to InTech's rights and permissions department (permissions@intechopen.com).
Violations are liable to prosecution under the governing Copyright Law.

Individual chapters of this publication are distributed under the terms of the Creative Commons Attribution 3.0 Unported License which permits commercial use, distribution and reproduction of the individual chapters, provided the original author(s) and source publication are appropriately acknowledged. More details and guidelines concerning content reuse and adaptation can be found at http://www.intechopen.com/copyright-policy.html.

Notice

Statements and opinions expressed in the chapters are these of the individual contributors and not necessarily those of the editors or publisher. No responsibility is accepted for the accuracy of information contained in the published chapters. The publisher assumes no responsibility for any damage or injury to persons or property arising out of the use of any materials, instructions, methods or ideas contained in the book.

Publishing Process Manager Iva Simcic
Technical Editor SPi Global
Cover InTech Design team

First published February, 2018
Printed in Croatia
Legal deposit, Croatia: National and University Library in Zagreb

Additional hard copies can be obtained from orders@intechopen.com

Antibody Engineering , Edited by Thomas Böldicke
p. cm.
Print ISBN 978-953-51-3825-9
Online ISBN 978-953-51-3826-6

We are IntechOpen, the first native scientific publisher of Open Access books

3,300+
Open access books available

107,000+
International authors and editors

113M+
Downloads

151
Countries delivered to

Our authors are among the
Top 1%
most cited scientists

12.2%
Contributors from top 500 universities

WEB OF SCIENCE™

Selection of our books indexed in the Book Citation Index
in Web of Science™ Core Collection (BKCI)

Interested in publishing with us?
Contact book.department@intechopen.com

Numbers displayed above are based on latest data collected.
For more information visit www.intechopen.com

For EU product safety concerns:
IN TECH d.o.o., Prolaz Marije Krucifikse Kozulić 3, 51000 Rijeka, Croatia,
info@intechopen.com or visit our website at intechopen.com.

Meet the editor

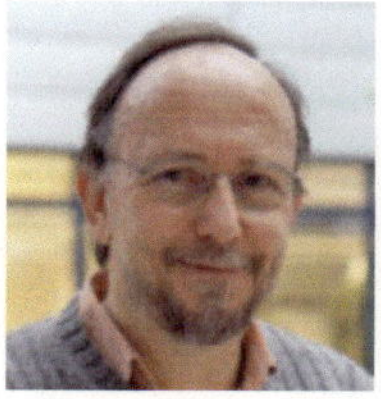

Thomas Böldicke received his PhD 1982 at the Max-Planck-Institut of Molecular Genetics, Berlin. He started his carrier as post doc at the German Research Centre for Biotechnology (GBF, Brunswick) in the Department of Genetics and Cell Biology by John Collins. Now he is senior scientist at the Helmholtz Centre for Infection Research (HZI, former GBF) and project leader intrabodies. 2011 he qualified as a professor in molecular biology and cell biology at the Technical University of Braunschweig, Germany. He is an expert in generating mouse and human hybridomas and in selecting and modifying recombinant antibodies. In the last decade he focused on the construction and characterization of intracellular antibodies. He has published 35 manuscripts.

Contents

Preface

Antibodies are most important molecules for therapy, diagnosis, and biological and medical research. For about 40 years, the hybridoma technology is used to generate mouse antibodies with high affinities. However, antibodies against nonimmunogenic, toxic, self-antigens and human/mouse cross-reactive epitopes cannot be obtained by this classical technique. Additionally, the mouse monoclonal antibodies elicit a strong immune response when applied in patients.

A breakthrough to solve these problems was the development of human antibody repertoires and *in vitro* antibody selection methods in the beginning of the nineties. In the following years, it was demonstrated that the generation of specific antibodies by the immune system could be imitated successfully *in vitro*. The development of antibodies, particularly human antibodies, could be dramatically improved. The human antibody repertoires and corresponding *in vitro* selection techniques are now used to generate and modify human antibodies against virtually every protein and desired epitope or conformation. This is the power and tasks of antibody engineering.

The most frequently *in vitro*–selected recombinant antibody format is the scFv, which can be converted into full-length antibodies or scFv-Fc proteins, both of which have similar characteristics. Engineering of the Fc region increases the half-life and improves the affinity of Fc domains for their receptors on immune effector cells or to complement. For specific applications, different antibody formats such as bispecific antibodies, minibodies, or diabodies can be generated. Furthermore, very stable single domain antibodies comprising only the variable domain of the heavy chain can be selected by phage display from camel- or shark-derived repertoires.

The first approved recombinant therapeutic antibodies were chimeric or humanized variants of mouse hybridoma antibodies. Today, fully human antibodies are selected from human antibody repertoires mainly against antigens involved in infectious diseases and cancer. However, the number of new mAbs validating new therapeutic targets is limited because therapeutic target discovery is very laborious. Affinity maturation of selected clones is important when low-affinity clones are selected from naive or synthetic libraries where the antibody genes have not been subjected to somatic hypermutation in contrast to immune libraries. New promising affinity maturation approaches include mammalian cell surface display of antibodies coupled with somatic hypermutation mediated by activation-induced cytidine deaminase (AID). Furthermore, affinity maturation based on incorporation of a random repertoire of microchip-synthesized CDRs into a known antibody framework has recently been demonstrated. However, affinity maturation based on introduction of random or site-directed mutations can be time-consuming because secondary libraries must be built up and screened.

By the end of 2016, over 50 fully human antibodies had been approved by the US Food and Drug Administration (FDA) or European Medicines Agency (EMA). Basically, they were selected by phage display or from transgenic mice comprising a large part of the human germ line antibody repertoire. Regarding phage display selection, most phase three and approved recombinant antibodies were selected from naïve single pot antibody libraries and only a very few were selected from synthetic or semisynthetic libraries. Besides phage display and yeast display, other *in vitro* display techniques have been established such as mRNA display, DNA display, bacterial display, mammalian cell surface display, and ribosomal display. In the future, it remains to be seen if the amount of new approved therapeutic antibodies from synthetic libraries as well as alternative *in vitro* display techniques will increase.

In addition to extracellular targeting of antigens, intracellular proteins can be targeted by intracellular antibodies (intrabodies), too. These intrabodies are essential to trace *in vivo* trafficking of proteins and to knock down proteins for revelation of protein functions. Due to their high specificity, they are able to target posttranslational modifications, interaction regions, conformers, splice variants, and isoforms without off target effects, which are a major problem of RNAi-mediated gene silencing. Some intrabodies have therapeutic potential against viral infections, brain diseases, or cancer. Anticancer intrabodies have been evaluated in xenograft tumor mouse models. Numerous preclinical studies and a smaller number of clinical trials have been investigated using therapeuticmRNA molecules that deliver the genetic information of genes and maybe this technique can be transferred to the delivery of intrabody mRNA in the future.

Antibodies against conformers of a protein are difficult to generate by the hybridoma technique because maintaining of a specific conformation in an immunized animal is difficult. But it can be done by *in vitro* selection of antibodies. Antibodies recognizing different conformers of signaling proteins are important to study cell signaling. In addition, for cancer treatment, antibodies that recognize active cell surface receptor conformers as well as antibodies that have the capability to differentiate cancer cells into nonmalignant cells are very valuable for the future. Finally, it has to be mentioned that new promising synthetic binders comprising variable non–immunoglobulin-binding sites embedded in a nonimmunoglobulin framework have been selected by the *in vitro* display systems generally used for selection of recombinant antibodies. For example, nonimmunoglobulin scaffolds are ankyrin repeat protein (DARPin), monobody, affibody, Kunitz domain, and anticalin. The main advantage is their stability. However, until now, no nonimmunoglobulin binder has been approved for application in patients.

This new antibody engineering book comprises current techniques to select and improve recombinant antibodies. Furthermore, single-domain antibodies, the problems of structural diversity of antibodies, unwanted immune reactions of recombinant antibodies, and bioinformatic approaches are demonstrated and discussed. The topics are presented by experts in the field of antibody engineering and are important for live science researchers and students and particularly for researches working with recombinant antibodies. A description of individual chapters is as follows:

Chapter 1 by O Backhauscomprises the generation of natural antibody diversity, which helps to understand the strategies of constructing immune, naive, and synthetic libraries. Construction of antibody libraries as well as *in vitro* and *in vivo* affinity maturation and de novo synthesis of antibody genes is described in **Chapter 2** by CC Lim et al. **Chapter 3** by LR Tsuruta et al. focuses on all known *in vitro* display techniques and antibody humanization by chain shuffling. **Chapter 4** by P Diebolder and A Krawczyk provides a detailed protocol for the selection of antiviral human antibodies from combinatorial immune phage display libraries. M Kato and Y Hanju compare in **Chapter 5** display screening with colony assays for antibody library screening. **Chapter 6** by T Sawa et al. deals with antibody-based immunotherapy against bacterial infections, particularly the construction of an scFv against PcrV, the cap structure in the translocational needle of the type III secretory apparatus of *P. aeruginosa.* The aimis to block bacterial toxin translocation. The following **Chapter 7** by A Chakrabarti describes purification of monoclonal antibodies by size exclusion chromatography. Two following chapters, **Chapters 8 and 9** by CH Leow et al. and A Steels et al., respectively, focus on the application and mechanism of single-domain antibodies, the most stable antibody format. **Chapter 10** by E Hifumi et al. describes isolation of the monomolecular structure of the constant region of a catalytic light chain.**Chapter 11** by V Karolina et al. comprises a review about immune-mediated skin reactions of anti-TNF alpha recombinant antibodies. Finally, **Chapter 12** by L Suneetha et al.demonstrates bioinformatic approaches for identification of pathogen-derived peptides involved in infectious diseases and discuss their potential as targets to elicit recombinant antibodies.

Antibody engineering facilitates the generation and modification of human antibodies against therapeutic antigens. Selected single clones can be modified and improved by engineering the variable binding domains and the Fc domains in the case of a full length antibody. New optimized recombinant antibodies are in development and will have extensive applications in the fields of immunology, biotechnology, diagnostics, and therapeutic medicine.

I want to express my thanks to the authors for very good collaboration, Ms. Iva Simcic, InTech's Publishing Process Manager for coordination through the entire book processing, my students for fruitful discussions, and Prof. Wulf Blankenfeldt for supporting my editorial work.

Thomas Böldicke
Helmholtz-Centre for Infection Research
Structure and Function of Proteins
Braunschweig, Germany

Chapter 1

Generation of Antibody Diversity

Oliver Backhaus

Additional information is available at the end of the chapter

http://dx.doi.org/10.5772/intechopen.72818

Abstract

Because of the huge diversity, the immunoglobulin repertoire cannot be encoded by static genes, which would explode the genomic capacity comprising about 20,000–25,000 human genes. The immunoglobulin repertoire is provided by the process of somatic germ line recombination, which is the only controlled alteration of the genomic DNA after meiosis. It takes place in mammalian B lymphocyte (B cells) precursors in the bone marrow. The genome germ line sequence of undeveloped B cells is organized in gene segments and compromise V (variable), D (diversity), and J (joining) gene segments constituting the variable domain of the heavy chain and only V and J genes for building up the variable domain of the light chain. The rearrangement of the variable region follows a strict order. The following processes that participate in the generation of antibody diversity were summarized—allelic, combinational, and junctional diversity, pairing of IgH and IgL, and receptor editing—which all together produce the primary antigen repertoire (pre-antigen stimulation). When a B cell encounters a foreign antigen, affinity maturation and class switch are induced. Thereby the antibody repertoire increases. The resulting secondary immunoglobulin repertoire reveals in humans at least 10^{11} specificities for different antigens.

Keywords: antibody diversity, somatic recombination, somatic hypermutation, class-switch recombination, allelic exclusion, B-cell receptor editing, pairing of VH and VL, germinal center

1. Introduction

The immune system is a complex system, comprising different organs and many specialized cell types, which are carrying out their development, maturation, and pathogen recognition at various sides in the body. The immune system has two major approaches to recognize and attack pathogens. The first is the innate immunity followed by the delayed adaptive immune response, based on specific antigen recognition receptors. The innate immune system is

INTECH
open science | open minds

© 2018 The Author(s). Licensee InTech. This chapter is distributed under the terms of the Creative Commons Attribution License (http://creativecommons.org/licenses/by/3.0), which permits unrestricted use, distribution, and reproduction in any medium, provided the original work is properly cited. (cc) BY

nonspecific and uses general pathogen recognition mechanisms, through pathogen-associated molecular patterns (PAMPs) recognized by cell surface or intracellular pattern recognition receptors (PRRs), such as toll-like receptors or NOD-like receptors (NLRs) and RIG-I-like receptors (RLRs) [1]. Cell types of the innate immunity are monocytes/macrophages, dendritic cells, mast cells, natural killer cells, granulocytes, B1 cells, and innate lymphoid cells (ILCs). Although it lacks specificity, it can react immediately on the invading pathogens and activates the adaptive immune system by presentation of the foreign antigen peptides.

The adaptive immune system needs to be activated and primed by the antigen and therefore acts delayed from the initial pathogen attack. It is based mainly on two cell types, the B cell and the T cell. Both cell types express specific receptors on their cell surface for pathogen recognition. Many different B- and T-cell clones exist in parallel inside the body, and each has a different receptor specificity to the antigen. These receptors were called B-cell receptor (BCR) and T-cell receptor (TCR). It is remarkable that despite the relatively small genome size of approximately 20,000–25,000 human genes [2, 3], the human body can produce an antibody repertoire which can recognize almost every possible antigenic structure. Of course, this cannot be achieved by encoding the antigen receptor specificity directly in the genome sequence.

The huge B-cell diversity is generated by a complex multistep process, starting in the bone marrow and ending up in the peripheral lymphoid tissues, such as lymph nodes, spleen, or mucosal lymphoid tissue. In the maturation of functional BCR or TCR, the antigen receptor genes were rearranged from many different possible gene segments to form a full receptor. In each step, the receptor is tested for functionality and excluded when it reveals self-antigen reactivity in order to prevent autoimmunity and making the immune system self-tolerant.

The B-cell maturation occurs inside the bone marrow before the B cells migrate to peripheral lymphoid tissues. On the contrary to B cells, T-cell progenitors migrate to the thymus to differentiate and to mature. After their maturation, B and T cells meet again in lymph nodes. In the germinal centers of the lymph node, antigens were presented to the B cells through antigen-presenting cells, particularly through follicular dendritic cells (FDC). In response to a foreign pathogen, B cells with the highest antigen affinity were selected from a pool of different BCR clones. This process is organized in a form of a repetitive cycle inside of the dark and light zone of a germinal center of the lymph node and is known as the cyclic reentry model (**Figure 4**).

An essential part of the cycle is the BCR affinity maturation of the B cells. It begins with the tight controlled somatic hypermutation (SHM), particularly in the variable regions of the light and heavy chain of the antigen receptor and is only active in the dark zone of the germinal center. This process creates BCRs with higher affinity, whereby the mutations which produced very low or nonfunctional receptors were excluded. Finally, high-affinity B cells differentiate either into plasma cells, which start to produce secreted antibodies with the same specificity as the BCR, or they differentiate into memory cells, conferring lifelong immunity.

This chapter will discuss in detail the different steps and processes, which contribute to the high diversity of B cells. Many steps are similar for the generation of T-cell receptor diversity and were not covered by this article.

http://dx.doi.org/10.5772/intechopen.72818

2. The primary antibody repertoire

2.1. Combinatorial diversity of immunoglobulins

Before immature naive B cells encounter a foreign antigen, their genomic sequence is rearranged by a well-controlled process, called somatic DNA recombination. This process is unique in lymphocytes, and except of the meiosis in the gametes, this is the only DNA recombination of somatic cells [4]. Before B cells leave the bone marrow to the secondary lymphatic organs, somatic DNA recombination takes place. The sum of all B lymphocytes in an individuum, producing different antibodies with different specificities and affinities, is designated as the antibody repertoire. In humans, the antibody repertoire consists of at least 10^{11} specificities [4]. The number varies and is limited by the total number of B cells and encountered antigens of an individuum. The immunoglobulin loci contain gene fragments to build up all immunoglobulin variable domains of the heavy and light chain. The different immunoglobulin loci are located on different chromosomes (Chr), the heavy chain on Chr14, the kappa light chain on Chr2, and the lambda light chain on Chr22. In contrast to the light chain loci, the heavy chain locus has several constant regions; each represents a different immunoglobulin isotype, e.g., IgM, IgD, IgG1, Ig2a, IgG2b, IgG3, IgE, and IgA in mice. The gene segments consist of different germ line sequences. For example, the variable gene locus of the heavy chain comprises 38–46 genes, which varies between individuals.

Besides different germ line segments, there exist a relative large number of pseudogenes of which some can undergo recombination leading to a nonfunctional variable region. An overview of the number of gene segments in the respective gene locus is given in **Table 1** (slightly modified from IMGT [5]).

The light chain loci have only variable (V) and joining (J) gene segments, whereby the heavy chain locus additionally has a diversity (D) gene segment, which lay between the V and J genes of the heavy chain variable region. One of each gene segment is randomly selected by the RAG1/RAG2 recombinase and joined together to form the variable region (**Figure 2c**) as shown as example with the variable region of the λ light chain. The recombination steps of the V region follow a strict order. The variable light chain recombines first with the V-J segments. Afterward the constant (C) domain is joined through RNA splicing of the primary RNA to the variable region. The construction of the V region of the heavy chain begins with

				Immunoglobulin (Ig) gene segments			
Gene locus	**Ig chain**	**Chromosomal location**	**Locus size (kb)**	**Variable (V)**	**Diversity (D)**	**Joining (J)**	**Constant (C)**
IGH	Heavy chain	14q32.33	1250	38–46	23	6	9
IGK	κ Light chain	2p11.2	1820[1]	34–38	0	5	1
IGL	λ Light chain	22q11.2	1050	29–33	0	4–5	4–5

[1]In one known haplotype, the locus size is reduced to 500 kb comprising only 17–19 IGκV genes.

Table 1. Number of functional human immunoglobulin gene segments in the heavy and light chain locus.

the recombination of the D and the J gene; then the V gene is joined to the DJ segment. Finally, the C domain is joined through RNA splicing of the primary RNA. **Figure 1** gives an overview of the respective steps of the V(D)J recombination for construction of the V region of the heavy chain immunoglobulin.

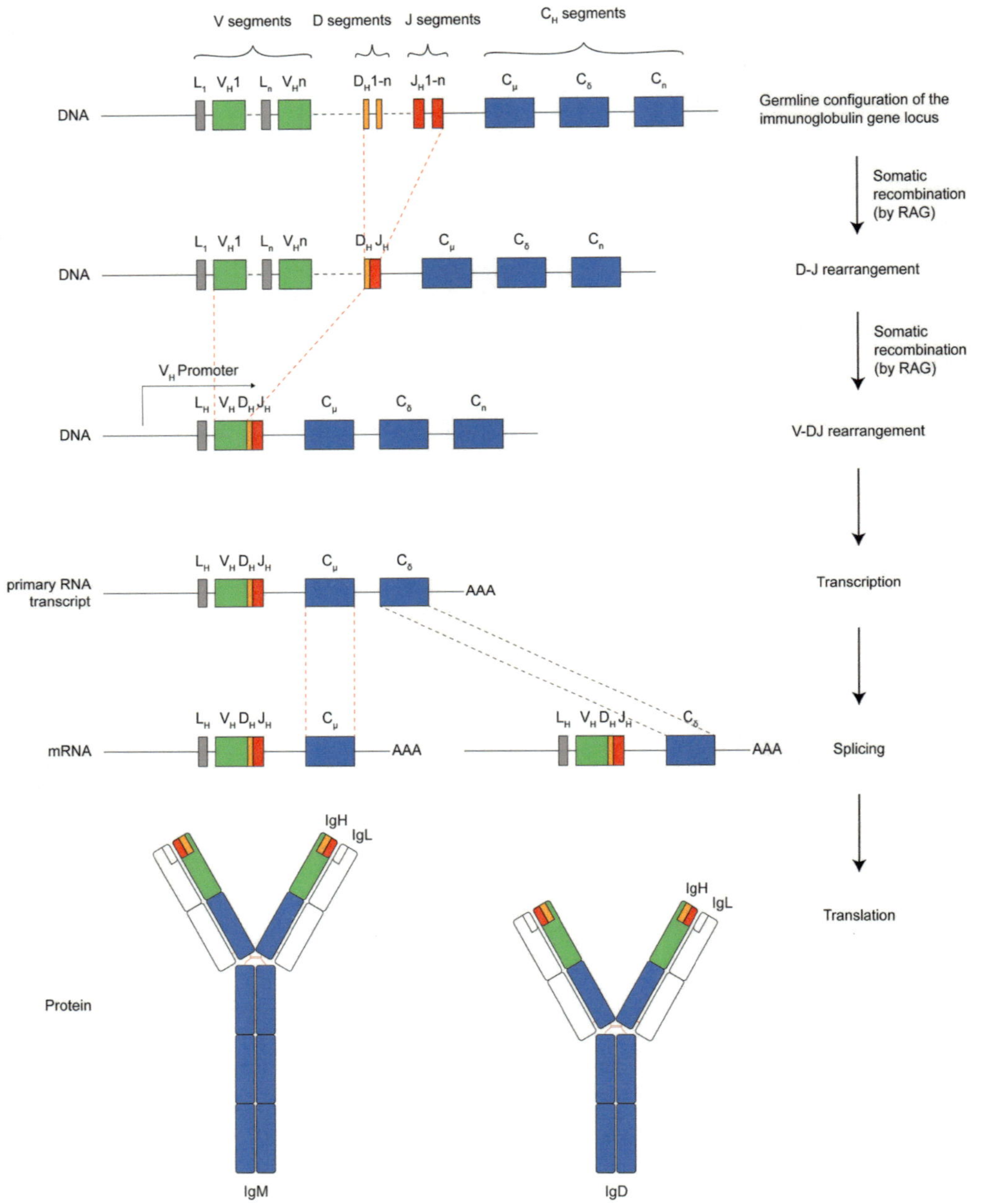

Figure 1. *V(D)J recombination of the heavy chain immunoglobulin (IgH) from germ line gene segments.* The immunoglobulin locus is organized in gene segments: the variable (V), diversity (D), and joining (J) and constant (C) gene segment. The variable (V) region comprising the V, D, and J gene segments is generated by random recombination of these sequences. L = leader sequence.

The figure illustrates the somatic recombination event of the antibody heavy chain in the bone marrow of developing B cells. At first, one of the D and J segments is randomly chosen and rearranged. In the following step, one of the variable gene segments is joined to form the V-D-J variable region. This process is catalyzed by the recombination activating gene 1/recombination activating gene 2 (RAG1/RAG2) recombinase. In the immature B cells in the bone marrow, the variable region is transcribed with the constant mu (C_μ) and the constant gamma (C_δ) chain, which produces two different mRNAs through alternative splicing which are finally translated into either IgM or IgD immunoglobulin.

The guided fashion of the recombination is mediated by recombinase signaling sequences (RSSs). The RSS is always directly adjacent to the coding region of the gene segments (**Figure 2A**). The nucleotide structure of the RSS is well defined and conserved (**Figure 2B**). A heptamer of seven conserved nucleotides is linked with a non-conserved linker sequence to a conserved nine-nucleotide nonamer [6–8]. The linker sequence is either 12 or 23 nucleotides long, and only a RSS with a 12 bp linker sequence can recombine with a 23 bp linker RSS, which is called the 12/23 rule. With the 12/23 rule, only corresponding gene segments can recombine. For instance, the V gene segments of the lambda light chain are always flanked downstream by a 23 bp RSS, and the genes of the J segments of the lambda light chain are always flanked upstream by a 12 bp RSS to the coding sequence. For the kappa light chain, it is the other way around, with the 12 bp RSS at the end of the V gene and the 23 bp RSS upstream of the coding sequence of the J gene. The heavy chain diversity gene segment is flanked by a 12 bp linker RSS from both sides and the V gene and the J gene segments with a 23 bp linker RSS upstream of the coding sequence, respectively. This allows only recombination in the desired V-D-J orientation, whereby during the recombination, the sequence between the chosen genes is excised and discarded. **Figure 2** shows the position and structure of recombinase signal sequences (RSSs) at the V, J, and D gene segments and RSS-guided RAG-dependent V-J rearrangement of the variable domain of the λ chain.

2.2. Junctional diversity of immunoglobulins

During V(D)J recombination the diversity of immunoglobulins is further increased by incorporation of additional nucleotides between the junctions of the V, D, and J gene segment of the heavy and V and J gene segment of the light chain. Especially the diversity of the CDR3 (complementarity-determining region), which has a huge influence on the antigen binding [9, 10], is affected with high frequency by this process, because of its position between the V and J gene segments in the heavy chain and between the V and J gene segments in the light chain. The CDR1 and CDR2 loops are not affected by junctional diversity, because of their position in the V gene segment of the heavy and light chain.

When two gene segments guided by the recombinase signaling sequences (RSSs) and the RAG1/RAG2 complex were brought together, the RAG complex excises the intervening DNA and produces short hairpins on both sides of the immunoglobulin gene segments (**Figure 3**). Then the Artemis/DNA-dependent protein kinase (DNA-PK) complex is recruited and cuts the DNA strand randomly at the site of the hairpin of both ends of the DNA strands [11–13]. This can produce palindromic DNA sequences at the side of the gene segment joint, and these nucleotides are called P nucleotides, because of its palindrome

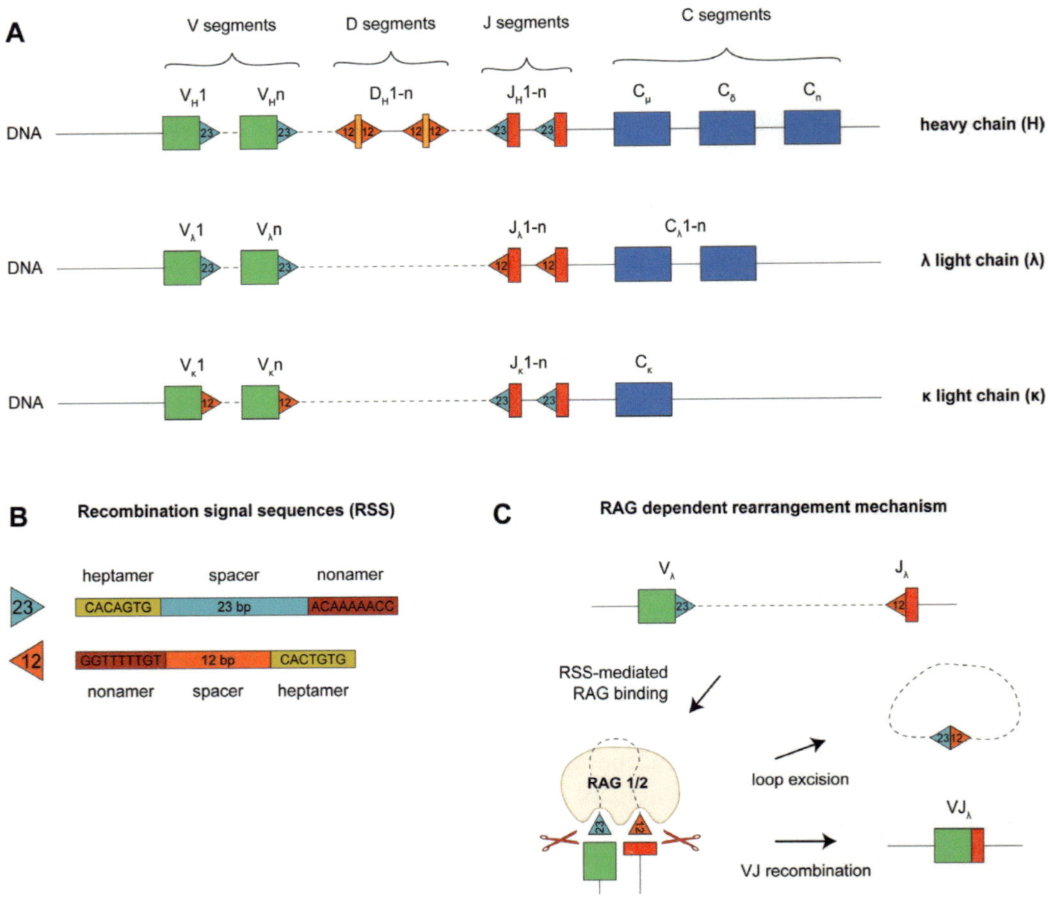

Figure 2. *Position and structure of recombinase signal sequences (RSSs) at the V, D, and J gene segments and RSS-guided RAG-dependent V-J λ rearrangement* (**A**). Schematic representation of the position and orientation of the different recombinase signal sequences (RSSs) at the V (variable), D (diversity), and J (joining) gene segments of the heavy (H) and of Vλ, Vκ, Jλ, and Jκ of the lambda (λ) and kappa (κ) locus. (**B**) Conserved nucleotide sequences of the two different RSSs. In each case, a conserved heptamer sequence and a conserved nonamer sequence encompass a non-conserved spacer sequence. Two different RSSs exist, which have either a 23 base pair (bp) spacer or a 12 base pair spacer. (**C**) The RAG1/RAG2 (recombination activating gene)-dependent rearrangement of the V region (here demonstrated with the variable domain of the λ chain) is mediated through a guided fashion by recombinase signal sequences (RSSs). The RAG1/RAG2 complex always binds a 23 bp spacer RSS together with a 12 bp spacer RSS and then mediates DNA cleavage between each gene segment (here Vλ and Jλ) and its heptamer. The sequence between the chosen genes are excised and discarded. The process described is called deletional joining and occurs when the two gene segments to be fused are in the same transcriptional orientation. However, in some instances, the two segments to be fused are in opposite transcriptional orientations in the germ line (inversional joining).

nature. Next, the terminal deoxynucleotidyl-transferase (TdT) adds further nucleotides at the single-stranded P nucleotide stretch [14]. The nucleotides were added randomly without any DNA template; hence they are called N nucleotides (non-template). After addition of a couple of N nucleotides, some base pairs between both single-stranded DNA stretches and the mismatched nucleotides were removed by an exonuclease; in this process the Artemis might be involved. The remaining gaps were filled by a DNA polymerase, and finally both

http://dx.doi.org/10.5772/intechopen.72818

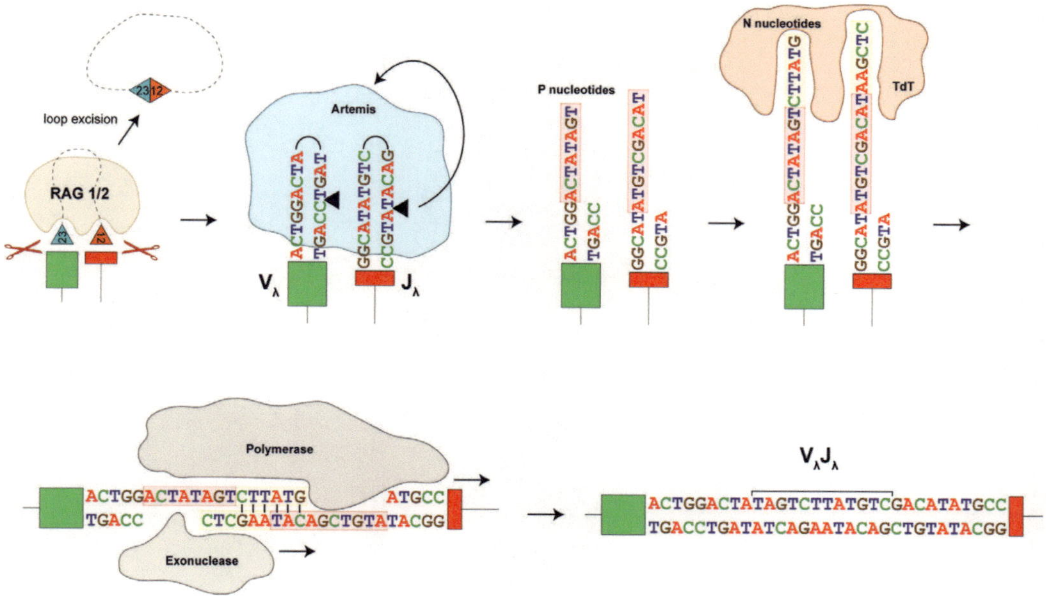

Figure 3. *Junctional diversity is produced by incorporation of additional nucleotides between the junctions of immunoglobulin germ line gene segments of the variable region.* After the RAG1/RAG2 (recombination activating gene) complex has removed the intervening DNA between two gene segments, in this case the V_λ and J_λ gene segment of the light chain, short hairpins were formed at both DNA blunted ends. Next, the Artemis is recruited and catalyzes a random single-stranded break at both DNA strands. This can produce in many cases a palindromic DNA sequence. These nucleotides are designated as P nucleotides. The single-stranded DNA is further extended by the addition of random nucleotides by the enzyme terminal deoxynucleotidyl-transferase (TdT). These nucleotides were named N nucleotides, because they are added without a DNA template. Some nucleotides at both single-stranded stretches match and can form hydrogen bonds (black lines). The mismatched DNA bases were removed by an exonuclease, and the remaining gaps were filled by a DNA polymerase and both DNA strands ligated. Underlined is the inserted sequence between the V_λ and J_λ gene segment.

DNA strands were joined together by the DNA ligase IV/X-ray repair cross-complementing protein 4 (XRCC4) complex.

The presence of N nucleotides is not equally distributed in the light and heavy chain [4]. The light chain has a remarkable lower appearance of N nucleotides in comparison to the heavy chain. The reason for this difference is the expression pattern of the terminal deoxynucleotidyl-transferase, which is much higher when the heavy chain is rearranged and already lower when subsequently the light chain is rearranged. The incorporation of additional nucleotides has not only beneficial effects, of cause the affinity of the antibody can be changed dramatically, but also missense mutations can be produced by violating the 3 bp codon structure, which can produce a frameshift in the coding sequence (non-productive rearrangements, see **Figure 3**).

2.3. Antibody diversity is further expanded by allelic exclusion, B-cell receptor editing, and pairing of VH and VL

In most cases, only one functional allele of an immunoglobulin gene is expressed. The other gene is transcripted in parallel, but usually only one of them can assemble into a functional

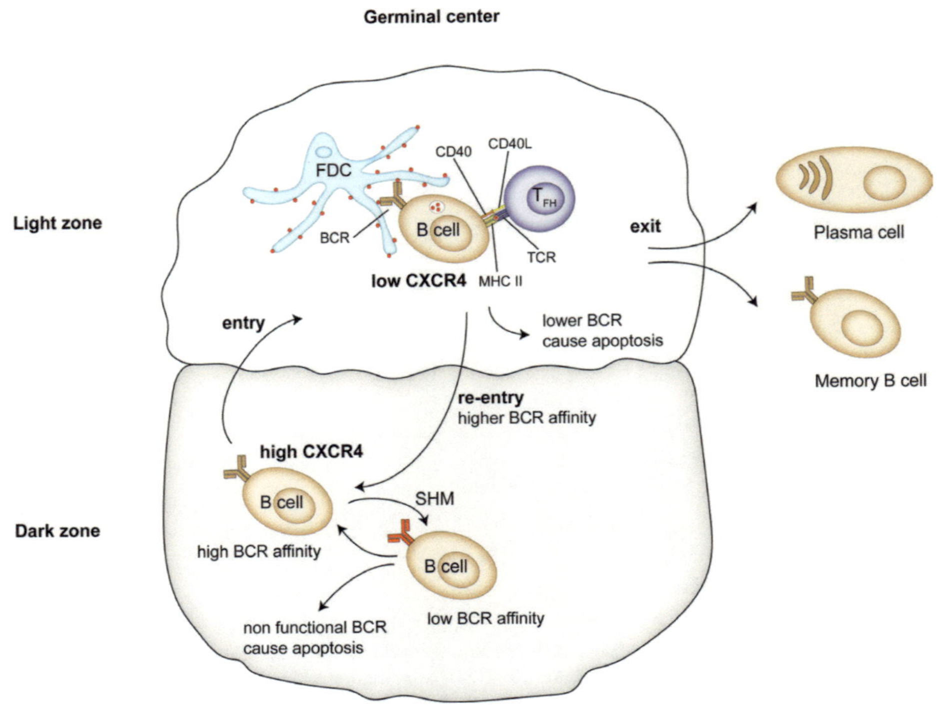

Figure 4. *Positive selection of high-affinity B cells in the lymph node germinal center.* B cells progress from the dark to the light zone. B cells in the dark zone highly express the chemokine receptor C-X-C chemokine receptor type 4 (CXCR4) and are undergoing somatic hypermutation of their variable-region genes. When they enter the light zone, CXCR4 expression is reduced. In the light zone, follicular dendritic cells (FDCs) present foreign antigens on their cell surface. B-cell clones, which have B-cell receptors (BCRs) with affinity to the antigen, can bind to it. The antigen/BCR complex is processed, and antigen peptides were presented through the MHC II for T-cell recognition. T_{FH} bind to the antigen presented on MHC II via its T-cell receptor and the B cell receives survival and proliferation signals through CD40-CD40L interaction and cytokines secreted by the corresponding T cells. B cell clones with low affinity die by apoptosis. B-cell clones which receive T_{FH} stimulation reenter the dark zone and upregulate CXCR4 expression. The affinity of the BCR is further increased by additional rounds of SHM, whereby B cells producing nonfunctional BCRs initiate apoptosis. B cells can repeat the cyclic affinity maturation until they express high-affinity BCR and finally leave the light zone for differentiation into antibody producing plasma cells. When B cells differentiate into plasma cells, they also switch their immunoglobulin class. Some B cells with lower affinity as plasma cells preferentially differentiate into memory B cells.

B-cell receptor (BCR) [15]. **Allelic exclusion** means that only clonally identical BCRs were expressed on the B-cell surface and not two different versions from two different alleles. In diploid organisms, such as mammals, two different copies of a gene are on a chromosome. For the immunoglobulin gene loci, only one allele is expressed on the B-cell surface. When V(D)J rearrangement did not produce a functional BCR, the second allele will be activated and tested. When this will also fail, the B cell will die by apoptosis; this process is called clonal deletion. The choice of two different immunoglobulin alleles further increases the antibody diversity [16].

The exact mechanism of allelic exclusion is not completely understood by now, but in general some important steps are known. During pre-B-cell development when the heavy and light chain rearrangement takes place in the bone marrow; only one allele is chosen for recombination, whereas the other will be silenced. When a functional heavy chain is produced, RAG1/RAG2 recombinase expression will be decreased, and RAG1/RAG2 is targeted for degradation [4]. Furthermore, the RAG1/RAG2 recombinase access to the heavy chain loci will be decreased. Later, when the light chain is rearranged, the prevented access to the heavy chain loci is sustained, and no further rearrangement or change of allele activity can occur.

Although some essential steps in the mechanism are known, the precise mechanism is still unknown and under controversial discussion [16].

When the production of a functional B-cell receptor fails, another immunoglobulin allele is tested, or the BCR could undergo additional rounds of V(D)J recombination, until a functional receptor will be produced or no further V, D, and J genes for recombination were available. Usually, V(D)J recombination ends when a functional BCR is produced. When a functional BCR exhibits reactivity against antigens of the own body (self-reactivity), a specialized mechanism attempts to rescue the functional BCR and tries to edit the self-reactive B-cell receptor. This mechanism is called **receptor editing** and is one of the key checkpoints and rescue mechanisms to ensure self-tolerance and to escape clonal deletion.

The idea of rendering self-reactive B cells by editing the BCR through continued recombination of the antibody genes was investigated by several groups between the late 1980s and early 1990s [17–20]. In one experiment, an H-2K^b MHC class I and an anti-H-2K^b antibody was expressed ectopically in transgenic mice [20]. They found that the anti-H-2K^b B cells were absent in the periphery, but B cells with the anti-H-2K^b were still in the bone marrow, trying to edit the BCR by high levels of RAG1/RAG2 recombinase [21]. About 25% of the functional antibodies are produced by receptor editing [22].

But there are reports that about 50% of B cells are initially self-reactive, and it is suggested that receptor editing is the main mechanism to confer self-tolerance [21], beside the clonal deletion of self-reactive B cells in the bone marrow and anergy of self-reactive B cells in the periphery. Anergy and deletion inactivate or remove self-reactive clones. Receptor editing is based on secondary Vκ → Jκ light chain rearrangements or, more rarely, by altering the variable region of heavy chains by the replacement of a VH gene segment in an established V_HDJ_H rearrangement.

In conclusion, the modification of the V region by receptor editing extents the antibody diversity and rescue some B cells from apoptosis especially when self-reactivity was observed.

The pairing of heavy and light chains is considered to contribute not to the same extent to the antibody diversity as the processes of somatic recombination and junctional diversity mentioned before. By combination of different variable regions of the light (VL) and the heavy chain (VH), the antibody repertoire is further expanded. Previous studies suggested that the combination of different VH and VL is completely by chance and no preference of V gene pairing was observed [23, 24]. But more recent publications, unveiled some preferred VH and VL gene pairings in human and mouse antibodies, by searching a newer and larger antibody database set (KabatMan dataset [25]) not available in the previous studies before [26]. The results revealed that pairing preference do exists but only for a small proportion of germ line immunoglobulin gene sequences.

3. The secondary antibody repertoire

3.1. Somatic hypermutation

After the assembly of the V region of the heavy and light chain and cell surface expression of a functional BCR, naive B cells migrate to the secondary lymphatic organs, for example, to the lymph nodes. In the germinal center of the lymph node, the primary antibody repertoire is further diversified by introducing mutations in the V domains of the heavy and light chain mediated by the activation-induced cytidine deaminase (AID) [27–29]. This enzyme is only expressed and active in germinal center-activated mature B cells and is the key enzyme for the somatic hypermutation (SHM). The anatomical structure of the germinal center in the lymph node is divided macroscopically in two parts, the light zone and the dark zone. Somatic hypermutation mediated by AID activity takes place in the dark zone. Cells which produce a nonfunctional B-cell receptor (BCR) upon mutation are dying by apoptosis, whereby the B cells with a functional BCR will migrate into the light zone. In the light zone, positive selected B cells with a low-affinity B-cell receptor were stimulated for survival, proliferation, and reentry to the dark zone for a next round of affinity maturation. At this point, after several rounds of affinity maturation, B cells can leave the germinal center and differentiate into antibody producing plasma cells or B memory cells. B cells with very low affinity are suffering for survival signals, and before they can reenter the dark zone, they die by apoptosis [30].

During the migration, B cells change their expression pattern depending on their location in the light or dark zone of the germinal center. The C-X-C chemokine receptor type 4 (CXCR4) is one of the classical markers, which changes the expression level in response of the migration to the other germinal zone. In the dark zone, the B-cell CXCR4 expression is strong and is reduced in the light zone. CXCL12 is a ligand of CXCR4 and expressed on the cell surface of reticular cells in the dark zone. The CXCL12/CXCR4 signaling of B cells in the dark zone is regarded as a homing signal to keep B cells in the dark zone, if CXCR4 expression is high [31, 32]. CXCR4 deficiency in germinal B cells restricted the B cells to the light zone, but the deletion is not sufficient alone for functional transition of dark zone B cells (centroblasts) to light zone B cells (centrocytes) [31].

The process of affinity maturation is also known as the cyclic reentry model (**Figure 4**). It starts with the introduction of mutations in the V region initiated by AID. The induced mutation rate is about one nucleotide per 10,000 nucleotides after each cell cycle division [4]. This is much higher than the normal mutation rate of about 10^{10} mutations per cell cycle. Only a slight change in one or a few amino acids in the CDRs or frameworks of the V region can change dramatically the antigen affinity and specificity. Mutations can have detrimental effects and produce lower affinity B-cell receptors, especially when the complementarity-determining regions (CDRs) are affected with mutations leading to antibodies which cannot anymore recognize the antigen-binding site. At this stage, negative selection of B cells occurs. When B cells are affected by negative changes and were not able to produce a functional receptor presented on the B cell surface or lost antigen affinity, cell death by apoptosis is initiated. Subsequently, phagocytic clearance of apoptotic B cells is executed by tingible body macrophages (TBM).

On the other hand, B-cell clones with a BCR of high affinity toward the antigen receive growth signals, for example, from the follicular T helper cells, and are expended. This principle is called positive selection. Selected B cells which have undergone affinity maturation are showing more mutations in the critical regions for the antigen binding, namely, the CDRs. A mutation in the CDR, which produces an amino acid change, very likely alters the antigen affinity.

B cells with sufficient affinity to the antigen which is presented by follicular dendritic cells (FDCs) in the light zone can capture it, process it, and present the antigen peptide via the major histocompatibility complex II (MHC II) to the T cells. Then, B-cell clones get survival and mitogenic signals through the T-cell receptor (TCR) recognition, CD40-CD40L interaction, and cytokine stimulation of T cells (**Figure 4**). As a consequence, B-cell receptors and CD40 cluster together and promote thereby positive selection signaling. Follicular dendritic cells present foreign antigens on their dendritic surface in form of iccosomes (immune complex-coated bodies) [33–35]. Iccosomes are antigen/antibody/complement complexes bound to Fc and complement receptors on FDCs. When B cells recognize antigens presented by iccosomes, they can take them up and process them for MHC II-mediated T-cell presentation. The efficiency and amount of iccosome uptake can also influence the fate of the B cell. B-cell clones with higher affinity for the antigen can capture more from the iccosome-presented antigen, which resulted in more representation of the processed antigen peptide on the B-cell surface, complexed in the MHC II molecule. Therefore, these clones get more surviving and proliferation signals in the light zone from the recognizing follicular T helper cell (T_{FH}).

The process of somatic hypermutation (SHM) has not only a cellular dimension; it also has a molecular dimension, which can be characterized by the details of the mechanism of SHM and affinity maturation. The central enzyme in SHM is the activation-induced cytidine deaminase (AID). AID catalyzes the deamination of the DNA nucleotide cytosine to uracil, which is usually only present in RNA molecules.

The expression of AID is tightly restricted to germinal center B cells; this protects other cells from somatic hypermutation. Furthermore, it cannot act on predominantly double-stranded genomic DNA. To protect the majority of the genomic DNA from mutation, AID has developed a clever mechanism [36–38]. AID can act specifically only on single-stranded DNA molecules. The genomic DNA is released during transcription as a single strand by the RNA polymerase, which granted access of the AID for deamination. The immunoglobulin V region genes are actively transcribed in germinal center B cells, and somatic hypermutation can occur. Beside of the immunoglobulin V region, also some other transcribed genes can be affected by AID, fortunately by a lower frequency. AID has not only the function of somatic hypermutation by acting on the immunoglobulin V region loci; it can also activate the immunoglobulin class-switching process by acting on the residues in switch regions.

The deamination of cytidine to uracil by AID is the initiation step of SHM or class-switch recombination (CSR). Further mutation of the DNA around the initial deamination is executed by two different DNA repair pathways [39–41]. For example, the DNA mismatch repair process recognizes the wrong base pairing of uracil (U) to guanosine (G). Mismatch repair proteins MSH2 and MSH6 (mutS homolog 2/6) detect the wrong U/G base pairing, which then recruits DNA nucleases to remove the uracil and the adjacent nucleotides. The following

DNA polymerase Polη has no exonuclease activity and is error prone in B cells. The polymerase preferentially misincorporates thymidine (T), regardless of the template sequence, which leads to a preference of adenosine (A)-thymidine (T) mutations at the original targeted cytosine and the adjacent nucleotides by the mismatch repair pathway.

Alternatively, in the base excision repair pathway, the uracil DNA glycosylase (UNG) cleaves the uracil nucleobase from the uridine and leaves an abasic site in the DNA strand. During the following DNA replication, a random DNA base will be inserted in the opposite DNA strand of the abasic nucleotide. This is mediated by an error-prone DNA polymerase used in translesion DNA synthesis for damaged DNA caused by UV radiation.

As mentioned before, AID can also initiate class-switch recombination, by acting of apurinic/apyrimidinic endonuclease 1 (APE1) upon UNG-mediated introduction of an abasic nucleotide in the switch region. APE1 cleaves the DNA strand at the abasic site and produces a single-strand nick. In the switch regions, upstream of the constant region genes, the DNA nick is further cleaved which produces a double-strand break (DSB). This leads to a joint of another constant region gene to the V region, produced by the double-strand break repair machinery.

3.2. Class-switch recombination

In naive B cells, which had already rearranged their V region by somatic DNA recombination, two antibody isotypes are co-expressed at the same time. The V region and the μ chain (IgM) together with the δ chain (IgD) were transcribed on the same RNA transcript. By alternative splicing, either the μ chain or the δ chain is chosen, which produces two different messenger RNAs (**Figure 1**). Upon antigen contact and B-cell activation, B cells switch their antibody isotypes from IgM/IgD to IgG, IgA, or IgE. This is achieved by a process called class-switch recombination (CSR) or isotype switching. The antibody isotype is changed by an exchange of the constant region of the heavy chain locus. Only the constant region is replaced by CSR, which means the V region stays the same, but class switch confers the antibody the ability to interact with different effector molecules by their fragment crystallizable (Fc) region (**Figure 5**).

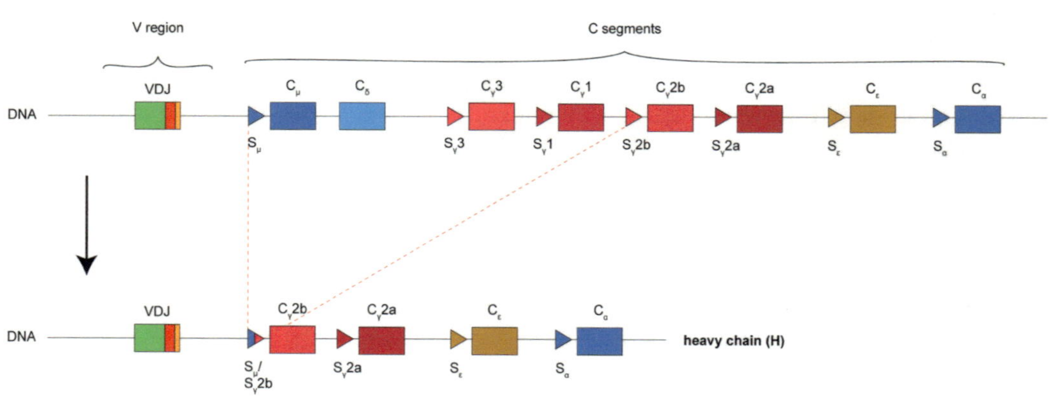

Figure 5. Mechanism of switch recombination from IgM to IgG2b.

Unlike in the parallel expression of IgM and IgD, the class switch is a chromosomal DNA rearrangement, leading to only one ultimate antibody isotype in the affected B cell. The process is guided by conserved switch region (S) upstream of the heavy chain constant genes, coding for the respective constant domains. The switch regions are repetitive stretches of DNA placed in introns upstream to the C region genes [28, 42]. The initial activation of CSR is done by the enzyme activation-induced cytidine deaminase (AID), which has also an essential role in the somatic hypermutation process. This produces a single-stranded DNA break (nick) at two switch regions, and the DNA between both switch sites were irreversible excised. The removal includes always the μ and δ chain constant region. Both DNA strands were brought together by the non-homologous end joining (NHEJ) mechanism; this rearranges the variable region with the constant region of the chosen immunoglobulin isotype. The decision which isotype will be produced is influenced by different cytokines, secreted by T cells [43, 44].

CSR is induced by the enzyme activation-induced cytidine deaminase (AID) acting on the switch regions (S) of the respective constant region gene. The non-homologous end joining (NHEJ) machinery joins the chosen constant gene segment to the V region (here C_y2b). The constant region gene, which is next to the V region, is then expressed together with the V(D)J gene sequence.

Author details

Oliver Backhaus

Address all correspondence to: olli.backhaus@googlemail.com

Institute of Pathology, University Clinic of RWTH Aachen, Aachen, Germany

References

[1] Kawai T, Akira S. The roles of TLRs, RLRs and NLRs in pathogen recognition. International Immunology. 2009;**21**(4):317-337. DOI: 10.1093/intimm/dxp017

[2] Stein LD. Human genome: End of the beginning. Nature. 2004;**431**(7011):915-916. DOI: 10.1038/431915a

[3] Pertea M, Salzberg SL. Between a chicken and a grape: Estimating the number of human genes. Genome Biology. 2010;**11**(5):206. DOI: 10.1186/gb-2010-11-5-206

[4] Murphy K et al. Janeway's Immunobiology. 8th ed. Vol. xix. New York: Garland Science; 2012. 868 p

[5] IMGT. The international ImMunoGeneTics information system: IMGT Repertoire (IG and TR) – Table Functional IG genes. Available from: http://www.imgt.org/IMGTrepertoire/LocusGenes/genetable/human/geneNumber.html [Accessed: February 19, 2017]

[6] Roth DB. V(D)J recombination: Mechanism, errors, and fidelity. Microbiology Spectrum. 2014;**2**(6):1-11. DOI: 10.1128/microbiolspec.MDNA3-0041-2014

[7] Ramsden DA, Baetz K, Wu GE. Conservation of sequence in recombination signal sequence spacers. Nucleic Acids Research. 1994;**22**(10):1785-1796

[8] Rodgers KK. Riches in RAGs: Revealing the V(D)J recombinase through high-resolution structures. Trends in Biochemical Sciences. 2017;**42**(1):72-84. DOI: 10.1016/j.tibs.2016.10.003

[9] Wu TT, Johnson G, Kabat EA. Length distribution of CDRH3 in antibodies. Proteins. 1993;**16**(1):1-7. DOI: 10.1002/prot.340160102

[10] Weitzner BD, Dunbrack Jr RL, Gray JJ. The origin of CDR H3 structural diversity. Structure. 2015;**23**(2):302-311. DOI: 10.1016/j.str.2014.11.010

[11] Ma Y et al. Hairpin opening and overhang processing by an Artemis/DNA-dependent protein kinase complex in nonhomologous end joining and V(D)J recombination. Cell. 2002;**108**(6):781-794

[12] Srivastava SK, Robins HS. Palindromic nucleotide analysis in human T cell receptor rearrangements. PLoS One. 2012;**7**(12):e52250. DOI: 10.1371/journal.pone.0052250

[13] Lu H, Schwarz K, Lieber MR. Extent to which hairpin opening by the Artemis: DNA-PKcs complex can contribute to junctional diversity in V(D)J recombination. Nucleic Acids Research. 2007;**35**(20):6917-6923. DOI: 10.1093/nar/gkm823

[14] Motea EA, Berdis AJ. Terminal deoxynucleotidyl transferase: The story of a misguided DNA polymerase. Biochimica et Biophysica Acta. 2010;**1804**(5):1151-1166. DOI: 10.1016/j.bbapap.2009.06.030

[15] Vettermann C, Schlissel MS. Allelic exclusion of immunoglobulin genes: Models and mechanisms. Immunological Reviews. 2010;**237**(1):22-42. DOI: 10.1111/j.1600-065X.2010.00935.x

[16] Mostoslavsky R, Alt FW, Rajewsky K. The lingering enigma of the allelic exclusion mechanism. Cell. 2004;**118**(5):539-544. DOI: 10.1016/j.cell.2004.08.023

[17] Gay D et al. Receptor editing: An approach by autoreactive B cells to escape tolerance. The Journal of Experimental Medicine. 1993;**177**(4):999-1008

[18] Tiegs SL, Russell DM, Nemazee D. Receptor editing in self-reactive bone marrow B cells. The Journal of Experimental Medicine. 1993;**177**(4):1009-1020

[19] Goodnow CC et al. Altered immunoglobulin expression and functional silencing of self-reactive B lymphocytes in transgenic mice. Nature. 1988;**334**(6184):676-682. DOI: 10.1038/334676a0

[20] Hartley SB et al. Elimination from peripheral lymphoid tissues of self-reactive B lymphocytes recognizing membrane-bound antigens. Nature. 1991;**353**(6346):765-769. DOI: 10.1038/353765a0

[21] Sukumar S, Schlissel MS. Receptor editing as a mechanism of B cell tolerance. Journal of Immunology. 2011;**186**(3):1301-1302. DOI: 10.4049/jimmunol.1090129

[22] Casellas R et al. Contribution of receptor editing to the antibody repertoire. Science. 2001;**291**(5508):1541-1544. DOI: 10.1126/science.291.5508.1541

[23] Brezinschek HP et al. Pairing of variable heavy and variable kappa chains in individual naive and memory B cells. Journal of Immunology. 1998;**160**(10):4762-4767

[24] de Wildt RM et al. Analysis of heavy and light chain pairings indicates that receptor editing shapes the human antibody repertoire. Journal of Molecular Biology. 1999;**285**(3):895-901. DOI: 10.1006/jmbi.1998.2396

[25] Johnson G, Wu TT. Kabat database and its applications: Future directions. Nucleic Acids Research. 2001;**29**(1):205-206

[26] Jayaram N, Bhowmick P, Martin AC. Germline VH/VL pairing in antibodies. Protein Engineering, Design & Selection. 2012;**25**(10):523-529. DOI: 10.1093/protein/gzs043

[27] Guikema JE et al. APE1- and APE2-dependent DNA breaks in immunoglobulin class switch recombination. The Journal of Experimental Medicine. 2007;**204**(12):3017-3026. DOI: 10.1084/jem.20071289

[28] Stavnezer J, Guikema JE, Schrader CE. Mechanism and regulation of class switch recombination. Annual Review of Immunology. 2008;**26**:261-292. DOI: 10.1146/annurev.immunol.26.021607.090248

[29] Rada C et al. Immunoglobulin isotype switching is inhibited and somatic hypermutation perturbed in UNG-deficient mice. Current Biology. 2002;**12**(20):1748-1755

[30] Mesin L, Ersching J, Victora GD. Germinal center B cell dynamics. Immunity. 2016;**45**(3):471-482. DOI: 10.1016/j.immuni.2016.09.001

[31] Bannard O et al. Germinal center centroblasts transition to a centrocyte phenotype according to a timed program and depend on the dark zone for effective selection. Immunity. 2013;**39**(5):912-924. DOI: 10.1016/j.immuni.2013.08.038

[32] Rodda LB et al. Phenotypic and morphological properties of germinal center dark zone Cxcl12-expressing reticular cells. Journal of Immunology. 2015;**195**(10):4781-4791. DOI: 10.4049/jimmunol.1501191

[33] Szakal AK, Kosco MH, Tew JG. A novel in vivo follicular dendritic cell-dependent iccosome-mediated mechanism for delivery of antigen to antigen-processing cells. Journal of Immunology. 1988;**140**(2):341-353

[34] Kranich J, Krautler NJ. How follicular dendritic cells shape the B-cell Antigenome. Frontiers in Immunology. 2016;**7**:225. DOI: 10.3389/fimmu.2016.00225

[35] Terashima K et al. Follicular dendritic cell and ICCOSOMES in germinal center reactions. Seminars in Immunology. 1992;**4**(4):267-274

[36] Chaudhuri J et al. Transcription-targeted DNA deamination by the AID antibody diversification enzyme. Nature. 2003;**422**(6933):726-730. DOI: 10.1038/nature01574

[37] Ramiro AR et al. Transcription enhances AID-mediated cytidine deamination by exposing single-stranded DNA on the nontemplate strand. Nature Immunology. 2003;**4**(5):452-456. DOI: 10.1038/ni920

[38] Sohail A et al. Human activation-induced cytidine deaminase causes transcription-dependent, strand-biased C to U deaminations. Nucleic Acids Research. 2003;**31**(12):2990-2994

[39] Wu X et al. Immunoglobulin somatic hypermutation: Double-strand DNA breaks, AID and error-prone DNA repair. Journal of Clinical Immunology. 2003;**23**(4):235-246

[40] Chen Z et al. AID-initiated DNA lesions are differentially processed in distinct B cell populations. Journal of Immunology. 2014;**193**(11):5545-5556. DOI: 10.4049/jimmunol.1401549

[41] Di Noia JM, Neuberger MS. Molecular mechanisms of antibody somatic hypermutation. Annual Review of Biochemistry. 2007;**76**:1-22. DOI: 10.1146/annurev.biochem.76.061705.090740

[42] Dunnick W et al. DNA sequences at immunoglobulin switch region recombination sites. Nucleic Acids Research. 1993;**21**(3):365-372

[43] Pinaud E et al. The IgH locus 3′ regulatory region: Pulling the strings from behind. Advanced Immunology. 2011;**110**:27-70. DOI: 10.1016/B978-0-12-387663-8.00002-8

[44] Shparago N et al. IL-10 selectively regulates murine Ig isotype switching. International Immunology. 1996;**8**(5):781-790

Chapter 2

High Affinity Maturated Human Antibodies from Naïve and Synthetic Antibody Repertoires

Chia Chiu Lim, Yee Siew Choong and Theam Soon Lim

Additional information is available at the end of the chapter

http://dx.doi.org/10.5772/intechopen.71664

Abstract

Recombinant human antibody technology has been the cornerstone of the uprising of biologics in the pharmaceutical industry. The introduction of various display technologies like phage, yeast, bacterial, ribosomal, mRNA, DNA display and mammalian cell surface display has allowed improved antibody generation programs. The ability to generate recombinant antibodies from available human antibody libraries by using *in vitro* display methods pave the way to select recombinant human antibodies against almost every antigen. The libraries are a close representation of the B-cell response elicited by the natural immune system. The introduction of various methods to fine tune the antibody affinities has made recombinant antibody technology highly sought after. The ability to engineer specific characteristics of each antibody by design is possible utilizing advanced *in vitro* strategies. This chapter will focus on the technologies commonly applied in antibody display technologies to engineer improved affinities.

Keywords: naïve- immune- and synthetic- antibody library, *in vitro* display systems, affinity maturation, *de novo* antibody gene synthesis, genome editing techniques

1. Introduction

The introduction of recombinant antibody technology has revolutionized and improved the way antibodies are being generated for various applications in research, diagnosis and therapy [1–4]. Antibodies have been the cornerstone for many biomedical advances in the past due to its high specificity and affinity to capture target antigens. The key characteristic of antibodies that makes it highly sought after is the defined specificity of the complementarity determining regions (CDR) of the variable domains against a specific target [5]. This specificity is programmed *in vivo* by a series of different molecular mechanisms such as V-D-J

INTECH
open science | open minds

© 2018 The Author(s). Licensee InTech. This chapter is distributed under the terms of the Creative Commons Attribution License (http://creativecommons.org/licenses/by/3.0), which permits unrestricted use, distribution, and reproduction in any medium, provided the original work is properly cited. (cc) BY

recombination of the heavy chain, V-J recombination of the light chain and somatic hypermutation [6, 7]. After primary immune response the $V_HD_HJ_H$ and V_LJ_L exons are randomly mutated, mainly in the CDRs, by somatic hypermutation leading to high affinity antibodies (see article of Oliver Backhaus in this book). These molecular processes have a profound effect on the way the genotype is delineated as the gene rearrangements will bring about multiple gene segment combinations. Additional mutagenesis is elicited through incorporation of additional nucleotides between the junctions of the V, D and J gene segment of the heavy chain and V and J gene segment of the light chain. These variations at the genotypic level have a direct influence on the phenotypic variation seen in terms of target specificity and affinity of the generated antibody [8, 9]. **Figure 1** shows the correlation between the genotypic variations and the phenotypic nature of the generated antibodies.

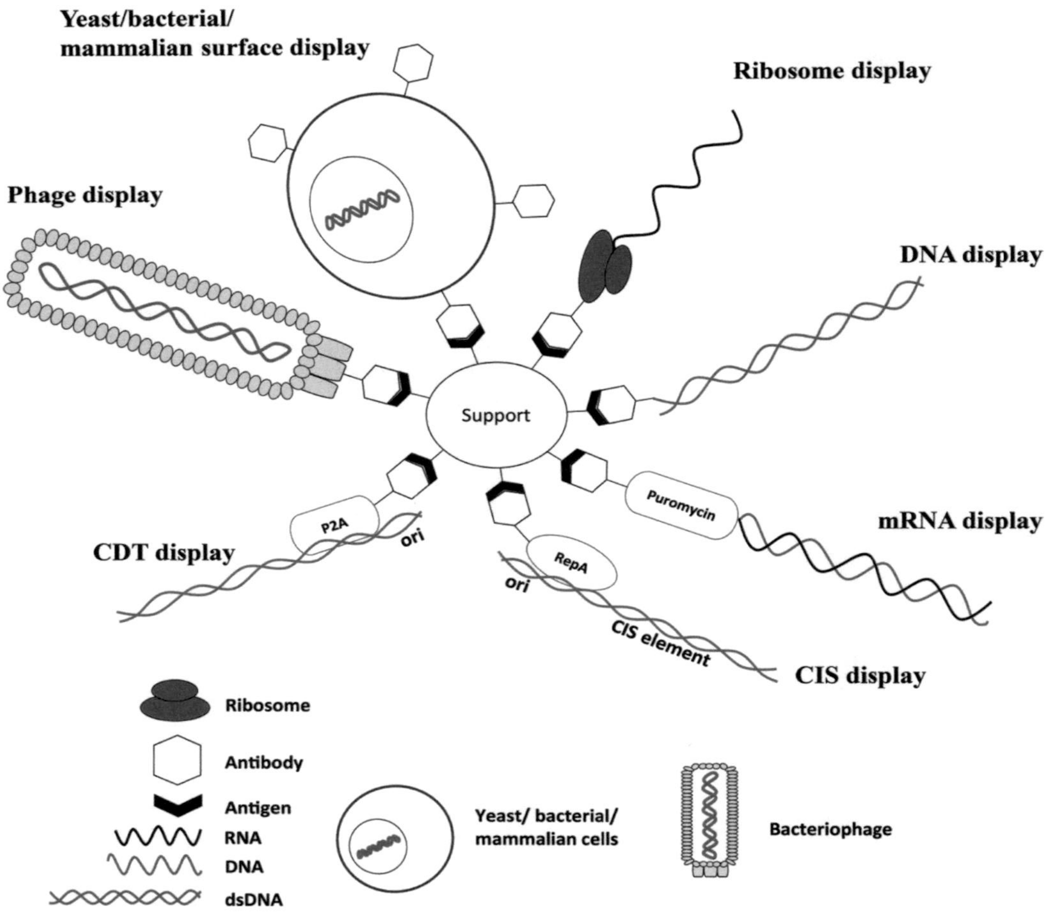

Figure 1. Illustration highlighting the different *in vitro* display technologies available.

The introduction of recombinant DNA technology and display technologies has allowed recombinant antibodies to be generated at a rapid pace. This is evident with the increase of recombinant antibodies going into clinical trials in the last 3 years [10, 11]. The general concept of display oriented techniques for antibody generation relies upon the ability to harness the natural or synthetic diversity of an antibody library [12]. As with most recombinant DNA approaches, the ability to customize or modify the genotype either at single base or amino acid level was now possible [13]. This opened many new avenues in the field of recombinant antibody technology to allow modification and customization of characteristics of the phenotype. The advent of display technologies allowed for selective isolation of specific phenotypes with their respective genotypic information to be retrieved together [14]. This means that it was now possible to replicate the *in vivo* antibody generation and maturation process *in vitro* [13]. The impact of antibody display technologies combined with affinity maturation strategies in the isolation and identification of high affinity antibodies is monumental in the way antibodies are made today.

1.1. Display technologies

The first display technology that was applied for the generation of recombinant antibodies was phage display. Although initially the technology was designed to display polypeptides, the robust nature of the method meant that larger proteins could also be displayed by bacteriophages [15, 16]. This allowed the introduction of antibody fragments to be presented on the surface of the phage particles for selection. Phage display takes advantage of the natural replication cycle of bacteriophages to fuse the antibody gene with the gene of a phage coat protein. This design allows the co-expression and translocation of the antibody fused coat protein during the phage packaging process to display the antibody proteins on the surface of mature phage particles. More importantly, this allowed for a physical linkage to be established between the genotype and phenotype [12].

Since the introduction of phage display, other display systems have been developed. This includes systems like yeast display, bacterial cell surface display, ribosomal display, mRNA display, DNA display and mammalian cell surface display [17]. **Figure 1** shows the alternative display systems used for antibody presentation. **Yeast display** has an additional feature compared to phage display when dealing with mammalian proteins. This is due to the application of the eukaryotic machinery to assimilate the display mechanism. In this system, the antibody gene is fused to the Aga2p agglutinin subunit found on the surface of yeast cells [18, 19]. In a similar fashion, **bacterial cell display** functions by displaying antibodies on the surface of Gram-negative or Gram-positive cells as a fusion to the flagella or outer membrane proteins [12, 16].

Ribosome display is a cell-free display approach where polysomes are stalled on mRNA templates and nascent antibody protein remains in complex with the ribosomes. The stalling of the ribosomes is done with the removal of a stop codon and a C-terminal peptide spacer is required to ensure proper folding of the protein [20]. This is critical as steric hindrance caused by the ribosomal tunnel can alter the folding of the protein leading to lower display efficiency [21]. A somewhat related method to ribosome display is **mRNA display**. In mRNA display systems, the interaction between the template and protein is covalently linked via puromycin. Puromycin functions to mimic the role of amino-acyl tRNA by attaching itself to a DNA primer affixed to the mRNA template. This allows puromycin to attach itself covalently to the nascent antibody protein based on the peptidyl transferase activity of the ribosome [12, 22].

Mammalian display approaches utilizes mammalian host cells like HEK293T and Chinese hamster ovary (CHO) cells to present a library of antibodies on the cell surface for selection [23]. The approach adapts a similar concept to that of yeast cell display [18]. It capitalizes on the transient expression of antibodies in which antibody encoding DNA introduced into the cells persist over days to consistently express antibodies. Transient expression systems are commonly used for single round selections from immune repertoires. A stable expression system with the integration of DNA to the host genome is inefficient because of multi-gene incorporation per cell making libraries difficult to resolve [24]. A suitable method to allow multi-round selection is by stable episomal vectors derived from viruses. Virus based vectors are used to infect mammalian cells to display the antibodies for selection making it suitable for large sized libraries [25]. A major advantage of mammalian cell systems is the ability to screen using full length IgG [26]. **DNA display** applied for the screening of peptides/proteins was originally based on streptavidin-fused peptides/proteins linked with their encoding DNAs via biotin in emulsion compartments [27]. However this method was not often used for recombinant antibody selection except some promising results with Fabs, and recently with bispecific diabody fragments have been reported [28, 29].

Other alternative DNA display systems are cis-activity based (CIS) and covalent display technology (CDT) display systems. CIS display uses the ability of the bacterial replication initiator protein, RepA to carry out a cis-activity. This means that RepA has the ability to bind the encoding DNA that was utilized. This activity is largely dependent on the presence of two non-coding regions 3′ to bind to the repA sequence. The actual mechanism is unknown but is believed to involve stalling of RNA polymerase during transcription at the CIS element allowing the nascent repA protein to non-covalently attach to its binding site of the template [30]. The covalent display technology (CDT) exploits the properties of the replication initiator protein from *E. coli* bacteriophage P2 [31]. A pool of DNA encoding antibody molecules is generated as a fusion to the P2A coding sequence [12]. The DNA pool is then transcribed and translated using cell free expression systems. The cis-activity of the P2A protein allows the DNA molecule to covalently tag with its own gene product [16, 17]. Ultimately, the recurring trend of all display systems is the ability of the system to allow the translation of antibody genes to produce a collection of antibody molecules that is physically fused to the encoding genes for selection.

Taking advantage of the different display systems, many different forms of libraries can be represented for antibody generation. There is no actual discrimination as to which method is best for antibody generation. All the display approaches highlighted are useful in different circumstances and has its own brand of unique features that makes some more suitable for a particular set of antigens. Ultimately, all the display systems are capable of isolating and identifying recombinant human monoclonal antibodies using a library of antibody genes [16]. The variation of the antibody sequences in the antibody gene repertoire (the diversity) will have a significant impact on the quality of antibodies generated. The antibody repertoire being presented on the various display platforms is in essence the basic antibody response divulged by the immune response system [32]. The multi-level process of antibody gene generation and maturation of the V-D-J gene segments will finally dictate the antibody characteristic being inherited to the display systems for recombinant antibody generation. This is evident as antibody V-D-J gene segments function as the basic building blocks of antibodies influencing the characteristics of the antibodies of an antibody gene repertoire [33]. Therefore, an understanding of the processes involved in antibody gene repertoire generation is vital to design engineering strategies for antibodies with improved affinities.

1.2. Generation of human antibody repertoires

The human antibody repertoire represents a diverse collection of immunoglobulin gene segments that encodes for heavy (V_H) and light chain (V_L) domains [34], forming an unique set of antigen-binding sites [35, 36]. The heavy chain (HC) locus is located at chromosome 14, comprises of V_H, D, J_H and C_H gene segments. The kappa light chain locus is found in chromosome 2 with the V_K, J_K and C_K gene segments. The lambda LC locus with the V_λ, J_λ, and C_λ gene segments are found on chromosome 22 [37].

The generation of a natural antibody repertoire is attributed to several natural mechanisms such as somatic recombination that is rearrangements of gene segments to form a single unique antibody gene sequence [38]. The V(D)J recombination process that takes place during B-cell development allows for combinatorial rearrangements of V (variable), D (diversity), and J (joining) gene segments of the heavy chain resulting in the formation of numerous possibilities [35, 39, 40], see also Backhaus O. this book. A similar process (the V_L-J_L rearrangement of the light chain) occurs at the light chain locus [39], see also Backhaus O. this book. This process is regulated by lymphocyte-specific RAG1 and RAG2 endonucleases that cleaves DNA at the recombination signal sequences (RSSs) resulting in blunt signal ends and hairpin coding ends. The ends are later joined by classical non-homologous end-joining (cNHEJ) pathway to ensure genomic stability [40, 41]. The outcome of recombination is an ordered fashion of V-D-J and V_L-J_L gene assembly that encodes the antibody binding site (variable region). Antibody diversity is further enhanced by junctional diversification, characterized by variability at the junctions due to insertions or/and deletions of few nucleotides during fusion of segments [38, 40].

An individual is expected to have at least 10^8 of antibody-producing B-cell clones that are responsive to unique antigens [42]. This natural repertoire is known as the naïve or primary repertoire, expresses cell surface IgM and has not undergone specialization by antigen encounter [37]. The antigen-binding site of an antibody consists of the surrounding framework regions and the complementarity determining regions (CDRs), CDR1, CDR2 and CDR3. CDR3 region are particularly important for antibody-antigen specificity [43]. The V(D)J and V(J) rearrangement of the antibody gene segments and somatic mutations will give rise to higher binding diversities to various antigens [35, 36].

Upon encountering new antigens, naïve B-cells are stimulated and become activated B-cells, undergo proliferation and differentiation. B-cell proliferation is also known as clonal expansion, in which an antibody B-cell clone specific to an antigen is selected and produced in large scale. This process takes place in secondary lymphoid organs such as lymph nodes and spleen, also referred to as germinal centers. The differentiation process generally involves somatic hypermutation (SHM) and class switch recombination (CSR). Somatic hypermutation introduced extensive point mutations in the variable (V) region gene, such as single base substitutions, insertions and deletions. Consequently, the V region exon is further diversified resulting in altered affinities against the target antigen [39, 41]. Class switch recombination replaces the constant region (C_H) gene of the HC resulting in class switching from IgM to IgE, IgA and IgG. The type of isotype used determines the methods for elimination of captured antigen by immunoglobulin or the location for antibody accumulation [37, 44, 45]. The combination of both mechanisms offers an improved diversity to the antibodies [46] and enables the selection for high affinity antibody-producing cells against a particular antigen. This process of improved affinity is known as affinity maturation of antibodies.

An essential element that mediates both SHM and CSR is the activation-induced cytidine deaminase [47]. AID is a protein exclusively expressed in activated B-cells in germinal centers but the exact function and mechanism of AID in SHM and CSR are not fully understood. However, several studies have been reported and shown that AID is capable of editing RNA and DNA deamination. AID deaminates cytidine residues to uracil residues on single-stranded DNA (ssDNA) at preferred "hotspots," described as DGYW motif. Such motif favors mutation and is ubiquitous throughout the genome. The maintenance of genome fidelity attempts to correct the "deamination error" by base excision repair and mismatch repair pathways, thereby producing mutations and double-stranded breaks [41, 45, 48].

The natural diversification processes has allowed for highly diverse antibody repertoires to be generated. This natural phenomenon is the basis of the unique ability of the immune system to counter any foreign infection. The ability to replicate or represent the *in vivo* repertoire in the laboratory is the basis of recombinant antibody technology. The need to reproduce this feature is achieved for example by the construction of antibody phage libraries. The robust nature of combinatorial technologies has enabled easy selection of monoclonal antibodies from highly diverse naïve, immune and synthetic repertoires by coupling it with biopanning processes [49].

Phage display enables the sorting and handling of large antibody libraries. Antibody phage libraries consist of a random collection of antibody variable genes being presented as a fusion to phage coat proteins. The antibody fragments can be expressed as a fusion protein on the surface of phages, without affecting the infectivity of phages [50]. Moreover, the displayed antibody molecules retains its antigen-antibody binding capabilities [51]. However, the challenge in generating high affinity antibodies is closely related to the quality of the library generated. Even so, the advancement of recombinant DNA technologies has allowed for downstream affinity maturation processes to be carried out for the improvement of antibody affinities post-selection [52, 53].

2. Antibody libraries

An antibody library is basically a physical collection of various antibody genes being represented in a single pool. Antibody molecules are divided into two sets of binding domains, the variable domain of the heavy chain (HC) and light chain [54] that either preferentially or concomitantly contributes to the binding affinity of the antibody to the target antigen [42]. Therefore, in order to replicate the diverse repertoire of antibodies afforded by the immune system, a random combinatorial mix of both the HC and LC repertoire is required. The source of the antibody repertoire has a profound influence on the type of antibody libraries being constructed as for example if you amplify the variable antibody genes from immune patients the immune response of different individuals in different health and disease states will have a definite impact on the diversity of the generated antibody repertoire. The diversity of naïve antibody repertoires will be reflected by random variations in the genetic information of the clones generated in the library [55]. This brings to light the different classification of antibody libraries that are essentially defined by the origin of the antibody repertoire. There are generally three different classes of antibody libraries namely the naïve, immune and synthetic antibody libraries applied for antibody display [56].

2.1. Naïve antibody libraries

The natural collection of immunoglobulins for antibody library generation is obtained from circulating B-cells in primary and secondary lymphoid tissues and blood. Naïve libraries are constructed from IgM mRNA of B-cells from healthy donors, non-immunized donors, isolated from peripheral blood lymphocytes, spleen, tonsils, and bone marrow. In some cases, the repertoire could also be retrieved from animal sources resulting in antibodies of different origins [57]. The diversity offered by a naïve repertoire is undeniably vast, whereby the antibody fragments are PCR amplified randomly from the antibody cDNA of non-antigen stimulated B-cells as well as those B-cells that have been resided in the immune system due to earlier infections [58, 59]. A single naïve library (also known as single pot library, generated from several donors) can be used to generate antibodies against all types of antigens, peptides, toxins, as well as self-antigens (typically important in the area of cancer and autoimmune disease therapeutics). Some of the antibodies are generated against red cell antigens, haptens, tumor necrosis factor (TNF) [15]. The clonal diversity exhibited by B-cells enables the generation of a range of antibodies against a wide variety of antigens. The characteristics of a naïve repertoire mainly result in modest affinity and polyreactivity antibodies. Due to the polyreactive nature of a naïve library, it is important to generate a larger library to increase success rates for obtaining high affinity antibodies against multiple antigens by successive rounds of selection. The main advantage of a naïve library is the ability to screen for antibodies against any antigens. This comes with a huge drawback, in which the antibodies are of lower affinities than from immunized clones [56, 60]. However, this issue can be solved and improved by affinity maturation *in vitro* to yield high affinity antibody against a specific antigen. Other shortcomings that can affect the library quality are inconsistent levels of variable antibody gene expression and the limitation of IgM to exhibit diversity, as well as increase chances of cross-reactivity [15]. To improve library quality, one of the method is to randomize the CDR regions of the variable genes while maintaining the original frameworks of the naïve library, this results in further diversification and modifications, becoming a semi-synthetic library [60].

2.2. Immune antibody libraries

The source of antibody genes for immune library generation is mainly focused on using IgG mRNA from disease-infected individuals or cancer patients. This may include patients with acute infections, recovery stage or patients which have recovered from a particular disease or infection [15]. In addition to that, cancer derived material can also be used as a source [61]. The unique characteristic of an immune repertoire is that the sample material is obtained from activated B-cells, where affinity maturation has taken place during antigen encounter [47]. Thus, it is easier to obtain high affinity binders specific to an antigen from immune libraries in comparison to naïve libraries due to the biased nature of the repertoire post-exposure of the antigen. The size of an immune library need not be as large as naïve libraries per se, but it can also be applied for other targets but may not be suitable for self-antigens [56, 62]. The obvious limitation of an immune library is the possibility of generating immune libraries of human donors against various targets. Therefore, the application of immune libraries from humans is mainly confined to disease-infected individuals [60] or cancer patients [61]. The biased nature of the library repertoire also means that the library is mainly useful against the antigen used for immunization. Therefore new libraries are required when dealing with targets of different diseases [62]. However, it is also possible for immune libraries to successfully enrich antibodies against non-related targets of the disease of origin. This indirectly indicates the influence of B-cell memory during immune responses that provides an extended breath of protection for individuals.

2.3. Synthetic antibody libraries

The main difference between naïve and immune libraries with synthetic libraries is the source of the repertoire used to build the library. While both naïve and immune libraries are amplified from a natural source, synthetic libraries are designed *in silico* and the repertoire is generated in controlled conditions [49, 56]. The artificial repertoire is generated from the diversity afforded by the randomization of the CDR using synthetic approaches [63]. The basic design of most synthetic libraries is the randomization of various CDRs using degenerated oligonucleotides. The freedom afforded by synthetic libraries is the possibility of pre-defined designs of the framework and the degree of randomization of the CDRs. The design pattern is generated based on bioinformatics analysis using existing experimental data on antibody epitopes, antigen-antibody interactions, affinity maturation designs, variable gene segments recombination, and structural predictions on variable regions to yield desirable synthetic repertoires. These studies provide insights to the hypervariable regions on amino acid predominance and variabilities [60]. The hypervariable regions (CDR loops) have been shown to exhibit some amino acid biases. In particular, certain residues (G, P, S, N, H, L, and Y) are predominantly found on CDR loops that are associated with improved antigen binding [64]. Designing CDR sequences that mimic the natural diversity can help circumvent selection of low affinity binders. The two major synthetic antibody libraries available, HuCAL® and n-CoDeR® are based on two separate platforms. Their models will be discussed further as case studies.

2.3.1. Case study of synthetic antibody libraries: HuCAL®

A novel concept of synthetic human library construction, named Human Combinatorial Antibody Library (HuCAL) uses more than one framework sequence to construct the library. The HuCAL construction is based on modular consensus frameworks, consisting of seven V_H and seven V_L consensus sequences to represent the major germline families, yielding 49 possible combinations of master genes [65]. The master genes are designed such that different frameworks promote different structural diversity of human antibodies while unfavorable residues that cause protein aggregation are removed. Furthermore, HuCAL is characterized by having unique restriction sites flanking all CDRs of the antibodies as well as usage of phage display and unique expression vectors. This allows for a seamless conversion to different antibody formats, for instance scFv and Fab [66, 67].

In HuCAL, the CDR3 regions are designed to exhibit natural amino acid composition and distribution as well as length variation at each position for each framework. The CDR is synthesized using trinucleotide mixtures (TRIM technology), which offers the elimination of stop codons and redundant amino acid residues in order to optimize CDR design for downstream production of encoded antibodies. TRIM technology uses trinucleotide phosphoramidites to add three bases at a time to a growing single strand of synthetic DNA [68]. The addition of three bases allows for the design and pre-determination of specific codons to be added. In addition to codon optimization for *E. coli*, improved accuracy of antibody design would then be possible. This ultimately improves the functional library size of HuCAL as well as the diversity by having higher number of clones with correct assembly, devoid of frameshifts, stop codons and deletions [69].

There have been different versions of the HuCAL library being constructed over the years, each with different characteristics. The initial HuCAL focuses on the scFv library construction using 49 master genes, resulting in high expression levels of HuCAL-scFv antibodies (2×10^9 clones) and nanomolar range of affinities to several antigens tested, such as haptens, DNA, peptides, and proteins [69]. HuCAL GOLD® is a synthetic Fab library, generated by diversifying six CDRs that mimics the natural diversity. Affinities of antibodies generated from this library are able to achieve picomolar range when tested on different target molecules [63]. The latest optimized version, HuCAL PLATINUM® has a more advantageous design focusing on the optimization of CDR3 sequences in the modular sequence in order to yield antibodies with improved folding and enhanced binding [70]. The optimization includes avoiding N-glycosylation sites and unproductive sequences to maximize the sequence space and availability. In addition, the library is improved to enhance antibody expression in both bacterial and mammalian expression systems. Sequence optimization on nucleotides has been extensively carried out during library construction, therefore Fab fragments and IgG formats can be expressed optimally in both bacterial and mammalian systems, respectively. The resulting library offers higher diversity than the HuCAL GOLD® library [64, 70].

2.3.2. Case study of synthetic antibody libraries: n-CoDeR®

The principle of the n-CoDeR® library is based on the recombination of a single framework with multiple CDRs from non-immunized donors to generate functional diversity [71]. This approach allows the retrieval of CDR loops from immunoglobulin genes from different germline origins. All CDR loops are successfully recombined into one single V_H-V_L scaffold, while maintaining reactivity and functionality of the antibody fragments [72]. The underlying concept of constructing the n-CoDeR® library is the amplification of desired CDR loops from immunoglobulin cDNA with overlap extension and assembly being performed to place the CDRs into the single framework [73]. The use of CDR loops originating from the human immune system is said to be remarkable as the sequences obtained have undergone *in vivo* processing, thus such sequences are said to have undergone proof-reading and the functionality has been confirmed [74]. The resulting genetic diversity of this library is remarkably enormous (2×10^9), and has the potential to yield diversities equaling the human immune system [56].

This library appears to be a suitable candidate for therapeutic and diagnostic applications as it can generate functional antibody fragments against many types of antigens. Initially the approach of using a single framework to present various types of CDR loops was seemed risky due to the limitation in capacity. It was later proved to be successful with the isolation of antibodies specific to various types of antigens reaching affinities in the sub-nanomolar range. Another benefit afforded by this approach was the ability to select a single framework that can customize desirable characteristics and properties, as well as ensuring that antibodies can be generated which can be produced and folded in good condition [56]. Antibodies harnessed from the n-CoDeR® library are potentially advantageous for therapeutic purpose as they demonstrated a lower number of T-cell epitopes than normal antibodies. It indicates that self-reactivity is therefore circumvented and immunogenicity issues are reduced [72].

3. Affinity maturation strategies for recombinant antibodies

Recombinant antibodies obtained via combinatorial library technology from naïve or synthetic libraries have the advantage of increased diversity as a result of the large repertoire of the antibody genes. Antibodies isolated from combinatorial libraries against their respective targets sometimes may not exhibit the desired specificity and affinity. The increased affinity of an antibody is important to enhance its pharmacokinetics, efficacy and safety profile by enhancing the binding strength and function of an antibody [75]. Such optimizations can be achieved either by *in vitro* or *in vivo* affinity maturation strategies.

3.1. *In vitro* approaches toward affinity maturation of antibodies

There are several strategies that have been used to perform *in vitro* affinity maturation to improve recombinant antibody molecules. Mutagenesis is widely employed to introduce mutations into antibody sequences. Sequences of antibody are diversified by random mutations via methods such as error-prone PCR or through site-directed mutations, where mutations are assigned to specific positions in CDRs or framework regions as well as mutational hot spots by using PCR and degenerate primers [76]. In addition, *de novo* synthesis of DNA offers the most straightforward modification procedure to further diversify the antibody sequences as a whole.

Random mutagenesis is a non-systematic mutagenesis method that can be performed in the absence of information regarding the importance of structures and residues that contribute to antigen-antibody binding as well as affinity maturation of antibody [77]. The method introduces point mutations into antibody genes in a random fashion. The mechanisms involves: (1) transitions, where a purine or pyrimidine is substituted by another purine or pyrimidine, (2) transversions, where a purine is substituted by a pyrimidine, or *vice versa*, (3) deletions of one or more nucleotides from the gene sequence, (4) insertions of one or more nucleotides into a gene sequence, (5) inversions where double-stranded DNA segments of two base pairs or longer is rotated at 180° [78].

Error-prone PCR is a universal method used for the introduction of random mutations by capitalizing on the natural error rate of a low fidelity DNA polymerase, for example *Taq* polymerase that lacks 3′ to 5′ proofreading activity. Several parameters during PCR amplification govern the error rate of DNA polymerases in order to create ideal mismatches in the amplified product. The manipulation of the enzyme's fidelity can be performed by varying several parameters like: (1) concentration of *Taq* DNA polymerase, (2) concentration of divalent cations (Mn^{2+} and Mg^{2+}), (3) concentration of deoxyribonucleoside triphosphates (dNTPs), (4) polymerase extension time and the (5) number of PCR cycles [79, 80]. Upon amplification, the product must be ligated to a suitable plasmid and an additional step is required to recover the transformants that consist of the mutations. Error-prone PCR is a robust technique, whereby it can only introduce limited amount of base substitutions into the gene sequence. Therefore it is very useful to identify amino acid positions that are associated with function, affinity and specificity of antibodies for the method to be applied on [1]. The resulting libraries consist of a large amount of A to G and T to C transitions, thus causing high GC content amplification bias. This limitation can be circumvented by the addition of unbalanced ratios of nucleotides to reduce the amplification bias. A commercial DNA polymerase, Mutazyme® was introduced for error-prone PCR with reduced mutational bias which overcomes the issue of preferential nucleotide base selection by *Taq* DNA polymerase during amplification [78]. Error-prone

PCR has been performed across the entire coding region to promote enhanced binders by the introduction of additional interacting residues between ligands and targets, altering the three dimensional structure of the target contact regions or promoting the thermal stability of ligands [53]. This method is suitable for use in ribosome, mRNA, and DNA displays whereby PCR amplification step is required after each round of selection. Additional mutations can be introduced to potential binders during this stage and can be characterized in the following round of selection. This approach was successfully used in combination with DNA shuffling for the selection and affinity maturation of an anti-fluorescein scFv which achieve an affinity of 100 fM from a 10^7 yeast display library [81]. Another variant of error-prone PCR applies isothermal rolling circle amplification for gene diversification. It amplifies a circular DNA template by rolling circle mechanism, generating single-stranded DNA comprising of multiple tandem repeats [82]. To generate a randomly mutated sequence library, a wild-type sequence can be introduced into a plasmid followed by isothermal rolling circle amplification under error-prone conditions [78, 83].

Recombination provides another approach for gene modification and diversification. Mutational rearrangements are highly advantageous to identify and obtain beneficial mutational combinations otherwise absent in nature. Chain shuffling is a process that serves as a "mix and match" system to increase gene repertoires. Chain shuffling allows for one of the two antibody chains (heavy or light chains) to be paired with a repertoire of partner chains to generate a secondary library in order to produce higher affinity antibodies. The domain shuffling is a useful affinity maturation tool for antibodies as it mimics the *in vivo* SHM process [84]. While DNA shuffling generates chimeric libraries through random fragmentation of a pool of similar genes, reassembly of the fragments will result in template switching giving rise to sequence diversity. Application of DNA shuffling to different antibody genes leads to exchange of CDRs and frameworks. Affinity maturation can be achieved by using a single variable heavy chain domain or light chain domain from a known binder and mixing it with an array of diverse different heavy chain or light chain domains for an improved affinity.

Site-directed mutagenesis involves *in vitro* gene modifications that are targeted at a specific genetic locus or a segment of DNA sequence to study the sequence-structure-function of a gene candidate [85]. However, site-saturating mutagenesis will substitute specific sites against all possible amino acid residues. Hence, the importance of a specific amino acid residue towards the function of an antibody can be elucidated through this focused mutagenesis method [78, 86]. This can be applied for stability engineering of antibodies by determining the influence of different amino acids at strategic positions along the antibody structure. Site-directed mutagenesis can be performed through several different approaches. The availability of restriction nucleases and DNA ligases allows easy incorporation of mutagenic sequences into templates to construct recombinant DNAs [87]. The rapid development of oligonucleotide synthesis has also contributed to oligonucleotide-mediated mutagenesis method. Such approach is designed to consist of internal mismatches that complement the template DNA for directing point mutations or multiple mutations. For instance, a mutagenic primer anneals to a single-stranded DNA template, followed by extension with Klenow fragment of DNA polymerase I and is ligated with T4 DNA ligase. The resulting combination of mutant and wild-type DNA is produced when the heteroduplex DNA is transfected into competent *E. coli* [85]. Kunkel mutagenesis uses a circular, single-stranded DNA (ssDNA) template that incorporates uracil as template. The ssDNA is then annealed to the mutagenic primers to generate double-stranded DNA (dsDNA) that consists of the mutation. The dsDNA is then transfected into *E. coli* where the bacterial repair mechanisms will remove the parent strand (uracil-strand) while the recombinant clones predominate and propagate [88, 89].

Mutagenesis on a single-stranded DNA template (ssDNA) is labor intensive because the template requires subcloning and ssDNA rescue. Therefore, several commercial kits are available that utilizes double-stranded DNA (dsDNA) as template for site-directed mutagenesis with mutagenic primers. The QuickChange™ system (Stratagene) uses a pair of complementary oligonucleotides (forward and reverse) that consists of the desired mutations to amplify the whole plasmid with high fidelity polymerase, followed by removal of the parental DNA using *Dpn 1* endonuclease. The GeneTailor™ system (Invitrogen) is somewhat similar to QuickChange™, however it requires DNA methylase to methylate the DNA template prior to amplification. The GeneEditor™ system requires multiple transformations and ampicillin resistance cloning vectors for selecting mutants that has undergone mutagenesis [88, 90]. A major convenience for the GeneTailor™ and QuickChange™ system is the ability to carry out the mutagenesis without requiring additional vectors, host strains, or restriction sites.

Another variant of site-directed mutagenesis is a PCR-driven method termed as overlap extension PCR. This technique employs PCR to generate modified genes from cloned DNA with just a few simple steps. The segments of a target gene are amplified from a DNA template using two flanking master primers and two internal primers. The internal primers consist of the desired mutation and overlapping nucleotide sequences. Two rounds of PCR are carried out, first by amplifying the target genes with their respective pair of primers to create two gene fragments that share some overlapping sequences at the 3′ end. Subsequently, these double-stranded duplexes are denatured and annealed, resulting in two heteroduplexes with each strand consisting of the mutated site. Then DNA polymerase functions to extend the overlapping ends of each heteroduplexes. A second PCR is done with the use of two flanking master primers to amplify the entire modified gene [90, 91]. This method was recently employed by Kitzman et al. [92] to create massive single amino acid mutagenesis in a parallel fashion coupled with microarray-based DNA synthesis technology. This is particularly useful for assessing and screening of variants in libraries.

The increased understanding of molecular biology and specific functions of molecular biology enzymes has allowed the introduction of different approaches for mutagenesis. The combination of the different function of various enzymes has been utilized successfully to carry out directed evolution of antibody genes. Lambda exonuclease in nature functions to assist the repair of dsDNA breaks of viral DNA. It is a highly processive 5′→3′ dsDNA exonuclease which selectively degrades the phosphorylated chain of a duplex DNA to yield mononucleotides and ssDNA. A strategy that takes advantage of this feature of lambda exonuclease was applied for antibody gene mutagenesis. The formed ssDNA template will function as the template for *in vitro* antibody gene recombination. The ssDNA template is then hybridized with degenerate oligonucleotides and treated with Klenow Fragment to generate dsDNA templates of the hybridized products. This will result in a final dsDNA template that has incorporated the diversification introduced by the degenerate oligos at a specific site of the antibody gene. The method was successfully applied to carry out chain shuffling and mutagenesis of antibody clones [93]. However, a major bottleneck with these methods is their inability to allow directed mutagenesis with codon specificity.

The diversification of the antibody repertoire can also be realized by *in vitro* somatic hypermutation using the AID enzyme [94]. The AID enzyme is classified in the APOBEC family of cytidine deaminases that is able to catalyze the deamination of cytidine residues to uridine residues *in vitro* only on ssDNA, giving rise to thymine residues at the end of the replication events [95].

Typically, the cytidines are targeted at the mutational hotspot motif RGYW and AGY (R = A/G, Y = C/T, W = A/T). This motif is also the preferred region for mutations during *in vivo* somatic hypermutation [96, 97]. Reports revealed that *in vitro* cytidine deamination occurs in an orientation-dependent fashion, relying on the transcription to gain access to both template and non-template strands of DNA. Nevertheless, it is capable of introducing mutations into DNA and therefore applicable for gene diversification [98, 99]. AID-mediated mutagenesis serves as a useful method to enhance antibody affinities through sequence diversity by introducing point mutations, such as single amino acid substitutions or indels (insertions, deletions) specifically on the antibody CDR sequences. Nucleotide transversions and duplications are among the most complicated to design into a library but possible with the AID-mediated mutagenesis approach [34]. The AID enzyme is capable of generating indels which are localized in CDR regions, while affinity maturation through somatic mutation further improves the antibody binding and specificity [100]. *In vitro* expression of the AID enzyme is sufficient to initiate indels, hypermutations inside the CDRs and clonal expansion that is comparable to *in vivo* events for antibody evolution.

Studies have been carried out to analyze the amino acid diversities in the germline and mature antibody sequences. It was found that the number of germline hotspots decreases in high affinity antibodies, suggesting that hotspot-based somatic mutations occurred via *in vivo* affinity maturation [101]. Through the *in vitro* randomization of these short CDR regions that somewhat mimics the natural *in vivo* SHM sequences diversity is generated and results in *in vitro* affinity maturation. These hotspots are embedded in the codons of amino acids that are directly and indirectly involved in interactions with antigens. They can serve as the mutation targets in the human genome allowing for various mutagenesis to occur with the aid of the general mutator candidates being AID enzymes or other trans-acting hypermutation factors [102].

The diversity associated with the utilization of various sequences either in the CDR or framework is directly related to the affinity of the clones generated [5, 103]. The continuous development in molecular technologies has allowed the introduction of various approaches for gene modification. The design of the framework regions in the antibody gene also plays a contributing role in the improvement of the antibody affinity. This is due to the influence of the framework genes on the stability, solubility and affinity of the antibody [104]. The framework regions mainly in the neighboring regions of the CDRs have been known to also contribute to the binding characteristic of antibody clones [46].

3.2. *De novo* synthesis of antibody genes

Direct gene synthesis of modified sequences or *de novo* synthesis of DNA is ideal to create desired gene sequences based on iterative and comprehensive analyses with the aid of high throughput sequencing technology. There are few reasons why *de novo* synthesis of DNA is preferred in many instances. Firstly, engineering new functions normally requires great modifications to the genetic sequences therefore *de novo* synthesis is more preferred. Secondly, *de novo* gene synthesis allows specific design of DNA constructs. *De novo* synthesis enables to study the influence of new designed sequences on particular functions of corresponding expressed recombinant antibodies. The aim is to improve or modify phenotypic features of antibodies.

Lastly, targeted sequences from natural constructs are sometimes hard to access, therefore synthesis provides a more efficient alternative to retrieve the targeted sequences [105]. Currently, oligos are generated or synthesized automatically, employing solid-phase phosphoramidite chemistry. The principle behind phosphoramidite-based oligo synthesis encompasses a total of four key steps (deprotection, coupling, capping and oxidation) to add one base at a time to a growing oligo chain attached to a solid support.

Synthesis takes place individually in small columns. The purified oligos are then subjected to quality assessments. The automated process can generate up to 100 nmol of oligos at a time with low error rates in the region of one base error in 200 nucleotides [105, 106].

Besides conventional gene synthesis from oligo fragments using column-based synthesized oligos, array-based oligos can be used for gene synthesis as well. An array-based synthesis has the advantage of high throughput synthesis. The polymer array support by Affymetrix is synthesized chemically comprising photolabile protecting groups and photolithography. The photolithographic mask is able to direct UV light over the solid substrate and selectively deprotect and activate the 5′-hydroxyl group in the growing chain, in order for free nucleotides to be incorporated into the chain. The mask is designed for exposing targeted sites on the microarray, where incorporation of nucleotides occurs while masking other non-targeted sites. The oligo fragments are directly synthesized on the support surface, and can be recovered as a heterogenous pool of sequences. Today, several technologies have surpassed the need to use the masking technique. An ink-jet-based printing developed by Agilent allows picolitres of free nucleotides and activator to be spotted on targeted sites on one array. NimbleGen Systems uses the programmed automated micromirror device to activate specific sites on the array. Furthermore, CustomArray (CombiMatrix) utilizes semiconductor-based electrochemical acid production to deprotect desired nucleosides [107, 108].

Nevertheless, the NimbleGen and CustomArray oligo synthesis techniques suffer high error rates when trying to generate longer and multiple oligo strands in parallel. This is due to the side reactions such as depurination and inefficient addition of nucleotides that results in unwanted substitution and indels (insertion/deletion) errors, which greatly affects the overall quality of the synthesized product. Therefore purification steps utilizing polyacrylamide gel electrophoresis and high performance liquid chromatography are essential to remove erroneous sequences upon generating the intended DNA sequences [109].

The generated oligo fragments obtained after conventional or area-based synthesis are then used as raw substrates to construct larger synthetic fragments (usually few hundreds of base pairs), also known as gene synthesis. Using a ligation-based approach, the complementary overlapping fragments are joined enzymatically by the thermostable DNA ligases, producing larger DNA fragments under high stringency [110]. Another approach, known as polymerase cycling assembly (PCA)-based method, utilizes polymerase to elongate the originated overlapping oligo fragments into double-stranded fragments [111]. Ligation-based synthesis offer higher stringency, therefore error in sequences is less likely to be assembled, but the oligo synthesis are costly due to synthesis of longer fragments. The longer oligonucleotides will allow for better annealing and less steps in comparison to shorter oligonucleotdies. The final step would sometimes involve an additional Polymerase chain reaction (PCR) amplification step to yield more material for cloning. On the contrary, PCA-based methods are more cost-effective as it relies on overlapping short oligo fragments (15–25 nt) per gene synthesis. However, this approach promotes higher error rates due to the lack of error elimination during hybridization [112]. Also, target diversity can be introduced at the regions where the overlapping oligo fragments hybridizes [109].

Despite the fact that concentrations of individual oligos on the array are quite low and insufficient for priming, as well as the error rates of the oligo pools are higher as the column-based methods, there are successful examples that overcome these challenges. This is done with the use of programmable DNA microchips with an array of oligonucleotides and their selection [113]. To increase the concentration of oligonucleotides for gene synthesis, amplification of oligo fragments before assembly is required. Sequence errors can be detected via hybridization of the synthetized cleaved oligonucleotides to complementary oligonucleotides spanned on a second area. Lastly error-free fragments will be assembled into full-length sequences. However, this method is not feasible for assembling a large pool of oligos because of the risk of cross-hybridization based on the huge diversity. Another approach used selective oligonucleotide pool amplification directed by predesigned barcodes to generate and assemble particular DNA fragments that are required to make a full gene before the barcodes are digested prior to full gene assembly [114]. Recently, this approach was applied to construct few scFv gene libraries with degenerate oligonucleotides synthesized on two DNA microchips in parallel [115]. The humanized anti-ErbB2 antibody (HuA21) was targeted to diversify the CDR regions via a small perturbation mutagenesis method and was validated using deep sequencing by the Illumina platform. Finally, the mutant candidates were screened by phage display to select for high affinity binders [115, 116].

gBlocks gene fragments are readily usable short-to-medium length synthesized DNA fragments that contains particular desired gene modifications. gBlocks are dsDNA blocks that undergo controlled synthesis allowing various applications for antibody and protein engineering. The main application focuses specifically on gene construction and editing. gBlocks are constructed using gene fragment libraries (pools of short DNA fragments that comprise 18 consecutive N bases or K (G,T) bases). The synthesized product is then subjected to various quality control tests such as capillary electrophoresis (fragment length) and mass spectrometry (sequence composition) to verify the final product and reduce potential errors. For gene editing, gBlocks can introduce modifications such as deletion or insertion on relatively short stretches of DNA fragments. The primers are designed to target the region of the gene that is to be edited. Subsequently, the region will be cleaved and replaced by the gBlock [109]. This method has allowed the design and generation of antibody libraries [117, 118].

3.3. *In vivo* approaches towards affinity maturation of antibodies

Bacterial mutator strains, such as *Escherichia coli* mutants are shown to introduce random mutations, such as single-base substitutions with higher rates than wild type strains. The mutant strains are characterized by the absence of several DNA repair pathways, resulting in a high rate of mutations [78]. Affinity maturation via this approach involves two key steps; firstly, antibody genes are transformed and replicated in *E. coli* mutants to introduce random mutations. Next, screening of mutated antibody clones to identify highest affinity binders is done using display technologies. The affinity maturation process requires several rounds of mutation, selection and amplification in order to obtain high affinity mutants. Phage display technology is best coupled with *E. coli* mutator cells for *in vivo* mutation of antibody fragments due to the ease of application with phage and phagemid vectors [119]. The *E. coli* mutator cell such as *E. coli* mutD5-FIT consists of mutD mutation, F′ factor for Fd phage transfection and *supE* mutation. This mutant is able to express phage displayed antibody fragments, where antibody genes are fused to the N-terminus of gene III protein and are subsequently packaged to form a mature virus particle. Alternatively, another *E. coli* mutator strain, XLIRed carries mutD, mutL and mutS, while it is devoid of the F′ episome. This does not allow the cell to be applied for phage infection. However, this F′ deficient mutator cell can be converted to F′ mutator strain by mating with other *E. coli* strains with F′ episome [120, 121]. The choice of bacterial mutator strains are largely governed by downstream selection strategies that requires rational considerations. A human antibody fragment that targets the hapten 2-phenyl-5-oxazolone (phOx) was affinity matured by a factor 100 fold via *E. coli* mutD5 strain, whereby the mutations are extensively located in CDR loops and less in framework regions, which improve the binding affinity of the antibody to the target [122].

In vivo affinity maturation can also be performed via AID-mediated mutagenesis. It fits quite well with the robust mammalian cell display techniques for selection and affinity maturation of functional antibody clones. As an example, the cDNA of an anti-human complement protein C5 antibody is transfected into HEK293 cells together with the AID enzyme expression plasmid to initiate *in vitro* SHM. The antibody clones are identified and isolated by fluorescence-activated cell sorting (FACS) with fluorescence labeled antigen followed by iterative rounds of SHM to yield high affinity antibodies [34]. In mammalian, yeast and bacterial cell surface display it is essential to select and isolate the cells that are able to produce functional antibodies. Cell-based sorting such as high throughput flow cytometry, allows high throughput screening of cells per minute, analyzing the cells according to size, granularity and binding to fluorescence labeled antigens. The utmost reason for antibody engineering is the production of human monoclonal antibody in large scale, hence, it is crucial to implement a selection towards antibody expressing mammalian cells. Mammalian display allows for screening of eukaryotes-expressed full length antibodies with correct glycosylation [18, 123].

The advancement of genome editing technologies offers a new approach to create sequence diversity. In fact, cells can repair DNA damages intrinsically by joining two ends together or filling the gap with similar sequences. However, cells can also repair the break by using a new piece of DNA that has the desired mutation. This is the basis of *in vivo* genome editing technologies today [124]. Extensive functional genomics studies helps to provide the insights required that targeted DNA double-stranded breaks (DSBs). The DSBs can induce genome editing via homologous recombination (HR) in the presence of exogenous homology repair template, as well as error-prone non-homologous end-joining repair (NHEJ) pathway in the absence of repair template. These two pathways are versatile to allow precise genome modification [125]. To date, there are four major classes of engineered DNA binding proteins to target DSBs: meganucleases, zinc finger (ZF) nucleases, transcription activator-like effectors (TALEs) and RNA-guided DNA endonuclease Cas9 [124].

Meganucleases are derived from microbial mobile genetic elements that integrate nuclease and DNA binding domains. ZF nucleases (Cys_2His_2 bound to a single atom of zinc) are eukaryotic transcription factors that contain the DNA binding domain and is similar to a set of three fingers, with each finger contacting with 3 nucleotides of DNA [126]. TALEs are produced naturally by *Xanthomonas* sp. that consist of DNA binding domains with 30–35 tandem repeats, with each domain recognizing a single nucleotide of DNA. Specificity of TALEs is governed by the two amino acids that are known as the repeat-hypervariable diresidues [127]. Both ZF nucleases and TALEs require *Fok*I nuclease to direct the nucleolytic activity towards the genome locus for modifications. Recently, RNA-guided DNA endonuclease Cas9 is given much more attention due to its simplicity and versatile approach towards *in vivo* genome engineering. It is derived from type II bacterial adaptive immune system. The CRISPR-Cas9 mediated immunity is explicitly explained in Yang et al. [128]. The hallmark of this system is the short RNA guide that recognizes the target DNA through base pairing, forming a RNA-DNA complex, subsequently Cas9 creates DSB on the target sequence [129, 130] and a designed DNA fragment can be specifically incorporated.

While other approaches have their own limitations, the robustness of the CRISPR-Cas9 system sheds some light on direct endogenous genome editing on virtually any organism of choice. Meganuclease lacks target specificity, which is why it is not widely employed. However, ZF domains have a tendency to crosslink with neighboring protein -domains or -complexes resulting in lower binding efficiency towards DNA targets. Although TALEs require only one nucleotide for binding towards target, however the synthesis for novel TALEs is costly due to their repetitive sequences [125]. Nevertheless, these enzymes are constructed in customizable fashion to cater for the need of genome editing, as well as programming the enzymes for multiplex gene targeting [54]. Some model organisms were tested with the genome editing technologies, such as zebrafish, rats, mice, *Drosophila, C. elegans*. Some delivery methods of introducing these programmed enzymes into organisms are microinjections of stem cells with mRNA encoding the enzymes or direct transfection of an plasmid consisting of the enzyme cDNA into HEK293 cells [128, 131].

4. Conclusion

Naïve and synthetic human antibody repertoires are a very valuable source for the selection of antibodies against nearly any antigen. The role display technologies play in the quest to generate monoclonal antibodies from these libraries is obvious with the increasing number of antibody lead candidates going into clinical trials.

Affinity maturation of selected binders is now possible by expressing for example the AID enzyme during selection of antibodies using antibody mammalian cell surface display or by using a pool of microchip-synthesized CDRs incorporated into an antibody framework. Selection of naïve and synthetic recombinant antibodies combined with *in vitro* and *in vivo* affinity maturation techniques will have a profound effect on the generation of high affinity diagnostic and therapeutic human antibodies.

Acknowledgements

The authors would like to acknowledge the support from the Malaysian Ministry of Higher Education under the Higher Institution Centre of Excellence (HICoE) Grant (Grant no. 311/CIPPM/44001005).

Author details

Chia Chiu Lim[1], Yee Siew Choong[1] and Theam Soon Lim[1,2]*

*Address all correspondence to: theamsoon@usm.my

1 Institute for Research in Molecular Medicine, Universiti Sains Malaysia, Minden, Penang, Malaysia

2 Analytical Biochemistry Research Centre, Universiti Sains Malaysia, Minden, Penang, Malaysia

References

[1] Ducancel F, Muller BH. Molecular engineering of antibodies for therapeutic and diagnostic purposes. mAbs. 2012;**4**:445-457

[2] Smith AJ. New horizons in therapeutic antibody discovery: Opportunities and challenges versus small-molecule therapeutics. Journal of Biomolecular Screening. 2015;**20**:437-453

[3] Weiner GJ. Building better monoclonal antibody-based therapeutics. Nature Reviews Cancer. 2015;**15**:361-370

[4] Zhang X, Soori G, Dobleman TJ, Xiao GG. The application of monoclonal antibodies in cancer diagnosis. Expert Review of Molecular Diagnostics. 2014;**14**:97-106

[5] Klein F, Diskin R, Scheid JF, Gaebler C, Mouquet H, Georgiev IS, Pancera M, Zhou T, Incesu R-B, Fu BZ. Somatic mutations of the immunoglobulin framework are generally required for broad and potent HIV-1 neutralization. Cell. 2013;**153**:126-138

[6] Villaudy J, Schotte R, Legrand N, Spits H. Critical assessment of human antibody generation in humanized mouse models. Journal of Immunological Methods. 2014;**410**:18-27

[7] Weisser NE, Hall JC. Applications of single-chain variable fragment antibodies in therapeutics and diagnostics. Biotechnology Advances. 2009;**27**:502-520

[8] Bowers PM, Neben TY, Tomlinson GL, Dalton JL, Altobell L, Zhang X, Macomber JL, Wu BF, Toobian RM, McConnell AD. Humanization of antibodies using heavy chain complementarity-determining region 3 grafting coupled with in vitro somatic hypermutation. Journal of Biological Chemistry. 2013;**288**:7688-7696

[9] Briney B, Crowe J. Secondary mechanisms of diversification in the human antibody repertoire. Frontiers in Immunology. 2013;**4**:7

[10] Ecker DM, Jones SD, Levine HL. The therapeutic monoclonal antibody market. mAbs. 2015. Taylor & Francis

[11] Gottlieb AB, Krueger JG, Lundblad MS, Göthberg M, Skolnick BE. First-in-human, phase 1, randomized, dose-escalation trial with recombinant anti–IL-20 monoclonal antibody in patients with psoriasis. PLoS One. 2015;**10**:e0134703

[12] Galán A, Comor L, Horvatić A, Kuleš J, Guillemin N, Mrljak V, Bhide M. Library-based display technologies: Where do we stand? Molecular BioSystems. 2016;**12**:2342-2358

[13] Bradbury AR, Sidhu S, Dübel S, McCafferty J. Beyond natural antibodies: The power of in vitro display technologies. Nature Biotechnology. 2011;**29**:245-254

[14] Tizei PA, Csibra E, Torres L, Pinheiro VB. Selection platforms for directed evolution in synthetic biology. Biochemical Society Transactions. 2016;**44**:1165-1175

[15] Bazan J, Całkosiński I, Gamian A. Phage display—A powerful technique for immunotherapy: 1. Introduction and potential of therapeutic applications. Human Vaccines & Immunotherapeutics. 2012;**8**:1817-1828

[16] Ullman CG, Frigotto L, Cooley RN. In vitro methods for peptide display and their applications. Briefings in Functional Genomics. 2011;**10**:125-134

[17] Fitzgerald K. In vitro display technologies–new tools for drug discovery. Drug Discovery Today. 2000;**5**:253-258

[18] Doerner A, Rhiel L, Zielonka S, Kolmar H. Therapeutic antibody engineering by high efficiency cell screening. FEBS letters. 2014;**588**:278-287

[19] Nelson AL, Dhimolea E, Reichert JM. Development trends for human monoclonal antibody therapeutics. Nature Reviews Drug Discovery. 2010;**9**:767-774

[20] Schaffitzel C, Hanes J, Jermutus L, Plückthun A. Ribosome display: An in vitro method for selection and evolution of antibodies from libraries. Journal of Immunological Methods. 1999;**231**:119-135

[21] Goldflam M, Ullman CG. Recent advances toward the discovery of drug-like peptides de novo. Frontiers in Chemistry. 2015;**3**:8

[22] Sumida T, Yanagawa H, Doi N. In vitro selection of fab fragments by mRNA display and gene-linking emulsion PCR. Journal of Nucleic Acids. 2012;**2012**:9

[23] Tomimatsu K, Matsumoto S-E, Tanaka H, Yamashita M, Nakanishi H, Teruya K, Kazuno S, Kinjo T, Hamasaki T, Kusumoto K-I. A rapid screening and production method using a novel mammalian cell display to isolate human monoclonal antibodies. Biochemical and Biophysical Research Communications. 2013;**441**:59-64

[24] David JK, Peter MB, Marilyn RK, Robert AH. Mammalian cell display and somatic hypermutation in vitro for human antibody discovery. Current Drug Discovery Technologies. 2014;**11**:56-64

[25] Jäger V, Büssow K, Wagner A, Weber S, Hust M, Frenzel A, Schirrmann T. High level transient production of recombinant antibodies and antibody fusion proteins in HEK293 cells. BMC Biotechnology. 2013;**13**:52

[26] Bowers PM, Horlick RA, Kehry MR, Neben TY, Tomlinson GL, Altobell L, Zhang X, Macomber JL, Krapf IP, Wu BF. Mammalian cell display for the discovery and optimization of antibody therapeutics. Methods. 2014;**65**:44-56

[27] Yonezawa M, Doi N, Higashinakagawa T, Yanagawa H. DNA display of biologically active proteins for in vitro protein selection. The Journal of Biochemistry. 2004;**135**:285-288

[28] Nakayama M, Komiya S, Fujiwara K, Horisawa K, Doi N. In vitro selection of bispecific diabody fragments using covalent bicistronic DNA display. Biochemical and Biophysical Research Communications. 2016;**478**:606-611

[29] Sumida T, Doi N, Yanagawa H. Bicistronic DNA display for in vitro selection of Fab fragments. Nucleic Acids Research. 2009;**37**:e147-e147

[30] Odegrip R, Coomber D, Eldridge B, Hederer R, Kuhlman PA, Ullman C, FitzGerald K, McGregor D. CIS display: In vitro selection of peptides from libraries of protein–DNA complexes. Proceedings of the National Academy of Sciences of the United States of America. 2004;**101**:2806-2810

[31] Sergeeva A, Kolonin MG, Molldrem JJ, Pasqualini R, Arap W. Display technologies: Application for the discovery of drug and gene delivery agents. Advanced Drug Delivery Reviews. 2006;**58**:1622-1654

[32] Wada A. Development of next-generation peptide binders using in vitro display technologies and their potential applications. Frontiers in Immunology. 2013;**4**:6

[33] Arnaout R, Lee W, Cahill P, Honan T, Sparrow T, Weiand M, Nusbaum C, Rajewsky K, Koralov SB. High-resolution description of antibody heavy-chain repertoires in humans. PLoS One. 2011;**6**:e22365

[34] McConnell AD, Do M, Neben TY, Spasojevic V, MacLaren J, Chen AP, Altobell L III, Macomber JL, Berkebile AD, Horlick RA. High affinity humanized antibodies without making hybridomas; immunization paired with mammalian cell display and in vitro somatic hypermutation. PLoS One. 2012;**7**:e49458

[35] Georgiou G, Ippolito GC, Beausang J, Busse CE, Wardemann H, Quake SR. The promise and challenge of high-throughput sequencing of the antibody repertoire. Nature Biotechnology. 2014;**32**:158-168

[36] Robinson WH. Sequencing the functional antibody repertoire [mdash] diagnostic and therapeutic discovery. Nature Reviews Rheumatology. 2015;**11**:171-182

[37] Beerli RR, Rader C. Mining human antibody repertoires. mAbs. 2010;**2**:365-378

[38] Mathonet P, Ullman C. The application of next generation sequencing to the understanding of antibody repertoires. Frontiers in Immunology. 2013;**4**:265

[39] LeBien TW, Tedder TF. B lymphocytes: How they develop and function. Blood. 2008;**112**:1570-1580

[40] Roth DB. V(D)J recombination: Mechanism, errors, and fidelity. Microbiology Spectrum. 2014;**2**:11

[41] Hwang JK, Alt FW, Yeap L-S. Related mechanisms of antibody somatic hypermutation and class switch recombination. Microbiology Spectrum. 2015;**3**:22

[42] Lerner RA. Combinatorial antibody libraries: New advances, new immunological insights. Nature Reviews Immunology. 2016;**16**:498

[43] Li W, Prabakaran P, Chen W, Zhu Z, Feng Y, Dimitrov DS. Antibody aggregation: Insights from sequence and structure. Antibodies. 2016;**5**:19

[44] Li Z, Woo CJ, Iglesias-Ussel MD, Ronai D, Scharff MD. The generation of antibody diversity through somatic hypermutation and class switch recombination. Genes & Development. 2004;**18**:1-11

[45] Muramatsu M, Kinoshita K, Fagarasan S, Yamada S, Shinkai Y, Honjo T. Class switch recombination and hypermutation require activation-induced cytidine deaminase (AID), a potential RNA editing enzyme. Cell. 2000;**102**:553-563

[46] Sela-Culang I, Kunik V, Ofran Y. The structural basis of antibody-antigen recognition. Frontiers in Immunology. 2013;**4**:13

[47] Ahmad ZA, Yeap SK, Ali AM, Ho WY, Alitheen NBM, Hamid M. scFv antibody: Principles and clinical application. Clinical and Developmental Immunology. 2012;**2012**:15

[48] Shinkura R, Ito S, Begum NA, Nagaoka H, Muramatsu M, Kinoshita K, Sakakibara Y, Hijikata H, Honjo T. Separate domains of AID are required for somatic hypermutation and class-switch recombination. Nature Immunology. 2004;**5**:707-712

[49] Sidhu SS, Fellouse FA. Synthetic therapeutic antibodies. Nature Chemical Biology. 2006;**2**:682-688

[50] Pande J, Szewczyk MM, Grover AK. Phage display: Concept, innovations, applications and future. Biotechnology Advances. 2010;**28**:849-858

[51] Shukra AM, Sridevi NV, Chandran D, Maithal K. Production of recombinant antibodies using bacteriophages. European Journal of Microbiology and Immunology. 2014;**4**:91-98

[52] Chodorge M, Fourage L, Ravot G, Jermutus L, Minter R. In vitro DNA recombination by L-Shuffling during ribosome display affinity maturation of an anti-Fas antibody increases the population of improved variants. Protein Engineering Design and Selection. 2008;**21**:343-351

[53] Huang R, Gorman KT, Vinci CR, Dobrovetsky E, Gräslund S, Kay BK. Streamlining the pipeline for generation of recombinant affinity reagents by integrating the affinity maturation step. International Journal of Molecular Sciences. 2015;**16**:23587-23603

[54] Findlay GM, Boyle EA, Hause RJ, Klein JC, Shendure J. Saturation editing of genomic regions by multiplex homology-directed repair. Nature. 2014;**513**:120-123

[55] Schwimmer LJ, Huang B, Giang H, Cotter RL, Chemla-Vogel DS, Dy FV, Tam EM, Zhang F, Toy P, Bohmann DJ, Watson SR, Beaber JW, Reddy N, Kuan H-F, Bedinger DH, Rondon IJ. Discovery of diverse and functional antibodies from large human repertoire antibody libraries. Journal of Immunological Methods. 2013;**391**:60-71

[56] Ponsel D, Neugebauer J, Ladetzki-Baehs K, Tissot K. High affinity, developability and functional size: The holy grail of combinatorial antibody library generation. Molecules. 2011;**16**:3675

[57] Dobson C, Minter R, Hart-Shorrock C. Naive antibody libraries from natural repertoires. In: Phage Display in Biotechnology and Drug Discovery. 2nd ed. Boca Raton: CRC Press; 2015. pp. 455-494

[58] Hoehn KB, Fowler A, Lunter G, Pybus OG. The diversity and molecular evolution of B-cell receptors during infection. Molecular Biology and Evolution. 2016;**33**:1147-1157

[59] Paramithiotis E, Cooper MD. Memory B lymphocytes migrate to bone marrow in humans. Proceedings of the National Academy of Sciences. 1997;**94**:208-212

[60] Bahara NHH, Tye GJ, Choong YS, Ong EBB, Ismail A, Lim TS. Phage display antibodies for diagnostic applications. Biologicals. 2013;**41**:209-216

[61] Dantas-Barbosa C, de Macedo Brigido M, Maranhao AQ. Antibody phage display libraries: Contributions to oncology. International Journal of Molecular Sciences. 2012;**13**:5420

[62] Moon SA, Ki MK, Lee S, Hong M-L, Kim M, Kim S, Chung J, Rhee SG, Shim H. Antibodies against non-immunizing antigens derived from a large immune scFv library. Molecules and Cells. 2011;**31**:509-513

[63] Rothe C, Urlinger S, Löhning C, Prassler J, Stark Y, Jäger U, Hubner B, Bardroff M, Pradel I, Boss M. The human combinatorial antibody library HuCAL GOLD combines diversification of all six CDRs according to the natural immune system with a novel display method for efficient selection of high-affinity antibodies. Journal of Molecular Biology. 2008;**376**:1182-1200

[64] González-Muñoz A, Bokma E, O'Shea D, Minton K, Strain M, Vousden K, Rossant C, Jermutus L, Minter R. Tailored amino acid diversity for the evolution of antibody affinity. mAbs. 2012;**4**:664-672

[65] Rauchenberger R, Borges E, Thomassen-Wolf E, Rom E, Adar R, Yaniv Y, Malka M, Chumakov I, Kotzer S, Resnitzky D. Human combinatorial Fab library yielding specific and functional antibodies against the human fibroblast growth factor receptor 3. Journal of Biological Chemistry. 2003;**278**:38194-38205

[66] Krebs B, Rauchenberger R, Reiffert S, Rothe C, Tesar M, Thomassen E, Cao M, Dreier T, Fischer D, Höß A. High-throughput generation and engineering of recombinant human antibodies. Journal of Immunological Methods. 2001;**254**:67-84

[67] Prassler J, Steidl S, Urlinger S. In vitro affinity maturation of HuCAL antibodies: Complementarity determining region exchange and RapMAT technology. Immunotherapy. 2009;**1**:571-583

[68] Frigotto L, Smith ME, Brankin C, Sedani A, Cooper SE, Kanwar N, Evans D, Svobodova S, Baar C, Glanville J. Codon-precise, synthetic, antibody fragment libraries built using automated hexamer codon additions and validated through next generation sequencing. Antibodies. 2015;**4**:88-102

[69] Knappik A, Ge L, Honegger A, Pack P, Fischer M, Wellnhofer G, Hoess A, WoÈlle J, Plückthun A, Virnekäs B. Fully synthetic human combinatorial antibody libraries (HuCAL) based on modular consensus frameworks and CDRs randomized with trinucleotides. Journal of Molecular Biology. 2000;**296**:57-86

[70] Prassler J, Thiel S, Pracht C, Polzer A, Peters S, Bauer M, Nörenberg S, Stark Y, Kölln J, Popp A. HuCAL PLATINUM, a synthetic Fab library optimized for sequence diversity and superior performance in mammalian expression systems. Journal of Molecular Biology. 2011;**413**:261-278

[71] Benhar I. Design of synthetic antibody libraries. Expert Opinion on Biological Therapy. 2007;**7**:763-779

[72] Carlsson R, Söderlind E. n-CoDeR concept: Unique types of antibodies for diagnostic use and therapy. Expert Review of Molecular Diagnostics. 2001;**1**:102-108

[73] Söderlind E, Strandberg L, Jirholt P, Kobayashi N, Alexeiva V, Åberg A-M, Nilsson A, Jansson B, Ohlin M, Wingren C. Recombining germline-derived CDR sequences for creating diverse single-framework antibody libraries. Nature Biotechnology. 2000;**18**:852

[74] Tikunova N, Morozova V. Phage display on the base of filamentous bacteriophages: Application for recombinant antibodies selection. Acta Naturae (англоязычная версия). 2009;**1**:20-28

[75] Hoogenboom HR. Selecting and screening recombinant antibody libraries. Nature Biotechnology. 2005;**23**:1105-1116

[76] Thie H, Voedisch B, Dübel S, Hust M, Schirrmann T. Affinity maturation by phage display. In: Dimitrov AS, editor. Therapeutic Antibodies: Methods and Protocols. Totowa, NJ: Humana Press; 2009. pp. 309-322

[77] Marvin JS, Lowman HB. Antibody humanization and affinity maturation using phage display. In: Phage Display in Biotechnology and Drug Discovery. 2nd ed. Boca Raton: CRC Press; 2015. pp. 347-372

[78] Labrou NE. Random mutagenesis methods for in vitro directed enzyme evolution. Current Protein and Peptide Science. 2010;**11**:91-100

[79] Martineau P. Error-prone polymerase chain reaction for modification of scFvs. In: O'Brien PM, Aitken R, editors. Antibody Phage Display: Methods and Protocols. Totowa, NJ: Humana Press; 2002. pp. 287-294

[80] McCullum EO, Williams BAR, Zhang J, Chaput JC. Random mutagenesis by error-prone PCR. In: Braman J, editor. In Vitro Mutagenesis Protocols. 3rd ed. Totowa, NJ: Humana Press; 2010. pp. 103-109

[81] Boder ET, Midelfort KS, Wittrup KD. Directed evolution of antibody fragments with monovalent femtomolar antigen-binding affinity. Proceedings of the National Academy of Sciences. 2000;**97**:10701-10705

[82] Ali MM, Li F, Zhang Z, Zhang K, Kang D-K, Ankrum JA, Le XC, Zhao W. Rolling circle amplification: A versatile tool for chemical biology, materials science and medicine. Chemical Society Reviews. 2014;**43**:3324-3341

[83] Fujii R, Kitaoka M, Hayashi K. One-step random mutagenesis by error-prone rolling circle amplification. Nucleic Acids Research. 2004;**32**:e145-e145

[84] Marks JD. Antibody affinity maturation by chain shuffling. In: Antibody Engineering: Methods and Protocols. Vol. 248. Humana Press; 2004. pp. 327-343

[85] Carter P. Site-directed mutagenesis. Biochemical Journal. 1986;**237**:1

[86] Ruff AJ, Dennig A, Schwaneberg U. To get what we aim for–progress in diversity generation methods. FEBS Journal. 2013;**280**:2961-2978

[87] Smith M. Site-directed mutagenesis. Trends in Biochemical Sciences. 1982;**7**:440-442

[88] Huang R, Fang P, Kay BK. Improvements to the Kunkel mutagenesis protocol for constructing primary and secondary phage-display libraries. Methods. 2012;**58**:10-17

[89] Pai JC, Entzminger KC, Maynard JA. Restriction enzyme-free construction of random gene mutagenesis libraries in *Escherichia coli*. Analytical Biochemistry. 2012;**421**:640-648

[90] Carrigan PE, Ballar P, Tuzmen S. Site-directed mutagenesis. In: Disease Gene Identification: Methods and Protocols. Totowa, NJ: Humana Press; 2011. pp. 107-124

[91] Ho SN, Hunt HD, Horton RM, Pullen JK, Pease LR. Site-directed mutagenesis by overlap extension using the polymerase chain reaction. Gene. 1989;**77**:51-59

[92] Kitzman JO, Starita LM, Lo RS, Fields S, Shendure J. Massively parallel single-amino-acid mutagenesis. Nature Methods. 2015;**12**:203-206

[93] Lim BN, Choong YS, Ismail A, Glökler J, Konthur Z, Lim TS. Directed evolution of nucleotide-based libraries using lambda exonuclease. BioTechniques. 2012;**53**:357-364

[94] Halemano K, Guo K, Heilman KJ, Barrett BS, Smith DS, Hasenkrug KJ, Santiago ML. Immunoglobulin somatic hypermutation by APOBEC3/Rfv3 during retroviral infection. Proceedings of the National Academy of Sciences. 2014;**111**:7759-7764

[95] Wei L, Chahwan R, Wang S, Wang X, Pham PT, Goodman MF, Bergman A, Scharff MD, MacCarthy T. Overlapping hotspots in CDRs are critical sites for V region diversification. Proceedings of the National Academy of Sciences. 2015;**112**:E728-E737

[96] Wang M, Rada C, Neuberger MS. Altering the spectrum of immunoglobulin V gene somatic hypermutation by modifying the active site of AID. Journal of Experimental Medicine. 2010;**207**:141-153

[97] Yau KY, Dubuc G, Li S, Hirama T, MacKenzie CR, Jermutus L, Hall JC, Tanha J. Affinity maturation of a VHH by mutational hotspot randomization. Journal of Immunological Methods. 2005;**297**:213-224

[98] Chaudhuri J, Tian M, Khuong C, Chua K, Pinaud E, Alt FW. Transcription-targeted DNA deamination by the AID antibody diversification enzyme. Nature. 2003;**422**:726-730

[99] Keim C, Kazadi D, Rothschild G, Basu U. Regulation of AID, the B-cell genome mutator. Genes & Development. 2013;**27**:1-17

[100] Bowers PM, Verdino P, Wang Z, da Silva Correia J, Chhoa M, Macondray G, Do M, Neben TY, Horlick RA, Stanfield RL. Nucleotide insertions and deletions complement point mutations to massively expand the diversity created by somatic hypermutation of antibodies. Journal of Biological Chemistry. 2014;**289**:33557-33567

[101] Ho M, Pastan I. In vitro antibody affinity maturation targeting germline hotspots. In: Therapeutic Antibodies: Methods and Protocols. Vol. 525. Humana Press; 2009. pp. 293-308

[102] Li B, Zhao L, Wang C, Guo H, Wu L, Zhang X, Qian W, Wang H, Guo Y. The protein-protein interface evolution acts in a similar way to antibody affinity maturation. Journal of Biological Chemistry. 2010;**285**:3865-3871

[103] Almagro JC. Natural and man-made V-gene repertoires for antibody discovery. Frontiers in Immunology. 2012;**3**:18

[104] Tiller KE, Tessier PM. Advances in antibody design. Annual Review of Biomedical Engineering. 2015;**17**:191-216

[105] Kosuri S, Church GM. Large-scale de novo DNA synthesis: Technologies and applications. Nature Methods. 2014;**11**:499-507

[106] Lindner T, Kolmar H, Haberkorn U, Mier W. DNA libraries for the construction of phage libraries: Statistical and structural requirements and synthetic methods. Molecules. 2011;**16**:1625-1641

[107] Baker M. Microarrays, megasynthesis. Nature Methods. 2011;**8**:457

[108] Bumgarner R. Overview of DNA microarrays: Types, applications, and their future. In: Current Protocols in Molecular Biology. John Wiley & Sons, Inc.; 2001

[109] Yazdi SHT, Kiah HM, Garcia-Ruiz E, Ma J, Zhao H, Milenkovic O. DNA-based storage: Trends and methods. IEEE Transactions on Molecular, Biological and Multi-Scale Communications. 2015;**1**:230-248

[110] Au L-C, Yang F-Y, Yang W-J, Lo S-H, Kao C-F. Gene synthesis by a LCR-based approach: High-level production of leptin-L54 using synthetic gene in *Escherichia coli*. Biochemical and Biophysical Research Communications. 1998;**248**:200-203

[111] TerMaat JR, Pienaar E, Whitney SE, Mamedov TG, Subramanian A. Gene synthesis by integrated polymerase chain assembly and PCR amplification using a high-speed thermocycler. Journal of Microbiological Methods. 2009;**79**:295-300

[112] Ma S, Saaem I, Tian J. Error correction in gene synthesis technology. Trends in Biotechnology. 2012;**30**:147-154

[113] Tian J, Gong H, Sheng N, Zhou X, Gulari E, Gao X, Church G. Accurate multiplex gene synthesis from programmable DNA microchips. Nature. 2004;**432**:1050-1054

[114] Kosuri S, Eroshenko N, LeProust EM, Super M, Way J, Li JB, Church GM. Scalable gene synthesis by selective amplification of DNA pools from high-fidelity microchips. Nature Biotechnology. 2010;**28**:1295-1299

[115] Hu D, Hu S, Wan W, Xu M, Du R, Zhao W, Gao X, Liu J, Liu H, Hong J. Effective optimization of antibody affinity by phage display integrated with high-throughput DNA synthesis and sequencing technologies. PLoS One. 2015;**10**:e0129125

[116] Xu M, Hu S, Ding B, Fei C, Wan W, Hu D, Du R, Zhou X, Hong J, Liu H. Design and construction of small perturbation mutagenesis libraries for antibody affinity maturation using massive microchip-synthesized oligonucleotides. Journal of Biotechnology. 2015;**194**:27-36

[117] Allen S, Clore A. Tailed primer for cloned products used in library construction. 2016, Google Patents

[118] Cortina-Ceballos B, Godoy-Lozano EE, Téllez-Sosa J, Ovilla-Muñoz M, Sámano-Sánchez H, Aguilar-Salgado A, Gómez-Barreto RE, Valdovinos-Torres H, López-Martínez I, Aparicio-Antonio R, Rodríguez MH, Martínez-Barnetche J. Longitudinal analysis of the peripheral B cell repertoire reveals unique effects of immunization with a new influenza virus strain. Genome Medicine. 2015;**7**:124

[119] Coia G, Hudson PJ, Irving RA. Protein affinity maturation in vivo using *E. coli* mutator cells. Journal of Immunological Methods. 2001;**251**:187-193

[120] Irving RA, Kortt AA, Hudson PJ. Affinity maturation of recombinant antibodies using E. coli mutator cells. Immunotechnology. 1996;**2**:127-143

[121] Rasila TS, Pajunen MI, Savilahti H. Critical evaluation of random mutagenesis by error-prone polymerase chain reaction protocols, *Escherichia coli* mutator strain, and hydroxylamine treatment. Analytical Biochemistry. 2009;**388**:71-80

[122] Low NM, Holliger P, Winter G. Mimicking somatic hypermutation: Affinity maturation of antibodies displayed on bacteriophage using a bacterial mutator strain. Journal of Molecular Biology. 1996;**260**:359-368

[123] Zhou C, Jacobsen FW, Cai L, Chen Q, Shen D. Development of a novel mammalian cell surface antibody display platform. mAbs. 2010. Taylor & Francis

[124] Urnov FD. Biological techniques: Edit the genome to understand it. Nature. 2014;**513**:40-41

[125] Hsu PD, Lander ES, Zhang F. Development and applications of CRISPR-Cas9 for genome engineering. Cell. 2014;**157**:1262-1278

[126] Carroll D. Genome engineering with zinc-finger nucleases. Genetics. 2011;**188**:773-782

[127] Boch J. TALEs of genome targeting. Nature Biotechnology. 2011;**29**:135

[128] Yang L, Yang JL, Byrne S, Pan J, Church GM. CRISPR/Cas9-directed genome editing of cultured cells. Current Protocols in Molecular Biology. 2014:31.1. 1-31.1. 17

[129] He Z, Proudfoot C, Mileham AJ, McLaren DG, Whitelaw CBA, Lillico SG. Highly efficient targeted chromosome deletions using CRISPR/Cas9. Biotechnology and Bioengineering. 2015;**112**:1060-1064

[130] O'Connell MR, Oakes BL, Sternberg SH, East-Seletsky A, Kaplan M, Doudna JA. Programmable RNA recognition and cleavage by CRISPR/Cas9. Nature. 2014;**516**: 263-266

[131] Gaj T, Gersbach CA, Barbas CF. ZFN, TALEN, and CRISPR/Cas-based methods for genome engineering. Trends in Biotechnology. 2013;**31**:397-405

Chapter 3

Display Technologies for the Selection of Monoclonal Antibodies for Clinical Use

Lilian Rumi Tsuruta, Santos Mariana Lopes dos and Ana Maria Moro

Additional information is available at the end of the chapter

http://dx.doi.org/10.5772/intechopen.70930

Abstract

The development and improvement of strategies related to discovery technologies of monoclonal antibodies (mAbs) (phage display, yeast display, ribosome display, bacterial display, mammalian cell surface display, mRNA display, DNA display, transgenic animal, and human B-cell derived) opened perspectives for the screening and the selection of therapeutic antibodies for, theoretically, any target from any kind of organism. The implantation of a robust platform of antibody discovery technologies allows reaching this goal. Additionally to recombinant antibody selection, antibody engineering technologies were developed and explored to obtain desired characteristics of selected leading candidates such as high affinity, low immunogenicity, improved functionality, improved protein production, improved stability, and others. mAb humanization methods emerged as alternative for generating humanized variants of promising candidates obtained from non-human organism that could elicit an immune response. This chapter contains an overview of discovery technologies, mainly display methods and antibody humanization methods for the selection of therapeutic humanized and human mAbs that appeared along the development of these technologies and thereafter. The increasing applications of phage display technology will be highlighted in the antibody engineering area (affinity maturation, guided selection to obtain human antibodies) giving promising perspectives for the development of future therapeutics.

Keywords: phage display, yeast display, mRNA display, DNA display, bacterial display, mammalian cell surface display, ribosomal display, fully human mAbs, humanization, therapeutic mAbs

INTECH
open science | open minds

© 2018 The Author(s). Licensee InTech. This chapter is distributed under the terms of the Creative Commons Attribution License (http://creativecommons.org/licenses/by/3.0), which permits unrestricted use, distribution, and reproduction in any medium, provided the original work is properly cited. (cc) BY

1. Introduction

The sale of therapeutic monoclonal antibodies (mAbs) is increasing yearly in relation to other class of biological products [1], and pharmaceutical/biotechnological companies are pursuing all opportunities to develop this product. Therapeutic mAbs are indicated to diverse clinical conditions such as treatment of cancers, immune-mediated disorders and infectious diseases, among others. Every year, new mAbs are approved while a crescent number of other mAbs advance to the next phase of clinical study [2].

Generation of mAbs started with the discovery of the hybridoma technology by Köhler and Milstein [3] in 1975. The fusion of B cells from immunized animals with myeloma cells originated hybrid cells producing unlimited quantities of antibodies with unique specificities. The potential of this technique for clinical and diagnostic use became evident with the approval of the first therapeutic mAb 10 years later, Orthoclone OKT3 targeting the CD3 receptor present in T lymphocytes to control renal transplantation rejection [4]. The clinical success conducted immediately to the development of other mAbs derived from this technology. However, due to the non-conforming sequence of murine mAbs, the generation of an immune response in humans was observed and the use of higher and multiple doses for prolonged time was not possible. Murine mAbs can induce immunogenicity, human anti-mouse antibodies (HAMA, including human anti-idiotype antibodies) affecting the safety and therapeutic efficacy [5]. The evaluation of mAb immunogenicity is crucial during clinical trials and it is recommended by regulatory agencies.

With advances in the understanding of antibody structure and in molecular biology techniques, the field of antibody engineering emerged with objective to change antibody properties by altering its primary sequence. Antibody humanization techniques use antibody engineering approaches to produce antibodies with less immunogenicity and preservation of affinity and specificity of the parental antibody of non-human origin [6]. The first humanization technique led to the combination of variable region domains of a murine antibody with human constant region domains resulting in chimeric antibodies with 70% of human content [7]. Chimeric antibodies maintained the specificity of parental murine antibody and demonstrated decreased immunogenicity, however, they generated human anti-chimeric antibodies (HACA) in approximately 40% of patients [5]. Efforts to obtain mAbs with a minimum of immunogenicity resulted in the development of a technique where sequences responsible for the antibody specificity to the antigen called complementarity-determining regions (CDRs) were transplanted to human framework sequences. This technique was designated CDR grafting and generated humanized antibodies [8–10]. However, it was observed that most of the antibodies obtained by CDR grafting did not preserve the affinity of the parental murine antibody. This fact is due to the influence of the human framework on the structure of the transplanted mouse CDRs [11, 12]. Through 3-dimensional modeling, key residues were identified in the murine framework sequences that interacted with CDRs and the antigen representing the integrity of the antigen-binding site. In a maneuver of back mutating the identified critical framework residues to the mouse framework sequence, antibodies with affinities close to the parental murine antibody were obtained. Using this approach Zenapax® (daclizumab) was approved by FDA in 1997 for therapeutic use for the prevention of renal transplantation rejection [13]. Soon the antibody humanization technique became viable for the clinical application of mAbs of non-human origin. In relation to immunogenicity, approximately 9% of humanized antibodies induced human anti-humanized antibodies (HAHA) in different clinical trials [5]. A less frequent humanization technique aiming to retain the original antibody affinity by altering only the mouse surface-exposed residues of the framework (veneering) was used with success for an anti-NaPi2b oncologic antibody where the humanized version (Rebmab200) demonstrated a slightly improved affinity in relation to the murine version (MX35) [14, 15].

Concomitant to the utilization of antibody humanization techniques started the development of *in vitro* display technologies and the exploration of the molecular diversity of the antibody genes present in a determined library. The first technology available was phage display by presenting exogenous peptides on filamentous bacteriophage (phage) surfaces [16]. The peptide sequences were fused to the amino-terminus of the p3 protein of phages and the fusion protein was expressed on the phage surface, further purified by affinity through the binding to a specific antibody. Selected phages were amplified in bacteria. Then, a biopanning process, a classical cyclic procedure to select phage clones presenting peptides by affinity binding was described [17]. The occurrence of the phage display technology to select mAbs depended on the development of two techniques. Firstly, the expression of functional antibody fragments (scFv and Fab fragment) in the periplasm of *Escherichia coli* was reported [18, 19]. The second technique to mention is the PCR for amplification of antibody genes (heavy and light chains) from hybridomas, a pool of prokaryotic and eukaryotic cells transfected with antibody genes, human peripheral blood cells or tissues rich in B cells [20–22]. The amplification of human immunoglobulin genes directly from immune or naïve human materials opened the possibility to select human antibodies from these sources, either for diagnostic or clinical purposes. In phage display technology, amplified antibody genes are cloned into appropriate phage display vectors to construct the library. Antibody fragments present in the library are expressed on the phage surface and then are submitted to biopanning to select phages by the binding to a specific peptide epitope or antigen. After some cycles of biopanning, the phages encoding the antibody fragments are analyzed individually to select specific clones. Soluble antibody fragments are expressed allowing the characterization of the antibodies and isolation of lead clones [23, 24]. Using phage display technology, six human mAbs were approved for therapeutic use and other candidates are in advanced phases of clinical studies [25]. Other *in vitro* display technologies were developed such as yeast display, ribosome display, bacterial display, mRNA display, mammalian cell surface display and DNA display and, although mAbs with therapeutic potential were obtained by using these other *in vitro* display technologies, no one reached the clinical approval so far.

In the present chapter, we describe discovery technologies to select human therapeutic mAbs.

2. Display technologies to obtain recombinant monoclonal antibodies

In vitro display technologies such as phage display, yeast display, ribosome display, bacterial display, mammalian cell surface display, mRNA display and DNA display represent *in vitro* selection platforms of specific molecules presented in a determined library. These technologies are used mainly to isolate peptides and antibody fragments in scFv, single domain antibody (sdAb) or Fab fragment formats. These technologies mimic the *in vivo* process for antibody generation and have four key steps as it occurs *in vivo* inside the immune system: (1) generation (or cloning) of genotypic diversity; (2) linkage between the genotype and phenotype; (3) application of selective pressure and (4) amplification. This process was initially developed for the collection of recombinant antibody genes from B lymphocytes from immunized mice and naïve or infected humans. The immunoglobulin gene repertoire is cloned into a vector to provide the connection between the genotype and the phenotype of each antibody, and clones are selected through the binding to the specific antigen [26]. The isolated clones are expressed in sufficient amounts to characterize them and to select the best candidate.

The main advantage of the *in vitro* display technology is the possibility to obtain antibodies to any kind of targets and epitopes because the construction of a naïve or synthetic antibody repertoire is not dependent on an *in vivo* immune response. Even antibodies against self-antigens, toxic, unstable and non-immunogenic antigens could be isolated by selection from a combinatorial antibody library [25].

Phage display technology is one of the main platforms for generation of human therapeutic antibodies together with transgenic immunized mice, antibody humanization techniques and single B cell expression cloning [26, 27].

2.1. Phage display technology

Phage display technology was the first *in vitro* display technology developed by presenting an exogenous peptide on the filamentous phage surface [16].

The first antibody combinatorial library was constructed on a λ lytic bacteriophage vector that releases Fab fragments from the periplasm after cell lysis. The screening of Fab fragments was successfully done by transferring the material to nitrocellulose filters followed by binding to radiolabeled antigen [28]. The same methodology was applied for cloning a human antibody library and selection of specific antibodies [29]. The library was constructed from antibody genes of peripheral blood lymphocytes of individuals that had recently received a tetanus toxoid immunization.

Biopanning procedures to select antibody fragments/peptides presented on the phage surface are more efficient for clone screening, since it allows to isolate clones with defined specificity and affinity [17]. Phage display libraries were initially established by the construction of peptide libraries on filamentous phages [30–32], not lytic to bacteria, and recombinant phages are released at the time they are assembled in the bacterial membrane. The expression of scFvs on the filamentous phage surface was described, allowing antibody selection from the library through binding to the antigen [33, 34]. Fab fragments can be presented on the phage surface and, in this case, one antibody chain is fused to the phage p3 protein and directed in the periplasm and the other antibody chain is secreted directly in the periplasm where the Fab fragment is assembled [35–37]. The presentation of single domain antibodies (dAbs) on phage surfaces was also reported [38]. The p3 protein is expressed on the external phage surface, presented in five copies, being involved in the bacterial infection through the binding of bacterial F pilus with the N-terminus of p3 protein [39–41]. The p3 protein vector system is mostly used for the selection of scFv, Fab fragments and single domain antibodies. The advantages are explained in the next section.

2.1.1. *Vector systems to display exogenous molecules*

Phage was initially used as a cloning vector and exogenous genes were inserted in its genome. This system leads to multiple presentations of exogenous peptides fused with phage p3 or p8 protein, making it difficult to select specific antibodies due to the avidity effect [16]. Antibody fragment genes were fused to the N-terminus of p3 phage protein and it was observed that phages continued to be infective [33, 35]. Phagemid vectors emerged as alternative of direct cloning into the phage genome (**Figure 1**).

Phagemids are plasmids containing the intergenic region (IR) of filamentous phage. The IR allows replication of the phagemid mediated by helper phage and packing of phagemid single-strand DNA. Phagemid vectors present some advantages in relation to phage genome cloning: double-strand DNA is obtained for library construction, the copy number of the protein presented on the phage surface may be controlled, easy conversion to soluble protein production by insertion of an amber stop codon between recombinant protein and p3 protein [35], and higher stability due to the resistance of exogenous molecules toward deletions [43]. The main protein fusions presented by phagemids are minor p3 or major p8 coat proteins and phagemids contain g3 or g8 genes near to the cloning site of exogenous proteins. Phagemids efficiently express recombinant proteins; however, they do not amplify phages. When bacteria containing phagemids are infected by a helper phage, it is possible to amplify phages since the helper phage synthesizes all phage proteins. Helper phages are filamentous phages with inactive packing signal, replication-deficient origin and generally carry an antibiotic resistance gene. Helper phage superinfection leads to the expression of both wild type protein and fusion protein on the phage surface. During the phage assembly, there is a

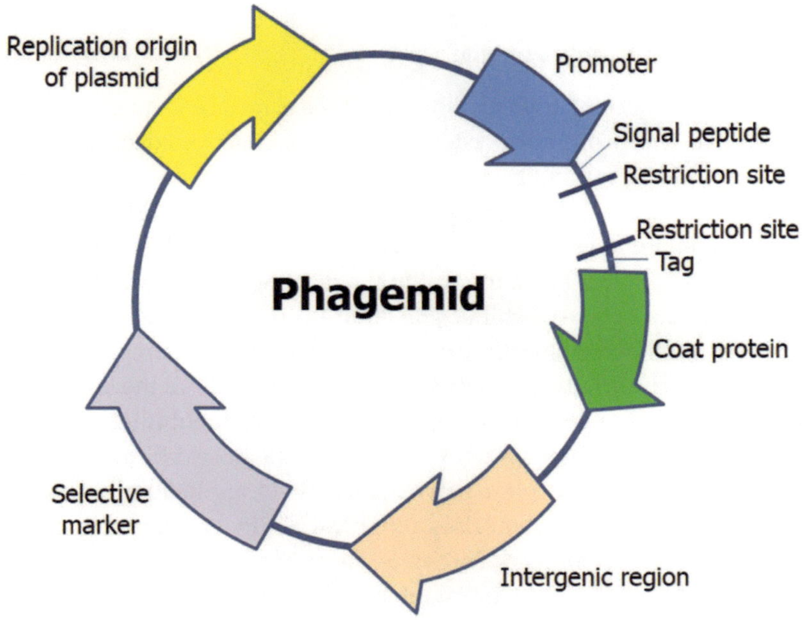

Figure 1. Scheme of phagemid vector used in phage display technology. Adapted from Qi et al. [42].

competition between the two proteins for virion incorporation. Phagemids are preferentially packed by helper phage due to the defective origin of the helper phage [44]. Phage p8 protein is the main surface protein, presenting 2700 copies per phage and has been used to present peptides [45–47] and antibody fragments [48–50]. The phage population using p8 fusion protein is multivalent, presenting approximately 900 peptides [46] and 24 Fab fragments [51] per phage particle. In the latter work, it was verified that the avidity effect of multiple copies on the phage surface did not allow selection of antibodies with high affinity. On the other hand, fusion proteins formed by antibody fragments and p3 proteins are presented in 1-3 copies because the expression of the fusion protein can be repressed by an inducible promoter.

Phage incorporates the fusion protein (antibody fragment and p3 protein) in the virion, while the wild-type p3 protein is produced by the helper phage. The presence of wild-type p3 protein is necessary for the bacteria infection. It was observed that when the N-terminal domain of p3 protein binds to bacteria F′ pili, the bacteria cell infected with the phage acquires immunity to the superinfection of other phages such as helper phage [23]. For this reason, the N-terminal domain of the p3 protein was deleted from fusion protein of the first phagemid vector presenting an Fab fragment, pComb3 [36] and other vectors presenting Fab fragments [37, 52].

2.1.2. Antibody library construction

Antibody gene combinatorial libraries with light and heavy chain genes can be constructed from various sources; human peripheral blood is the most used and spleen, lymph nodes and bone marrow are used if possible. The libraries do not represent the repertoire of antibody gene pairs because the heavy and the light chain genes are amplified separately and then paired randomly by PCR or cloning. This feature increases the diversity of the library and consequently the chance to obtain antibody clones with the desired specificity. Therefore, each antibody library represents a unique repertoire.

Basically, there are two kinds of antibody libraries to select recombinant antibodies: the library derived by a source which immune system had not been activated to recognize a specific antigen (*naïve*), and the immune library derived from donors who received immunization, have been infected or chronically diseased or suffer from cancer [26]. The immune library contains an affinity-matured antibody repertoire and therefore, higher affinity antibodies can be selected in comparison to a naïve library. In the development of human therapeutic antibodies, it is not possible to construct immune libraries to each disease due to ethical issues. Moreover, the construction of a specific library is laborious, high-costing and time-consuming to be considered for each antigen. The option in these cases has been the use of a naïve human library formed by the V, D-J-genes of the IgM repertoire from not intentionally immunized donors. The B cell repertoire can potentially contain also memory cells to previous immunization/infections of donors. In principle, a naïve library can be applied for mAb selection to any kind of antigen, since the library comprises a high variability of immunoglobulin genes and comprises antibody genes from many donors. Some antibodies isolated from a human naïve library presented good specificity to the target and low affinity being necessary to increase it for clinical applications [53]. Naïve human libraries later constructed presented larger sizes and higher affinity clones could be selected. As examples, we can cite Dyax (now Shire) [54], CAT [55, 56], XOMA [57] and HAL [58, 59] naïve human libraries. To increase the variability and size, human semi-synthetic and synthetic libraries [60–73] were constructed based on germline framework sequences, framework sequences of known antibody sequences, consensus framework sequences and human germline VH and VL gene segments. The diversity of antibody sequences was particularly introduced by randomization of CDR sequences, mainly CDR3. A semi-synthetic library was obtained by random mutation of the CDR3 sequence of the heavy chain from a single antibody clone [60] resulting in higher affinity derived clones. An alternative to randomization of CDRs was devised, introducing any codon combination at a specific position to obtain more nature-like antibodies [74] using two strategies: trinucleotide phosphoramidites [66, 68, 70] and Slonomics approaches [71, 72]. HuCAL, HuCAL GOLD and HuCAL PLATINUM libraries are examples of synthetic libraries obtained by trinucleotide phosphoramidites [66, 68, 70] and the Ylanthia library was constructed by the Slonomics method [72].

2.1.3. Antibody selection from library

The scheme of antibody phage display technology is shown in **Figure 2**. The selection of phages presenting specific antibodies occurs by the specific binding to the antigen by a biopanning process. Only phages expressing antibodies on the surface are amplified and after the biopanning process, the library is enriched with clones presenting moderate or high affinity to the antigen. In principle, only a single round of selection would be sufficient, however, unspecific binding of antibodies presented by phages limits the library enrichment and in practice, two to five rounds of a biopanning process are performed for antibody isolation. Enriched phages obtained at the first round can be amplified in bacteria culture and then submitted to subsequent rounds of biopanning process. Some methodologies were used to isolate phage clones presenting specific antibodies. Phages can be selected by antibody binding to the antigen coated in microplates [36, 53], to antigen-coupled to resins [33], in solution using biotinylated antigens [75], or to antigen present on a cell surface [76]. After antibody phages are bound to the antigen, they are washed and then eluted by soluble antigen [77], acid solution [36] or alkali solution [53].

After antibody clone selection, the candidates are expressed and characterized individually to evaluate their affinity and specificity. Phagemid vectors can display or secrete antibody fragments through incorporation of an amber stop codon between the antibody fragment gene and the p3 protein. Antibody fragments are displayed on the phage surface when the suppressor *E. coli* strain is transfected and antibodies can be expressed when the non-suppressor *E. coli* strain is used because the amber codon is read as stop codon in this case [35]. Another option would be the conversion from a phage display vector to an expression vector of a soluble antibody fragment [36] or recloning antibody genes to an expression vector [77].

In general, in the case of naïve or synthetic human antibody libraries, the antibody affinity is proportional to the library size and, in the case of naïve human antibody libraries, the dissociation constant (K_D) was in the 10^{-6} to 10^{-7} M range for small libraries [53] and in the order of 10^{-9} M for larger libraries [55, 57].

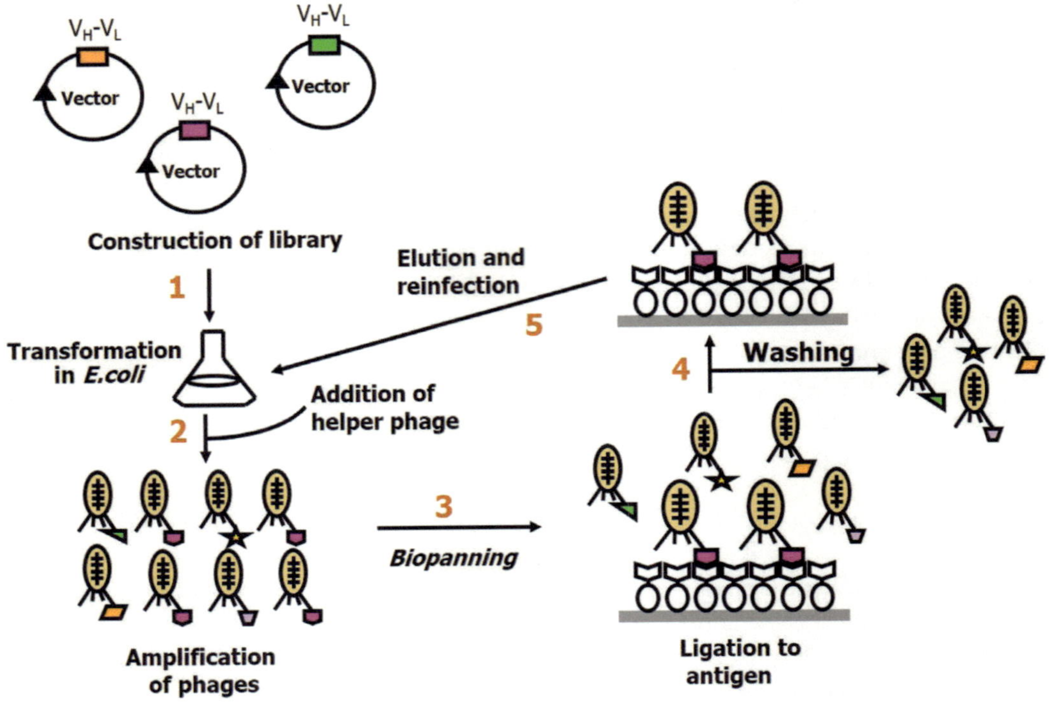

Figure 2. General scheme of phage display technology for selection of scFv fragments. (1) After scFv library construction, an aliquot is transformed in *E. coli* and grown up to OD_{600} of 0.6. (2) Helper phage is introduced to the culture and phages displaying antibody fragments are obtained. (3) Binding of scFvs displayed by phages to the antigen coated in wells of a microtiter plate. (4) Non-binding phages are washed away. (5) Phages are eluted and then reinfected into *E. coli* for a new round of antibody selection.

2.1.4. Affinity maturation of antibodies

The affinity of antibodies selected by naïve or synthetic phage display antibody libraries is generally adequate for research purposes; however they present low affinity for therapeutic applications. In these cases, selected clones should be submitted to the affinity maturation process [43]. Phage display technology allows the construction of a second antibody library originating from a selected clone, facilitating the selection of human antibodies for therapeutic use. Mutagenesis strategies have been applied to improve antibody affinity [23]. A point mutation library was constructed using error-prone PCR [78] simulating random point mutations generated by natural somatic mutation. This approach was used for anti-progesterone scFv fragments obtained from a naïve antibody library and the antibody affinity increased 30-fold. Other work constructed mutant scFv libraries against digoxigenin with low, moderate and high PCR error rate and showed that the highest antibody affinity improvement was related to higher mutation rates in the positions outside of the CDRs [79]. In addition, introduction of hot spot mutations in antibody germline sequences led to higher affinities of antibodies [80]. This approach presents advantage in relation to previous mutagenesis strategy due to the construction of smaller size libraries allowing parallel screening of multiple mutant libraries.

Mammalian cell surface display of antibody libraries coupled with *in vitro* somatic hypermutation (SHM) by the action of the activation-induced cytidine deaminase (AID) enzyme emerged as an interesting approach for affinity maturation of human antibodies [81–83]. In mammalian cell surface display, full-length and glycosylated IgGs are displayed by a transmembrane domain on the cell surface and antibody clones are isolated by screening techniques such as magnetic bead selection followed by *in vitro* SHM induction of clones which had been selected further by flow cytometry [82]. *In vitro* SHM has the ability to reproduce the *in vivo* human antibody maturation in non-B cells and introduces both point mutations and insertion/deletion to the antibody sequence in the region related to antigen contact [83]. One special characteristic of AID is that this enzyme acts preferentially toward germline hotspot motifs (WRCH) present in the antibody DNA sequence, specifically in the variable domains, and promotes point mutations at high rates in amino acid residues which change the antibody binding features [83].

2.1.5. Guided selection technique for antibody humanization

The technique of guided selection has the advantage of allowing selection of a human-nature antibody from a non-human original antibody sequence without the analysis of the antibody structure using *in vitro* display technology. Two publications demonstrated the viability of this technique using an "in series" process by different approaches [84, 85]. One publication used a rodent heavy chain (MAb32), Fd fragment, as a template and ligated it into a vector containing a human light chain repertoire [84]. A phage repertoire was selected by the antigen and the isolated human light chains were paired to a repertoire of human heavy chains. The selection of phages by the antigen was performed again and a human antibody clone was obtained recognizing the N-terminal region of the mouse antibody's target and demonstrating a similar affinity constant as the original clone. [84]. Figini et al. constructed a hybrid library combining the light chain of a murine anti-hapten antibody and the human heavy chain repertoire, from which human heavy chain sequences were isolated based on the light-heavy chain pairing ability to combine and bind to the antigen. The selected sequences were paired to the human light chain repertoire to obtain the human antibody [85].

Humira (adalimumab), an anti-TNF-α mAb, was isolated using this technique by an "in parallel" process, and it represents the first fully human antibody and also the first mAb derived by phage display technology approved by FDA in 2002 [86]. This anti-TNF-α mAb was obtained using the rodent antibody sequence (variable domains of heavy and light chains) as a template. Initially, two hybrid libraries were constructed; one formed by pairing the murine heavy chain sequence and a human light chain variable domain repertoire, and the second library was composed of the murine light chain sequence paired to a human heavy chain variable domain repertoire. Both hybrid libraries were selected against TNF-α and the antibody clones were isolated. The human antibody sequences obtained by the screening of each library were combined and the resulting library was reselected against the antigen. A human anti-TNF-α antibody was obtained and, after submitting to CDR mutagenesis, the high affinity D2E7 mAb was isolated with main indications for rheumatoid arthritis and Crohn's disease [86]. One disadvantage of the guided selection technique is that the construction of hybrid libraries can result in changes of the paratope altering the antibody fine specificity as observed previously [50, 87, 88]. This phenomenon was observed by using an "in series" process of guided selection technique for human interferon γ receptor 1 (IFNGR-1) [89]. To obtain a human antibody with the same paratope of the original rodent antibody, a variation of this technique was performed by the preservation of the CDR3 sequence of the heavy chain from the non-human template sequence [90, 91].

2.1.6. Advantages of phage display technology

Antibody phage display technology is more utilized in the discovery of therapeutic mAbs than any other display technologies due to many advantages: (1) it was the first display technology developed so the methodology is well-established; (2) it uses the low cost *E. coli* expression system; (3) it is possible to construct large naïve libraries for selection of human antibodies against most antigens and desired epitopes; (4) selection process is versatile with the ability to determine the epitope of the antibody; (5) it can be used for affinity maturation of antibodies; and (6) antibody humanization by guided selection technique to obtain human antibodies is possible [25, 92]. As disadvantages, it can be mentioned: (1) selection of an antibody with low affinity from naïve and synthetic libraries that implies that *in vitro* affinity maturation for therapeutic application is recommendable; and (2) low antibody expression in *E. coli* for some isolated antibody sequences.

2.2. Yeast display

The yeast display technology uses yeast cells to present exogenous peptides or antibody fragments on the cell surface. In this technology, exogenous molecules are fused to the a-agglutinin adhesion receptor of *Saccharomyces cerevisiae* which is localized on the yeast surface and the cell repertoire can be screened by flow cytometry [93]. A-agglutinin receptor acts as adhesion molecule that stabilizes cell-cell interactions and promotes fusion between an "a" and α haploid cell to obtain a diploid cell. This receptor is composed of the Aga1 and Aga2 protein. Aga1 protein is secreted and binds covalently to b-glucan present in the extracellular matrix of the yeast cell wall. Aga2 protein binds to Aga1 protein through two disulfide bonds and the antibody fragment is fused to the C-terminal end of Aga2 protein (**Figure 3**) [94]. Aga1 protein and the fusion protein are expressed by induction of the GAL1 promoter with galactose [95]. ScFv is the most frequent antibody format displayed on yeast surface. Other formats include Fab fragment, whole IgG and single domain antibodies [38, 96].

The library is constructed by cloning the antibody genes into the yeast display vector and has smaller size than phage display libraries. After yeast transformation and growth, antibody expression is induced and then flow cytometry screening is performed with specific ligands to enrich binders of the library. After about three rounds of antibody selection, the enriched library is transformed in *E. coli* for analysis of plasmid DNA by sequencing [96].

Yeast display technology is used to improve the ligand affinity of scFv fragments and thermal stability of proteins [97–99] and also to isolate novel antibodies with suitable affinity and specificity [94]. One advantage of this technology is the characterization of binding properties such as affinity of one clone displaying an antibody fragment on the yeast surface without sub-cloning, expression and purification steps [94]. The display level is diverse and the binding

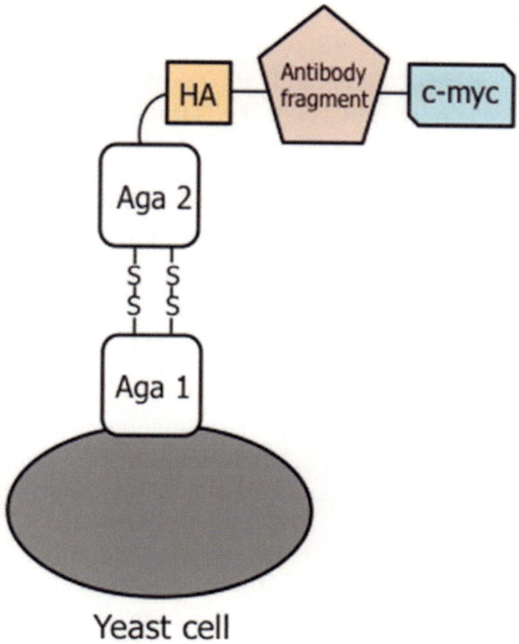

Figure 3. Scheme of the a-agglutinin receptor of yeast cell surface presenting a recombinant antibody fragment as fusion protein with Aga2 protein. Hemagglutinin (HA) tag is fused to the C-terminal end of the Aga2 protein followed by antibody fragment and c-myc tag that is fused to the C-terminal end of the recombinant antibody fragment. The presentation of the fusion protein can be monitored by anti-tags antibodies and/or binding to antigen labeled with fluorophore. Adapted from Boder and Wittrup [93].

avidity is reduced due to the cell sorting potential of flow cytometry. Yeast cells can be sorted according to the antibody binding range to the antigen and also by antibody expression range on the yeast surface through labeling the cell with fluorophore-conjugated antigen and with reagents to identify epitope of tags [94]. Boder's group used kinetic screening for a yeast display library containing random mutations and they isolated scFv clones with high affinity (48 fM) [100]. A naïve human scFv library composed by more than 10^9 clones was constructed by yeast display technology; antibody clones were firstly selected by magnetic bead screening followed by flow cytometry screening, isolating antibodies with an affinity of nM range [101]. Magnetic bead screening was applied to remove yeast cells not presenting antibody fragments like the biopanning process used in the phage display technology. As a consequence, the yeast display library size became suitable for the antibody selection by flow cytometry [96].

The construction of a yeast display vector displaying a Fab fragment was reported [102] and a single vector presenting two expression cassettes with the GAL1 promoter was used. The heavy chain fragment was expressed as a fusion protein to the N-terminal end of Aga2 protein and the light chain gene was expressed as a soluble fragment, resulting in a Fab fragment assembled on the yeast surface. The affinity matured library allowed the selection of high affinity antibodies.

A novel approach combining phage and yeast display technologies was tested to select Fab fragments against antigen 85 of *Mycobacterium tuberculosis* [103]. Initially, a large naïve scFv library was selected by antigen binding using phage display technology. The enriched library with compatible size to flow cytometry screening was cloned into yeast display vector and highly specific antibodies were obtained. This strategy could be applied to any antigen and will serve as an alternative approach to isolate high affinity antibodies.

The major advantage of yeast display technology is the library screening using flow cytometry that allows defining specific parameters to select antibodies displayed on yeast surface. Yeast displaying antibodies can be sorted by binding to fluorescently-conjugated antigen and it is possible to separate clones quantitatively using binding affinity or dissociation kinetics parameters. Yeast cells can display about 10^5 antibodies and the expression range can be evaluated also by binding of epitope tags using fluorophore-labeled reagents [104].

Another advantage is that this platform uses yeast and therefore presents post-translational modifications like existing in the mammalian system but not present in bacteria. Post-translational modifications include glycosylation of antibodies, appropriate protein folding in the endoplasmic reticulum in the presence of chaperones and improved solubility of the product [96, 104].

In comparison to phage display technology, a yeast display platform has a limitation of the library size, due to lower efficiency of yeast transformation [96, 104]. Efforts to circumvent this problem led to the improvement of yeast transformation efficiency, allowing the construction of libraries with 10^{10} clones [105]. Another disadvantage of this platform is the multivalent display of antibodies on yeast surface and the selection based on avidity parameters [96, 104].

Among cell surface display-based technologies, we mentioned yeast and mammalian display technologies in this chapter. A prokaryotic system such as bacterial cell surface display (either Gram-negative or Gram-positive bacteria) has also been developed with the selection of high affinity binders [106–108]. The library screening is performed through the binding of the protein displayed on the cell surface to a specific fluorescently labeled ligand and analyzed mainly by flow cytometry as occurs in other cell surface display technologies. An *E. coli* display system was first extensively studied for antibody fragment isolation, then variations of this methodology were developed by genetic engineering [108–110], and full-length IgG was also displayed on bacteria [111]. There are few works considering Gram-positive bacterial cell surface display. A Gram-positive *Staphylococcus* display system was investigated [108, 112] and high affinity small proteins known as affibody molecules were selected using this system [113, 114], opening an attractive perspective for future development.

2.3. mRNA and ribosome display technologies

mRNA display technology emerged together with ribosome display technology as a revolutionary *in vitro* display platform to obviate cell transformation steps. Both technologies are centered in a fully cell-free strategy to select specific binders with great potential for diagnostic and clinical use.

The characteristics of mRNA display and ribosome display technology allows construction of libraries much larger than other *in vitro* display technologies because it avoids the library size limitation of phage and yeast display technologies which are dependent on the efficiency of cell transformation steps. Another advantage of this technology is the extensive use of PCR that contributes to the introduction of more diversity to the library by mutations. The mRNA and ribosome display platform can be applied for selection of novel molecules, including antibody fragments, and for affinity maturation of antibodies [115].

During ribosome display, an antibody repertoire is constructed *in vitro* comprising mRNA, ribosome and translated antibody fragment [116]. The vector used contains no stop codon so that the translated antibody fragment is not released from ribosome and mRNA. After biopanning and ribosome disruption, mRNA is isolated and RT-PCR follows. Then, the cDNAs of the antibody fragments are amplified by PCR to obtain DNA for the next round of selection.

One special feature of mRNA display technology is the use of an adaptor molecule between the mRNA and translated proteins that binds them covalently forming a very stable complex to thermal and physicochemical stress that could be present during the selection step [117, 118]. In mRNA display technology, DNA molecules are initially *in vitro* transcribed to mRNA, then mRNA is translated and covalently ligated to the translated protein through puromycin, an adaptor molecule. The number of mRNA-protein complexes formed determines the functional library size. After the translation, the ribosome forms a peptide bond between the puromycin and the C-terminal residue of the polypeptide and the complex obtained is purified from the ribosome. It is followed by cDNA synthesis of the mRNA-protein complex by reverse transcription so that the library composed of cDNA/mRNA-protein complexes is build. This library is submitted to affinity selection by incubation with the target using affinity chromatography or immunoprecipitation techniques. The enriched library is recovered and mRNA hydrolysis at high pH is performed to release the cDNAs. These cDNAs are amplified by PCR to obtain DNA molecules for another round of selection and specific binders are isolated [115]. mRNA display technology presents monovalent complexes during selection and thus specific binders can be selected without interference of avidity parameters [119]. Furthermore, the diversity of libraries generated by mRNA or ribosome display can be increased by involving error-prone PCR, DNA shuffling and using an error-prone RNA-dependent RNA polymerase during *in vitro* transcription [115].

Using ribosome display, scFv fragments and Fab fragments with high affinities have been selected [120–124]. The construction of an affinity matured library for antibody mimics using mRNA display with the selection of high affinity molecules was described by Xu's group [125]. In relation to antibody fragments, mRNA display technology was used for the selection of an anti-fluorescein antibody in scFv format [126] and also for Fab fragments [127]. The selection of Fab fragments was possible by combination of mRNA display technology and emulsion PCR.

2.4. DNA display technology

DNA display technology is another complete *in vitro* display platform using a cell free system that was initially developed for the selection of peptides linked to their coding DNA present in a library [128–130]. Doi and Yanagawa established *in vitro* transcription and translation reactions in an emulsion compartment—STABLE (Streptavidin-biotin linkage in emulsions) [128]. A random decapeptide library comprising fusion proteins formed by the peptides and streptavidin-His (STA-His, His tag fused to the C-terminus of Streptavidin) was synthesized and ligated to the biotinylated DNA by a stable bond. The library was submitted to affinity selection using nickel resin. Isolated DNAs were cloned into a vector, amplified and sequenced. A limited affinity selection efficiency was observed so that the method needed improvement [128]. The selection of diverse anti-FLAG Tag peptides from a peptide-DNA library was performed using monoclonal antibody anti-FLAG M2 [129]. The same group also demonstrated that folded proteins can be displayed on the DNA display platform by the introduction of linkers between streptavidin and fused proteins [130]. It could be shown that the GST gene could be enriched by this method by the selection of the DNA-protein conjugates with glutathione-coupled beads. The application of DNA display technology to select Fab fragments using the STABLE method was described later [131]. The selection of a Fab fragment gene was performed using a new approach: randomized hydrophobic core in the constant region with heat treatment application for selective pressure.

Advantages of this technology compared to other cell free *in vitro* display technologies such as ribosome and mRNA display is that RNase-free conditions are not needed for the selection step because a reverse transcription step is unnecessary. Furthermore, the removal of a stop codon between nucleic acid and peptide is not necessary. DNA display technology is simpler than other fully *in vitro* display technologies, with lesser steps [128–130]. One disadvantage of this technology is its novelty, devoid of a robust platform and knowledge in comparison to other *in vitro* display technologies.

3. Approved therapeutic monoclonal antibodies

By the end of 2016, 20 fully human mAbs were approved for therapeutic use by the US Food and Drug Administration (FDA) and often approved by the European Medicines Agency (EMA) too. The approved fully human mAbs are derived basically from two technologies: phage display or transgenic mice expressing human antibody genes [132, 133]. Among approved mAbs, five were generated by phage display with selection of antigen-specific binders from two different libraries, Cambridge Antibody Technology - CAT (MedImmune, subsidiary of AstraZeneca) based on scFv fragments or Dyax Corp's human Fab fragment libraries [25, 134]. The other 15 mAbs were developed in transgenic mice, with integrated human immunoglobulin loci.

Considering the therapeutic mAbs approved which used phage display technology to acquire the human antibody composition, there are examples of different targets for immune intervention: two (adalimumab and belimumab) are in use for autoimmune diseases, one (raxibacumab) is for control of *Bacillus anthracis* infection and two others (ramucirumab and necitumumab) address growth factor receptors for cancer treatment.

The first fully human mAb approved for therapy in 2002 (FDA) and 2003 (EMA)—adalimumab (Humira®, AbbVie Inc., formerly Abbott Laboratories)—was generated by phage display technology [25, 134]. Adalimumab is an anti-TNFα mAb developed in 1993 through a collaboration between BASF Bioresearch Corporation and CAT using an anti-TNF murine antibody (MAK195) from BASF as a template for guided selection of human antibody V-domains with CAT's antibody phage display technology [25]. Adalimumab was first approved for treatment of rheumatoid arthritis (RA) under the brand name Humira (human monoclonal antibody in rheumatoid arthritis) [25, 135]. Besides RA, adalimumab is currently used in the treatment of plaque psoriasis, ulcerative colitis, Crohn's disease, non-infectious uveitis, hidradenitis suppurativa, psoriatic arthritis, juvenile idiopathic arthritis and ankylosing spondylitis [136].

Nine years after the approval of the first human mAb developed by phage display technology (adalimumab), in 2011 belimumab (Benlysta, GSK) was approved for the treatment of systemic lupus erythematosus [25, 134, 137]. Belimumab was selected using CAT library as a result of the collaboration between CAT and Human Genome Sciences (now GlaxoSmithKline), and targets the soluble form of human B-lymphocyte stimulator (BLyS) [25, 134]. Under a license to use the CAT library, Human Genome Sciences (now GSK) discovered Raxibacumab (Abthrax) also using phage display. Raxibacumab binds the *Bacillus anthracis* protective antigen (PA) and was approved by FDA in 2012 for the prophylaxis and treatment of anthrax [25, 134, 138, 139].

In addition to the three previously described antibodies, which were discovered using scFv-fragment CAT library by antibody phage display, two mAbs—ramucirumab and necitumumab—were derived from the same technology but from a different library, a human Fab-fragment library constructed by de Haard and colleagues at Dyax [25, 134]. Ramucirumab (Cyramza, Eli Lilly) is an anti-VEGFR-2 (vascular endothelial growth factor receptor 2) mAb approved for the treatment of cancer (gastric or gastroesophageal junction, non-small cell lung and colorectal) in 2014 [140]. Necitumumab (Portrazza, Eli Lilly) targets epidermal growth factor receptor (EGFR) and blocks binding to epidermal growth factor (EGF) [25, 134]. This mAb gained first marketing approval for FDA and EMA in 2015 and 2016, respectively, for the treatment of non-small cell lung cancer [25, 141, 142].

Ranibizumab (Lucentis, Genentech), an anti-VEGF-A (vascular endothelial growth factor A) Fab fragment, was generated by the humanization of the murine mAb A4.6.1 [134]. Based on a random mutation library, clones were selected by phage display [143]. Afterward, an alanine scanning study and information of the crystal structure of the Fab-VEGF complex were used for affinity maturation [144, 145]. This mAb was approved in the US in 2006 for the treatment of age-related macular degeneration [25, 134], and posteriorly for the treatment of macular edema after retinal vein occlusion, diabetic macular edema and diabetic retinopathy [25].

4. Future perspectives of the development of recombinant antibodies

This chapter is focused on fully human therapeutic mAbs, mainly those derived from phage display technologies. Other technologies emerged in recent years for the obtainment of human mAbs with high promises of success, derived directly from human B lymphocytes by two main approaches, immortalization of memory B cells by polyclonal stimulation followed by EBV transformation and/or the capture and sorting of memory B cells or plasmablasts followed by amplification of the mAb variable chains expressed by the single B cell, which can be transfected to mammalian cells [27]. The natural pairing of rearranged heavy chain and light chains regions can be found only in B cells. Display technologies add complexity to the repertoire by pairing light and heavy chains by chance. A very promising new class of antibodies consists of single domain antibodies from camels and sharks comprising only one variable domain of the heavy chain [146, 147]. These molecules are stable, non-aggregating molecules both *in vitro* and *in vivo*. Carrying the ability to bind antigens intracellularly as intrabodies inside the nucleus or cytosol makes them an important platform for antigen trafficking and knockdown, meaning a promise for the future [38].

It draws attention when analyzing the therapeutic mAbs in the market that the majority of them target cancer and autoimmune diseases, while some are directed to other conditions and very few are directed to infectious diseases treatment. It is also more astonishing since the first use of antibodies in immunotherapy fought against infectious diseases by the end of the nineteenth century. One obvious reason is that bacterial infections can be treated with antibiotics and many can be prevented by vaccination. Viral infections, on the other hand, are more complicated to treat by vaccination or treatment with antibodies as some viruses exhibit high mutation rates.

Broadly neutralizing mAbs to influenza viruses can be used to probe *in vitro* vaccine candidates and provide useful information for understanding data generated by preliminary *in vivo* studies, contributing to a universal influenza virus vaccine strategy [148, 149]. The identification of new conserved epitopes resulted from analysis with two broadly neutralizing mAbs, specific for the HA2 subunit of influenza virus belonging to different clades. Both mAbs were generated by phage display from B cells of an influenza vaccinated individual [150] and from a "non-immune" human antibody library [151]. Contrary to the disadvantages listed for phage display libraries, these are high affinity mAbs, in the range of nanomolar and picomolar, respectively.

Generation of mAbs by phage display technology was a breakthrough since this technology opened possibilities to isolate human antibodies for any kind of epitope/antigen without immunization. The success of this technology can be observed by the approval of some drugs, mAbs and other kinds of proteins, and many more are under clinical studies at different stages. There are some candidates for Phase 3 clinical trial, bringing promises of new drugs in the near future [25, 134]. As a perspective for infectious diseases, this technology should be more widely applied for rapid screening of antibodies for diagnostic or therapeutic purposes based on immune or naïve human libraries when epidemic infectious disease breaks without an available drug for its treatment. Other perspective concerns the combinatorial library construction. Recently, the human antibody repertoire derived from blood of human naïve or immunized donors has been intensively analyzed by next-generation sequencing [152, 153]. Advances in the knowledge of the human antibody repertoire would help in the designing of antibody libraries and for antibody maturation of existing human libraries, making possible the selection of mAbs with higher affinity for clinical use.

Author details

Lilian Rumi Tsuruta*, Mariana Lopes dos Santos and Ana Maria Moro

*Address all correspondence to: lilian.tsuruta@butantan.gov.br

Lab Biopharmaceuticals in Animal Cells, Instituto Butantan, São Paulo, SP, Brazil

References

[1] Aggarwal RS. What's fueling the biotech engine-2012 to 2013. Nature Biotechnology. 2014;**32**(1):32-39

[2] Reichert JM. Antibodies to watch in 2017. MAbs. 2017;**9**(2):167-181

[3] Kohler G, Milstein C. Continuous cultures of fused cells secreting antibody of predefined specificity. Nature. 1975;**256**(5517):495-497

[4] Norman DJ, Shield CF3rd, Barry J, Henell K, Funnell MB, Lemon J. A U.S. clinical study of Orthoclone OKT3 in renal transplantation. Transplantation Proceedings. 1987;**19**(2 Suppl 1):21-27

[5] Hwang WY, Foote J. Immunogenicity of engineered antibodies. Methods. 2005;**36**(1):3-10

[6] Almagro JC, Fransson J. Humanization of antibodies. Frontiers in Bioscience: A Journal and Virtual Library. 2008;**13**:1619-1633

[7] Morrison SL, Johnson MJ, Herzenberg LA, Oi VT. Chimeric human antibody molecules: Mouse antigen-binding domains with human constant region domains. Proceedings of the National Academy of Sciences of the United States of America. 1984;**81**(21):6851-6855

[8] Jones PT, Dear PH, Foote J, Neuberger MS, Winter G. Replacing the complementarity-determining regions in a human antibody with those from a mouse. Nature. 1986; **321**(6069):522-525

[9] Verhoeyen M, Milstein C, Winter G. Reshaping human antibodies: Grafting an antilysozyme activity. Science. 1988;**239**(4847):1534-1536

[10] Riechmann L, Clark M, Waldmann H, Winter G. Reshaping human antibodies for therapy. Nature. 1988;**332**(6162):323-327

[11] Queen C, Schneider WP, Selick HE, Payne PW, Landolfi NF, Duncan JF, et al. A humanized antibody that binds to the interleukin 2 receptor. Proceedings of the National Academy of Sciences of the United States of America. 1989;**86**(24):10029-10033

[12] Caldas C, Coelho V, Kalil J, Moro AM, Maranhão AQ, Brígido MM. Humanization of the anti-CD18 antibody 6.7: An unexpected effect of a framework residue in binding to antigen. Molecular Immunology. 2003;**39**(15):941-952

[13] Tsurushita N, Hinton PR, Kumar S. Design of humanized antibodies: From anti-Tac to Zenapax. Methods. 2005;**36**(1):69-83

[14] Lopes dos Santos M, Yeda FP, Tsuruta LR, Horta BB, Pimenta Jr AA, Degaki TL, et al. Rebmab200, a humanized monoclonal antibody targeting the sodium phosphate transporter NaPi2b displays strong immune mediated cytotoxicity against cancer: A novel reagent for targeted antibody therapy of cancer. PLoS One. 2013;**8**(7):e70332.

[15] Lindegren S, Andrade LN, Back T, Machado CM, Horta BB, Buchpiguel C, et al. Binding affinity, specificity and comparative biodistribution of the parental murine monoclonal

antibody MX35 (anti-NaPi2b) and its humanized version Rebmab200. PLoS One. 2015;**10**(5):e0126298

[16] Smith GP. Filamentous fusion phage: Novel expression vectors that display cloned antigens on the virion surface. Science. 1985;**228**(4705):1315-1317

[17] Parmley SF, Smith GP. Antibody-selectable filamentous fd phage vectors: Affinity purification of target genes. Gene. 1988;**73**(2):305-318

[18] Better M, Chang CP, Robinson RR, Horwitz AH. *Escherichia coli* secretion of an active chimeric antibody fragment. Science. 1988;**240**(4855):1041-1043

[19] Skerra A, Pluckthun A. Assembly of a functional immunoglobulin Fv fragment in *Escherichia coli*. Science. 1988;**240**(4855):1038-1041

[20] Larrick JW, Danielsson L, Brenner CA, Abrahamson M, Fry KE, Borrebaeck CA. Rapid cloning of rearranged immunoglobulin genes from human hybridoma cells using mixed primers and the polymerase chain reaction. Biochemical and Biophysical Research Communications. 1989;**160**(3):1250-1256

[21] Orlandi R, Gussow DH, Jones PT, Winter G. Cloning immunoglobulin variable domains for expression by the polymerase chain reaction. Proceedings of the National Academy of Sciences of the United States of America. 1989;**86**(10):3833-3837

[22] Sastry L, Alting-Mees M, Huse WD, Short JM, Sorge JA, Hay BN, et al. Cloning of the immunological repertoire in *Escherichia coli* for generation of monoclonal catalytic antibodies: Construction of a heavy chain variable region-specific cDNA library. Proceedings of the National Academy of Sciences of the United States of America. 1989;**86**(15):5728-5732

[23] Burton DR, Barbas CF3rd. Human antibodies from combinatorial libraries. Advances in Immunology. 1994;**57**:191-280

[24] Winter G, Griffiths AD, Hawkins RE, Hoogenboom HR. Making antibodies by phage display technology. Annual Review of Immunology. 1994;**12**:433-455

[25] Frenzel A, Schirrmann T, Hust M. Phage display-derived human antibodies in clinical development and therapy. MAbs. 2016;**8**(7):1177-1194

[26] Hoogenboom HR. Selecting and screening recombinant antibody libraries. Nature Biotechnology. 2005;**23**(9):1105-1116

[27] Wilson PC, Andrews SF. Tools to therapeutically harness the human antibody response. Nature Reviews Immunology. 2012;**12**(10):709-719

[28] Huse WD, Sastry L, Iverson SA, Kang AS, Alting-Mees M, Burton DR, et al. Generation of a large combinatorial library of the immunoglobulin repertoire in phage lambda. Science. 1989;**246**(4935):1275-1281

[29] Persson MA, Caothien RH, Burton DR. Generation of diverse high-affinity human monoclonal antibodies by repertoire cloning. Proceedings of the National Academy of Sciences of the United States of America. 1991;**88**(6):2432-2436

[30] Cwirla SE, Peters EA, Barrett RW, Dower WJ. Peptides on phage: A vast library of peptides for identifying ligands. Proceedings of the National Academy of Sciences of the United States of America. 1990;**87**(16):6378-6382

[31] Scott JK, Smith GP. Searching for peptide ligands with an epitope library. Science. 1990;**249**(4967):386-390

[32] Devlin JJ, Panganiban LC, Devlin PE. Random peptide libraries: A source of specific protein binding molecules. Science. 1990;**249**(4967):404-406

[33] McCafferty J, Griffiths AD, Winter G, Chiswell DJ. Phage antibodies: Filamentous phage displaying antibody variable domains. Nature. 1990;**348**(6301):552-554

[34] Breitling F, Dübel S, Seehaus T, Klewinghaus I, Little M. A surface expression vector for antibody screening. Gene. 1991;**104**(2):147-153

[35] Hoogenboom HR, Griffiths AD, Johnson KS, Chiswell DJ, Hudson P, Winter G. Multi-subunit proteins on the surface of filamentous phage: Methodologies for displaying antibody (Fab) heavy and light chains. Nucleic Acids Research. 1991;**19**(15):4133-4137

[36] Barbas CF3rd, Kang AS, Lerner RA, Benkovic SJ. Assembly of combinatorial antibody libraries on phage surfaces: The gene III site. Proceedings of the National Academy of Sciences of the United States of America. 1991;**88**(18):7978-7982

[37] Garrard LJ, Yang M, O'Connell MP, Kelley RF, Henner DJ. Fab assembly and enrichment in a monovalent phage display system. Bio/Technology. 1991;**9**(12):1373-1377

[38] Boldicke T. Single domain antibodies for the knockdown of cytosolic and nuclear proteins. Protein Science. 2017

[39] Lubkowski J, Hennecke F, Pluckthun A, Wlodawer A. The structural basis of phage display elucidated by the crystal structure of the N-terminal domains of g3p. Nature Structural Biology. 1998;**5**(2):140-147

[40] Lubkowski J, Hennecke F, Pluckthun A, Wlodawer A. Filamentous phage infection: Crystal structure of g3p in complex with its coreceptor, the C-terminal domain of TolA. Structure. 1999;**7**(6):711-722

[41] Holliger P, Riechmann L. A conserved infection pathway for filamentous bacteriophages is suggested by the structure of the membrane penetration domain of the minor coat protein g3p from phage fd. Structure. 1997;**5**(2):265-275

[42] Qi H, Lu H, Qui HJ, Petrenko V, Liu A. Phagemid vectors for phage display: Properties, characteristics and construction. Journal of Molecular Biology. 2012;**417**:15

[43] Bradbury AR, Marks JD. Antibodies from phage antibody libraries. Journal of Immunological Methods. 2004;**290**(1-2):29-49

[44] Vieira J, Messing J. Production of single-stranded plasmid DNA. Methods in Enzymology. 1987;**153**:3-11

[45] Il'ichev AA, Minenkova OO, Tat'kov SI, Karpyshev NN, Eroshkin AM, Ofitserov VI, et al. The use of filamentous phage M13 in protein engineering. Molekuliarnaia Biologiia. 1990;**24**(2):530-535

[46] Greenwood J, Willis AE, Perham RN. Multiple display of foreign peptides on a filamentous bacteriophage. Peptides from *Plasmodium falciparum* circumsporozoite protein as antigens. Journal of Molecular Biology. 1991;**220**(4):821-827

[47] Felici F, Castagnoli L, Musacchio A, Jappelli R, Cesareni G. Selection of antibody ligands from a large library of oligopeptides expressed on a multivalent exposition vector. Journal of Molecular Biology. 1991;**222**(2):301-310

[48] Chang CN, Landolfi NF, Queen C. Expression of antibody Fab domains on bacteriophage surfaces. Potential use for antibody selection. Journal of Immunology. 1991;**147**(10):3610-3614

[49] Huse WD, Stinchcombe TJ, Glaser SM, Starr L, MacLean M, Hellstrom KE, et al. Application of a filamentous phage pVIII fusion protein system suitable for efficient production, screening, and mutagenesis of F(ab) antibody fragments. Journal of Immunology. 1992;**149**(12):3914-3920

[50] Kang AS, Jones TM, Burton DR. Antibody redesign by chain shuffling from random combinatorial immunoglobulin libraries. Proceedings of the National Academy of Sciences of the United States of America. 1991;**88**(24):11120-11123

[51] Kang AS, Barbas CF, Janda KD, Benkovic SJ, Lerner RA. Linkage of recognition and replication functions by assembling combinatorial antibody Fab libraries along phage surfaces. Proceedings of the National Academy of Sciences of the United States of America. 1991;**88**(10):4363-4366

[52] Soderlind E, Simonsson AC, Borrebaeck CA. Phage display technology in antibody engineering: Design of phagemid vectors and in vitro maturation systems. Immunological Reviews. 1992;**130**:109-124

[53] Marks JD, Hoogenboom HR, Bonnert TP, McCafferty J, Griffiths AD, Winter G. By-passing immunization. Human antibodies from V-gene libraries displayed on phage. Journal of Molecular Biology. 1991;**222**(3):581-597

[54] de Haard HJ, van Neer N, Reurs A, Hufton SE, Roovers RC, Henderikx P, et al. A large non-immunized human Fab fragment phage library that permits rapid isolation and kinetic analysis of high affinity antibodies. The Journal of biological chemistry. 1999;**274**(26):18218-18230

[55] Vaughan TJ, Williams AJ, Pritchard K, Osbourn JK, Pope AR, Earnshaw JC, et al. Human antibodies with sub-nanomolar affinities isolated from a large non-immunized phage display library. Nature Biotechnology. 1996;**14**(3):309-314

[56] Lloyd C, Lowe D, Edwards B, Welsh F, Dilks T, Hardman C, et al. Modelling the human immune response: Performance of a 1011 human antibody repertoire against a broad

panel of therapeutically relevant antigens. Protein Engineering, Design & Selection. 2009;**22**(3):159-168

[57] Schwimmer LJ, Huang B, Giang H, Cotter RL, Chemla-Vogel DS, Dy FV, et al. Discovery of diverse and functional antibodies from large human repertoire antibody libraries. Journal of Immunological Methods. 2013;**391**(1-2):60-71

[58] Hust M, Meyer T, Voedisch B, Rülker T, Thie H, El-Ghezal A, et al. A human scFv antibody generation pipeline for proteome research. Journal of Biotechnology. 2011;**152**(4):159-170

[59] Kugler J, Wilke S, Meier D, Tomszak F, Frenzel A, Schirrmann T, et al. Generation and analysis of the improved human HAL9/10 antibody phage display libraries. BMC Biotechnology. 2015;**15**:10

[60] Barbas CF3rd, Bain JD, Hoekstra DM, Lerner RA. Semisynthetic combinatorial antibody libraries: A chemical solution to the diversity problem. Proceedings of the National Academy of Sciences of the United States of America. 1992;**89**(10):4457-4461

[61] Hoogenboom HR, Winter G. By-passing immunisation. Human antibodies from synthetic repertoires of germline VH gene segments rearranged in vitro. Journal of Molecular Biology. 1992;**227**(2):381-388

[62] Griffiths AD, Williams SC, Hartley O, Tomlinson IM, Waterhouse P, Crosby WL, et al. Isolation of high affinity human antibodies directly from large synthetic repertoires. The EMBO journal. 1994;**13**(14):3245-3260

[63] Nissim A, Hoogenboom HR, Tomlinson IM, Flynn G, Midgley C, Lane D, et al. Antibody fragments from a 'single pot' phage display library as immunochemical reagents. The EMBO Journal. 1994;**13**(3):692-698

[64] Pini A, Viti F, Santucci A, Carnemolla B, Zardi L, Neri P, et al. Design and use of a phage display library. Human antibodies with subnanomolar affinity against a marker of angiogenesis eluted from a two-dimensional gel. The Journal of Biological Chemistry. 1998;**273**(34):21769-21776

[65] Soderlind E, Strandberg L, Jirholt P, Kobayashi N, Alexeiva V, Aberg AM, et al. Recombining germline-derived CDR sequences for creating diverse single-framework antibody libraries. Nature Biotechnology. 2000;**18**(8):852-856

[66] Knappik A, Ge L, Honegger A, Pack P, Fischer M, Wellnhofer G, et al. Fully synthetic human combinatorial antibody libraries (HuCAL) based on modular consensus frameworks and CDRs randomized with trinucleotides. Journal of Molecular Biology. 2000; **296**(1):57-86

[67] Silacci M, Brack S, Schirru G, Marlind J, Ettorre A, Merlo A, et al. Design, construction, and characterization of a large synthetic human antibody phage display library. Proteomics. 2005;**5**(9):2340-2350

[68] Rothe C, Urlinger S, Lohning C, Prassler J, Stark Y, Jager U, et al. The human combinatorial antibody library HuCAL GOLD combines diversification of all six CDRs according

to the natural immune system with a novel display method for efficient selection of high-affinity antibodies. Journal of Molecular Biology. 2008;**376**(4):1182-1200

[69] Yang HY, Kang KJ, Chung JE, Shim H. Construction of a large synthetic human scFv library with six diversified CDRs and high functional diversity. Molecules and Cells. 2009;**27**(2):225-235

[70] Prassler J, Thiel S, Pracht C, Polzer A, Peters S, Bauer M, et al. HuCAL PLATINUM, a synthetic Fab library optimized for sequence diversity and superior performance in mammalian expression systems. Journal of Molecular Biology. 2011;**413**(1):261-278

[71] Zhai W, Glanville J, Fuhrmann M, Mei L, Ni I, Sundar PD, et al. Synthetic antibodies designed on natural sequence landscapes. Journal of Molecular Biology. 2011;**412**(1): 55-71

[72] Tiller T, Schuster I, Deppe D, Siegers K, Strohner R, Herrmann T, et al. A fully synthetic human Fab antibody library based on fixed VH/VL framework pairings with favorable biophysical properties. MAbs. 2013;**5**(3):445-470

[73] de Kruif J, Terstappen L, Boel E, Logtenberg T. Rapid selection of cell subpopulation-specific human monoclonal antibodies from a synthetic phage antibody library. Proceedings of the National Academy of Sciences of the United States of America 1995;**92**(9):3938-3942

[74] Shim H. Synthetic approach to the generation of antibody diversity. BMB Reports. 2015;**48**(9):489-494

[75] Hawkins RE, Russell SJ, Winter G. Selection of phage antibodies by binding affinity. Mimicking affinity maturation. Journal of Molecular Biology. 1992;**226**(3):889-896

[76] Marks JD, Ouwehand WH, Bye JM, Finnern R, Gorick BD, Voak D, et al. Human antibody fragments specific for human blood group antigens from a phage display library. Bio/Technology. 1993;**11**(10):1145-1149

[77] Clackson T, Hoogenboom HR, Griffiths AD, Winter G. Making antibody fragments using phage display libraries. Nature. 1991;**352**(6336):624-628

[78] Gram H, Marconi LA, Barbas CF3rd, Collet TA, Lerner RA, Kang AS. vitro selection and affinity maturation of antibodies from a naive combinatorial immunoglobulin library. Proceedings of the National Academy of Sciences of the United States of America. 1992;**89**(8):3576-3580

[79] Daugherty PS, Chen G, Iverson BL, Georgiou G. Quantitative analysis of the effect of the mutation frequency on the affinity maturation of single chain Fv antibodies. Proceedings of the National Academy of Sciences of the United States of America. 2000;**97**(5):2029-2034

[80] Ho M, Kreitman RJ, Onda M, Pastan I. vitro antibody evolution targeting germline hot spots to increase activity of an anti-CD22 immunotoxin. The Journal of Biological Chemistry. 2005;**280**(1):607-617

[81] Bowers PM, Horlick RA, Neben TY, Toobian RM, Tomlinson GL, Dalton JL, et al. Coupling mammalian cell surface display with somatic hypermutation for the discovery and maturation of human antibodies. Proceedings of the National Academy of Sciences of the United States of America. 2011;**108**(51):20455-20460

[82] Bowers PM, Horlick RA, Kehry MR, Neben TY, Tomlinson GL, Altobell L, et al. Mammalian cell display for the discovery and optimization of antibody therapeutics. Methods. 2014;**65**(1):44-56

[83] King DJ, Bowers PM, Kehry MR, Horlick RA. Mammalian cell display and somatic hypermutation in vitro for human antibody discovery. Current Drug Discovery Technologies. 2014;**11**(1):56-64

[84] Jespers LS, Roberts A, Mahler SM, Winter G, Hoogenboom HR. Guiding the selection of human antibodies from phage display repertoires to a single epitope of an antigen. Bio/Technology. 1994;**12**(9):899-903

[85] Figini M, Marks JD, Winter G, Griffiths AD. In vitro assembly of repertoires of antibody chains on the surface of phage by renaturation. Journal of Molecular Biology. 1994;**239**(1):68-78

[86] Osbourn J, Groves M, Vaughan T. From rodent reagents to human therapeutics using antibody guided selection. Methods. 2005;**36**(1):61-68

[87] Zebedee SL, Barbas CF3rd, Hom YL, Caothien RH, Graff R, DeGraw J, et al. Human combinatorial antibody libraries to hepatitis B surface antigen. Proceedings of the National Academy of Sciences of the United States of America. 1992;**89**(8):3175-3179

[88] Ohlin M, Owman H, Mach M, Borrebaeck CA. Light chain shuffling of a high affinity antibody results in a drift in epitope recognition. Molecular Immunology. 1996;**33**(1):47-56

[89] Watzka H, Pfizenmaier K, Moosmayer D. Guided selection of antibody fragments specific for human interferon gamma receptor 1 from a human VH- and VL-gene repertoire. Immunotechnology: An International Journal of Immunological Engineering. 1998;**3**(4):279-291

[90] Beiboer SH, Reurs A, Roovers RC, Arends JW, Whitelegg NR, Rees AR, et al. Guided selection of a pan carcinoma specific antibody reveals similar binding characteristics yet structural divergence between the original murine antibody and its human equivalent. Journal of Molecular Biology. 2000;**296**(3):833-849

[91] Klimka A, Matthey B, Roovers RC, Barth S, Arends JW, Engert A, et al. Human anti-CD30 recombinant antibodies by guided phage antibody selection using cell panning. British Journal of Cancer. 2000;**83**(2):252-260

[92] Zhao A, Tohidkia MR, Siegel DL, Coukos G, Omidi Y. Phage antibody display libraries: A powerful antibody discovery platform for immunotherapy. Critical Reviews in Biotechnology. 2016;**36**(2):276-289

[93] Boder ET, Wittrup KD. Yeast surface display for screening combinatorial polypeptide libraries. Nature Biotechnology. 1997;**15**(6):553-557

[94] Feldhaus MJ, Siegel RW. Yeast display of antibody fragments: A discovery and characterization platform. Journal of Immunological Methods. 2004;**290**(1-2):69-80

[95] Gera N, Hussain M, Rao BM. Protein selection using yeast surface display. Methods. 2013;**60**(1):15-26

[96] Sheehan J, Marasco WA. Phage and yeast display. Microbiology Spectrum. 2015;**3**(1):17 AID-0028-2014

[97] Shusta EV, Kieke MC, Parke E, Kranz DM, Wittrup KD. Yeast polypeptide fusion surface display levels predict thermal stability and soluble secretion efficiency. Journal of Molecular Biology. 1999;**292**(5):949-956

[98] Shusta EV, Holler PD, Kieke MC, Kranz DM, Wittrup KD. Directed evolution of a stable scaffold for T-cell receptor engineering. Nature Biotechnology. 2000;**18**(7):754-759

[99] Orr BA, Carr LM, Wittrup KD, Roy EJ, Kranz DM. Rapid method for measuring ScFv thermal stability by yeast surface display. Biotechnology Progress. 2003;**19**(2):631-638

[100] Boder ET, Midelfort KS, Wittrup KD. Directed evolution of antibody fragments with monovalent femtomolar antigen-binding affinity. Proceedings of the National Academy of Sciences of the United States of America. 2000;**97**(20):10701-10705

[101] Feldhaus MJ, Siegel RW, Opresko LK, Coleman JR, Feldhaus JM, Yeung YA, et al. Flow-cytometric isolation of human antibodies from a nonimmune Saccharomyces cerevisiae surface display library. Nature Biotechnology. 2003;**21**(2):163-170

[102] van den Beucken T, Pieters H, Steukers M, van der Vaart M, Ladner RC, Hoogenboom HR, et al. Affinity maturation of Fab antibody fragments by fluorescent-activated cell sorting of yeast-displayed libraries. FEBS Letters 2003;**546**(2-3):288-294.

[103] Ferrara F, Naranjo LA, Kumar S, Gaiotto T, Mukundan H, Swanson B, et al. Using phage and yeast display to select hundreds of monoclonal antibodies: Application to antigen 85, a tuberculosis biomarker. PLoS One. 2012;**7**(11):e49535

[104] Boder ET, Raeeszadeh-Sarmazdeh M, Price JV. Engineering antibodies by yeast display. Archives of Biochemistry and Biophysics. 2012;**526**(2):99-106

[105] Benatuil L, Perez JM, Belk J, Hsieh CM. An improved yeast transformation method for the generation of very large human antibody libraries. Protein Engineering, Design & Selection. 2010;**23**(4):155-159

[106] Georgiou G, Stathopoulos C, Daugherty PS, Nayak AR, Iverson BL, Curtiss R 3rd. Display of heterologous proteins on the surface of microorganisms: From the screening of combinatorial libraries to live recombinant vaccines. Nature Biotechnology. 1997;**15**(1):29-34

[107] Samuelson P, Gunneriusson E, Nygren PA, Stahl S. Display of proteins on bacteria. Journal of Biotechnology. 2002;**96**(2):129-154

[108] Lofblom J. Bacterial display in combinatorial protein engineering. Biotechnology Journal. 2011;**6**(9):1115-1129

[109] Francisco JA, Campbell R, Iverson BL, Georgiou G. Production and fluorescence-activated cell sorting of *Escherichia coli* expressing a functional antibody fragment on the external surface. Proceedings of the National Academy of Sciences of the United States of America. 1993;**90**(22):10444-10448

[110] Daugherty PS, Chen G, Olsen MJ, Iverson BL, Georgiou G. Antibody affinity maturation using bacterial surface display. Protein Engineering. 1998;**11**(9):825-832

[111] Mazor Y, Van Blarcom T, Mabry R, Iverson BL, Georgiou G. Isolation of engineered, full-length antibodies from libraries expressed in *Escherichia coli*. Nature Biotechnology. 2007;**25**(5):563-565

[112] Samuelson P, Hansson M, Ahlborg N, Andreoni C, Gotz F, Bachi T, et al. Cell surface display of recombinant proteins on Staphylococcus carnosus. Journal of Bacteriology. 1995;**177**(6):1470-1476

[113] Lofblom J, Wernerus H, Stahl S. Fine affinity discrimination by normalized fluorescence activated cell sorting in staphylococcal surface display. FEMS Microbiology Letters. 2005;**248**(2):189-198

[114] Kronqvist N, Lofblom J, Jonsson A, Wernerus H, Stahl S. A novel affinity protein selection system based on staphylococcal cell surface display and flow cytometry. Protein Engineering, Design & Selection. 2008;**21**(4):247-255

[115] Lipovsek D, Pluckthun A. In-vitro protein evolution by ribosome display and mRNA display. Journal of Immunological Methods. 2004;**290**(1-2):51-67

[116] Pluckthun A. Ribosome display: A perspective. Methods in Molecular Biology. 2012; **805**:3-28

[117] Roberts RW, Szostak JW. RNA-peptide fusions for the in vitro selection of peptides and proteins. Proceedings of the National Academy of Sciences of the United States of America. 1997;**94**(23):12297-12302

[118] Nemoto N, Miyamoto-Sato E, Husimi Y, Yanagawa H. In vitro virus: Bonding of mRNA bearing puromycin at the 3'-terminal end to the C-terminal end of its encoded protein on the ribosome in vitro. FEBS Letters. 1997;**414**(2):405-408

[119] Josephson K, Ricardo A, Szostak JW. mRNA display: From basic principles to macrocycle drug discovery. Drug Discovery Today. 2014;**19**(4):388-399

[120] Hanes J, Schaffitzel C, Knappik A, Pluckthun A. Picomolar affinity antibodies from a fully synthetic naive library selected and evolved by ribosome display. Nature Biotechnology. 2000;**18**(12):1287-1292

[121] Zhou L, Mao WP, Fen J, Liu HY, Wei CJ, Li WX, et al. Selection of scFvs specific for the HepG2 cell line using ribosome display. Journal of Biosciences. 2009;**34**(2):221-226

[122] Zhao HY, Zhang YZ, Xiao CL. Advances in the study of affinity selection-ultrafiltration/HPLC-MS. Yao Xue Xue Bao. 2009;**44**(10):1084-1088

[123] Luo Y, Xia Y. Selection of single-chain variable fragment antibodies against fenitrothion by ribosome display. Analytical Biochemistry. 2012;**421**(1):130-137

[124] Stafford RL, Matsumoto ML, Yin G, Cai Q, Fung JJ, Stephenson H, et al. In vitro Fab display: A cell-free system for IgG discovery. Protein Engineering, Design & Selection. 2014;**27**(4):97-109

[125] Xu L, Aha P, Gu K, Kuimelis RG, Kurz M, Lam T, et al. Directed evolution of high-affinity antibody mimics using mRNA display. Chemistry & Biology. 2002;**9**(8):933-942

[126] Fukuda I, Kojoh K, Tabata N, Doi N, Takashima H, Miyamoto-Sato E, et al. In vitro evolution of single-chain antibodies using mRNA display. Nucleic Acids Research. 2006;**34**(19):e127

[127] Sumida T, Yanagawa H, Doi N. In vitro selection of fab fragments by mRNA display and gene-linking emulsion PCR. Journal of Nucleic Acids. 2012;**2012**:371379

[128] Doi N, Yanagawa H. STABLE: Protein-DNA fusion system for screening of combinatorial protein libraries in vitro. FEBS Letters. 1999;**457**(2):227-230

[129] Yonezawa M, Doi N, Kawahashi Y, Higashinakagawa T, Yanagawa H. DNA display for in vitro selection of diverse peptide libraries. Nucleic Acids Research. 2003;**31**(19):e118

[130] Yonezawa M, Doi N, Higashinakagawa T, Yanagawa H. DNA display of biologically active proteins for in vitro protein selection. Journal of Biochemistry. 2004;**135**(3):285-288

[131] Sumida T, Doi N, Yanagawa H. Bicistronic DNA display for in vitro selection of Fab fragments. Nucleic Acids Research. 2009;**37**(22):e147

[132] Lonberg N. Fully human antibodies from transgenic mouse and phage display platforms. Current Opinion in Immunology. 2008;**20**(4):450-459

[133] Bruggemann M, Osborn MJ, Ma B, Hayre J, Avis S, Lundstrom B, et al. Human antibody production in transgenic animals. Archivum Immunologiae et Therapiae Experimentalis (Warsz). 2015;**63**(2):101-108

[134] Nixon AE, Sexton DJ, Ladner RC. Drugs derived from phage display: From candidate identification to clinical practice. MAbs. 2014;**6**(1):73-85

[135] Scheinfeld N. Adalimumab (HUMIRA): A review. Journal of Drugs in Dermatology. 2003;**2**(4):375-377

[136] Humira (Adalimumab). Abbvie Inc. 2016 Available from: https://www.humira.com/ [Accessed: Jan 24, 2017]

[137] Benlysta (Belimumab), GSK 2016 Available from: http://www.benlysta.com/ [Accessed: Jan 24, 2017]

[138] Mazumdar S. Raxibacumab. MAbs. 2009;**1**(6):531-538

[139] Raxibacumab. ABthrax – Prescribing Information. GSK; 2016 Available from: https://www.gsksource.com/pharma/content/dam/GlaxoSmithKline/US/en/Prescribing_Information/Raxibacumab/pdf/RAXIBACUMAB-PI-PIL.PDF [Accessed: Jan 24, 2017]

[140] Cyramza (Ramucirumab), Eli Lilly 2016 Available from: http://www.cyramzahcp.com/ [Accessed: Jan 24, 2017]

[141] Reichert JM. Antibodies to watch in 2016. MAbs. 2016;**8**(2):197-204

[142] Garnock-Jones KP. Necitumumab: First global approval. Drugs. 2016;**76**(2):283-289

[143] Baca M, Presta LG, O'Connor SJ, Wells JA. Antibody humanization using monovalent phage display. The Journal of Biological Chemistry. 1997;**272**(16):10678-10684

[144] Muller YA, Chen Y, Christinger HW, Li B, Cunningham BC, Lowman HB, et al. VEGF and the Fab fragment of a humanized neutralizing antibody: Crystal structure of the complex at 2.4 A resolution and mutational analysis of the interface. Structure. 1998;**6**(9):1153-1167

[145] Chen Y, Wiesmann C, Fuh G, Li B, Christinger HW, McKay P, et al. Selection and analysis of an optimized anti-VEGF antibody: Crystal structure of an affinity-matured Fab in complex with antigen. Journal of Molecular Biology. 1999;**293**(4):865-881

[146] Muyldermans S. Nanobodies: Natural single-domain antibodies. Annual Review of Biochemistry. 2013;**82**:775-797

[147] Zielonka S, Empting M, Grzeschik J, Konning D, Barelle CJ, Kolmar H. Structural insights and biomedical potential of IgNAR scaffolds from sharks. MAbs. 2015;**7**(1):15-25

[148] Burioni R, Canducci F, Mancini N, Clementi N, Sassi M, De Marco D, et al. Monoclonal antibodies isolated from human B cells neutralize a broad range of H1 subtype influenza A viruses including swine-origin Influenza virus (S-OIV). Virology. 2010;**399**(1):144-152

[149] Krause JC, Tsibane T, Tumpey TM, Huffman CJ, Basler CF, Crowe Jr JE. A broadly neutralizing human monoclonal antibody that recognizes a conserved, novel epitope on the globular head of the influenza H1N1 virus hemagglutinin. Journal of Virology 2011;**85**(20):10905-10908

[150] Ekiert DC, Bhabha G, Elsliger MA, Friesen RH, Jongeneelen M, Throsby M, et al. Antibody recognition of a highly conserved influenza virus epitope. Science. 2009;**324** (5924):246-251

[151] Sui J, Hwang WC, Perez S, Wei G, Aird D, Chen LM, et al. Structural and functional bases for broad-spectrum neutralization of avian and human influenza A viruses. Nature Structural & Molecular Biology. 2009;**16**(3):265-273

[152] DeKosky BJ, Lungu OI, Park D, Johnson EL, Charab W, Chrysostomou C, et al. Large-scale sequence and structural comparisons of human naive and antigen-experienced antibody repertoires. Proceedings of the National Academy of Sciences of the United States of America. 2016;**113**(19):E2636-E2645

[153] DeWitt WS, Lindau P, Snyder TM, Sherwood AM, Vignali M, Carlson CS, et al. A public database of memory and naive B-cell receptor sequences. PLoS One. 2016;**11**(8):e0160853

Detailed Protocols for the Selection of Antiviral Human Antibodies from Combinatorial Immune Phage Display Libraries

Philipp Diebolder and Adalbert Krawczyk

Additional information is available at the end of the chapter

http://dx.doi.org/10.5772/intechopen.70139

Abstract

Broadly, neutralizing antiviral antibodies holds great promise for improving treatment opportunities for patients suffering from viral infections (e.g., human immunodeficiency virus [HIV], hepatitis B virus [HBV], cytomegalovirus [CMV], Rabies, Ebola, Zika) leading to serious health disorders or even to death without effective antiviral treatment. The potential of antibodies in host protection against lethal viral infections has been demonstrated in numerous animal models and is best exemplified by the protection conferred to neonates by maternal antibodies. Over the past few decades, virus-neutralizing human monoclonal antibodies (nAbs) have been isolated from humans successfully cured of disease using a wide range of recently developed antibody isolation technologies. In this chapter, we present an approach for isolating recombinant human nAbs from combinatorial gene libraries being cloned from individuals who have recovered from viral infections. The presented protocols describe the selection and screening of antiviral single-chain antibody fragments (scFvs) from phage display immune libraries. This technology represents a well-established, high-throughput approach allowing fast selection of broadly neutralizing, antiviral antibodies. The protocols for generating and selecting antigen-specific scFvs can be applied for the selection of scFvs against any target.

Keywords: recombinant human monoclonal antibodies, broadly neutralizing antiviral antibodies, antibody phage display, combinatorial immune libraries, high-throughput screening

1. Introduction

Antibodies are powerful tools for the prophylaxis and treatment of viral infections. The use of antibodies against severe, life-threatening infections began in the 1890s when Robert Koch

INTECH
open science | open minds

© 2018 The Author(s). Licensee InTech. This chapter is distributed under the terms of the Creative Commons Attribution License (http://creativecommons.org/licenses/by/3.0), which permits unrestricted use, distribution, and reproduction in any medium, provided the original work is properly cited. (cc) BY

demonstrated that administration of sheep antiserum against diphtheria toxin to a girl dying from diphtheria infection led to her rapid recovery and survival [1]. On that basis, numerous attempts to treat potentially deadly viral diseases such as influenza, severe acute respiratory syndrome (SARS), or Ebola by administrating sera from survivors have successfully been undertaken [2]. Further improvements led to the development of polyclonal hyperimmunoglobulin G (IgG) preparations, consisting of purified antibodies from seropositive donors [3]. Several hyperimmunoglobulins against human cytomegalovirus (CMV), hepatitis B virus (HBV), rabies, and other viral infections are available on the market. Although polyclonal preparations provide strong antiviral activity, the major disadvantage of such hyperimmunoglobulin preparations is that they include a high amount of nonspecific antibodies and only a low proportion of neutralizing antibodies. The development of hybridoma technology by Köhler & Milstein in 1975 revolutionized science and medicine and led to the isolation of numerous monoclonal antibodies [4]. Since the commercialization of the first therapeutic monoclonal antibody product in 1986, this class of therapeutics has grown significantly [5]. In 2016, 5 of the top 20 pharmaceuticals were therapeutic antibody drugs [6]. The vast majority of monoclonal antibodies is approved for the treatment of cancers, multiple sclerosis, or rheumatoid arthritis [7]. However, numerous potent human or humanized antiviral antibodies against H5N1 influenza virus, human immunodeficiency virus (HIV), herpes simplex virus (HSV), human cytomegalovirus (CMV), hepatitis C virus (HCV), Ebola virus, severe acute respiratory syndrome (SARS) virus, and other viral infections are in preclinical development, clinical studies, or even approved for antiviral treatment [2, 7–12]. Antibodies mostly neutralize free viruses by targeting the initial stages of virus infection described as the binding of free virions to permissive target cells followed by entry and replication [2]. Neutralizing antibodies not only provide new tools for prophylaxis and therapy of viral diseases, but also identify conserved epitopes that may be used to design new vaccines capable of conferring broader protection [11]. However, enveloped viruses such as HIV-1, HSV-1/2, CMV, and measles can also move between adjacent cells without diffusing through the extracellular environment (cell-to-cell spread). This mechanism facilitates rapid viral dissemination, promotes immune evasion from the host's immune response, and enhances the progression of disease [13]. We recently described a murine monoclonal antibody (mAb) capable of inhibiting the cell-to-cell spread of HSV. This antibody proved to be highly effective in the prevention of drug-resistant HSV infections in highly immunodeficient NOD/SCID mice indicating the enormous potential of antibody blocking mechanisms crucial for the virus spread [12]. Due to these unique features, this antibody was humanized for clinical applications and is now being tested in phase I and II trials. Besides the generation of antiviral antibodies by humanization approaches, neutralizing antibodies can also be isolated from humans cured of viral infections, such as SARS or Ebola [9, 14]. Various methods have been developed for the isolation of antibodies from humans including B-cell immortalization and single-cell expression cloning [15]. Among these approaches, high-throughput screening of phage-displayed antibody libraries has become one of the leading technologies for generating human therapeutic antibodies (**Figure 1**) [16]. Nowadays, very large phage display libraries from naive (IgM) B-cell repertoires (>10^{10} independent clones) are widely used for the selection of human antibodies against a broad panel of targets including human self-antigens to identify high-affinity binders. However, these antibodies are not affinity-matured by the human immune system. Hence, the preparation of combinatorial immune libraries from immunized or infection cured donors can deliver a broader range of highly functional antibodies, even from smaller libraries (i.e., potent antiviral antibodies with broadly neutralizing efficacies). For instance, the selection of combinatorial immune repertoires (>10^8 independent clones) from HSV seropositive donors resulted in a broad panel of various high-affinity binders with partly HSV-neutralizing properties [17, 18].

Although various other *in vitro* selection platforms have been developed during the last decades (e.g., ribosome display and yeast display), phage display using filamentous phages is predominantly used for library generation since it is robust, inexpensive, and allows the automation of the selection and screening process. Due to the limitation in the production of full-length IgG antibodies in *Escherichia coli*, only smaller antibody fragments (e.g., scFvs or Fabs) can be efficiently expressed within the *E. coli* periplasm as functional proteins. Several systems

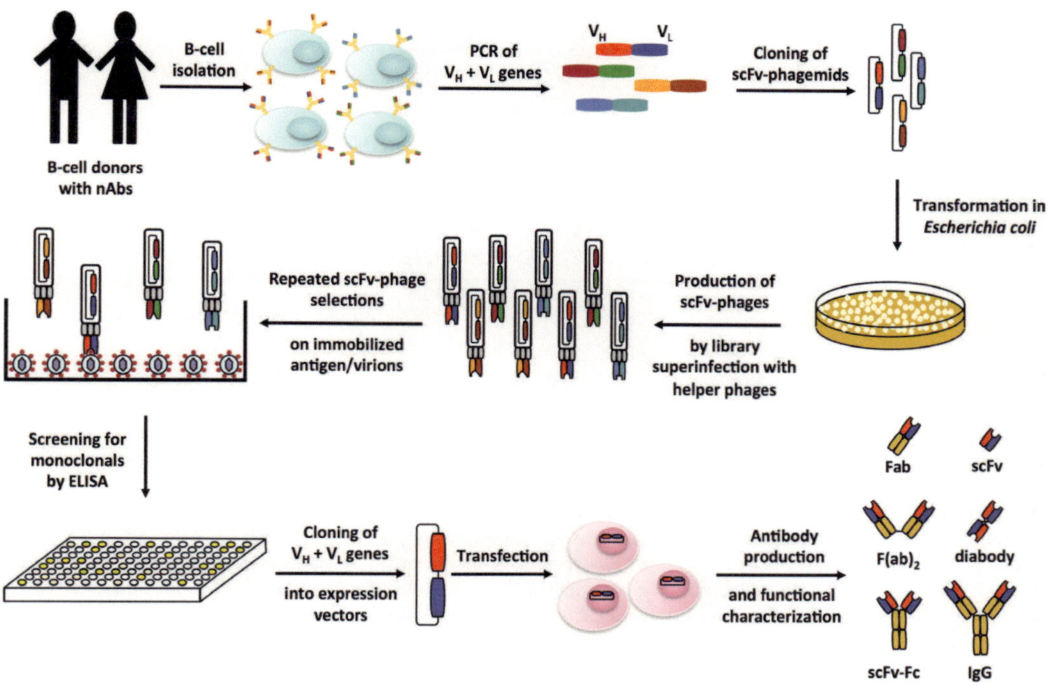

Figure 1. Isolation of human neutralizing antiviral antibodies (nAbs) by phage display technique. Lymphocytes comprising B-cells from humans harboring neutralizing antibodies with unique features, e.g., Ebola disease survivors are isolated from blood, spleen, lymph nodes, or bone marrow by standard techniques (e.g., PBMCs by Ficoll density gradient centrifugation). Lymphocytes RNA is prepared and transcribed into single-stranded cDNA that is used as the source for PCR amplification of the variable heavy (VH) and light chain (VL) genes. Variable genes are randomly cloned into phagemid vectors as scFv antibody fragments prior to electroporation of phagemids into *E. coli* bacteria to produce combinatorial immune libraries. Library glycerol stocks are then used for the generation of a bacterial culture that is superinfected with a helper phage to produce phages presenting different scFvs on their surface. Specific binding scFv-phages are enriched over several selection rounds by stringent washing and elution using antigen/virions immobilized on immunotubes. After screening for monoclonal binders on ELISA plates, the best specific binders are directly produced as monovalent scFvs in bacteria cultures or cloned into appropriate expression vectors for the production of Fab, or various bivalent antibody formats prior to functional analysis (e.g., virus neutralization capacity and affinity).

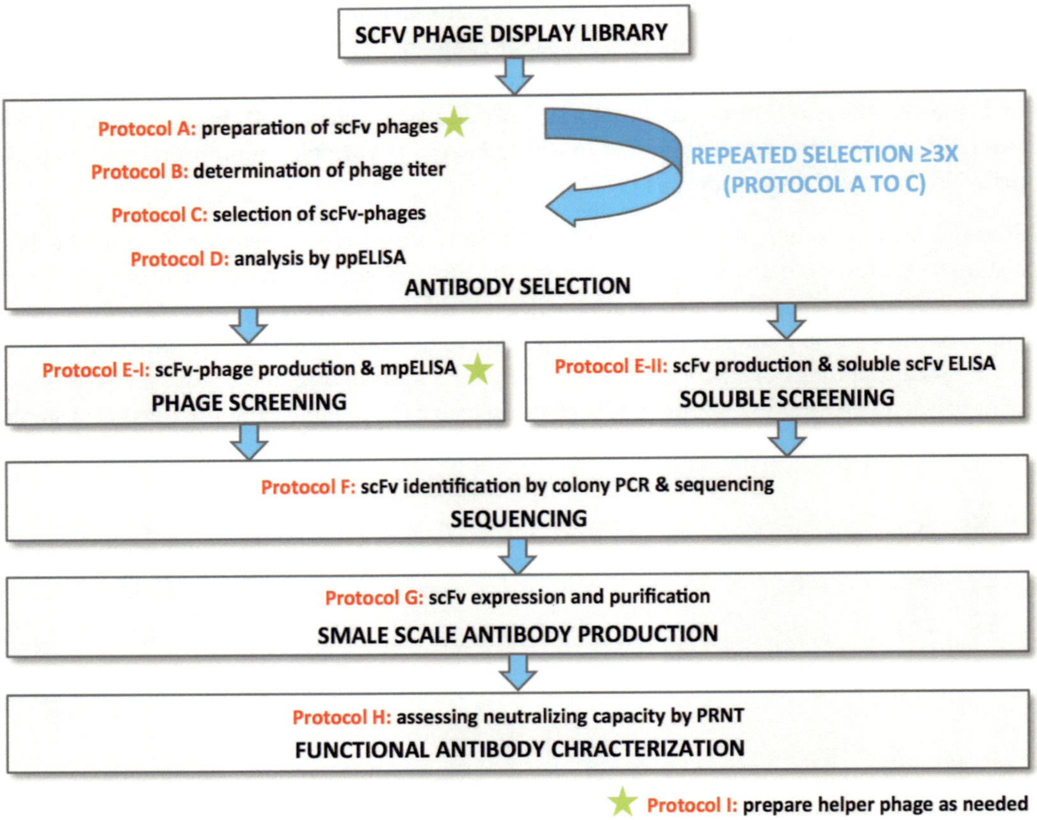

Figure 2. Workflow of the selection and screening procedure. For the selection of antigen-specific scFv-phages, log-phase library cultures are packed by superinfection with helper phages (for the preparation of helper phages, see Protocol I) that provide all proteins necessary for phage propagation (see Protocol A). After IPTG induction, expressed scFv-pIII fusions are inserted within the produced phages leading to the presentation of scFv antibody fragments on the phage surface. After determination of phage titer (see Protocol B), specific binding scFv-phages are enriched over several selection rounds by stringent washing and elution on recombinant antigen/virions that have been immobilized onto immunotubes (see Protocol C). Successful enrichment of specific binding scFv-phages can be analyzed by polyclonal phage ELISA (ppELISA) (see Protocol D) prior to screening of monoclonal antibodies as scFv-phages by monoclonal phage ELISA (mpELISA) (see Protocol E-I) or as soluble scFvs (see Protocol E-II). After the identification of bacterial colonies encoding for full-length scFvs by colony PCR and sequencing (see Protocol F), soluble scFvs can be produced in the periplasm of bacteria (see Protocol G) or variable antibody genes can be cloned into mammalian expression vectors to produce Fab or various bivalent antibody fragments. Finally, antibody fragments can be analyzed for their neutralizing activity in functional assays like the plaque reduction neutralization test (PRNT) (see Protocol H).

for displaying antibody fragments on the phage surface have been developed over time using different vectors and phage coat proteins for display. The most common type (3 + 3 system) is based on phagemid vectors where the antibody gene fragments are cloned as fusions with the pIII phage gene. Cloning of the antibody gene repertoires can be done by using different strategies in one, two, or three independent steps where the variable light and heavy chain genes are PCR-amplified and randomly combined into reliable phagemid vectors. In the-one step cloning strategy, the VH and VL genes are separately amplified with an overlapping, additional linker sequence and combined by assembly PCR [19]. In the two-step cloning strategy, mostly the VL gene repertoire is cloned first into the phagemid followed by insertion of the VH repertoire into the VL phagemid [17, 18, 20–22]. In the three-step cloning strategy, two separate VH and VL libraries are prepared before exercising one repertoire and including it into the phagemid containing the other repertoire [23]. After electroporation of the phagemids into electrocompetent *E. coli* bacteria, the antibody libraries are grown on selection plates and stored as frozen bacterial glycerol stocks. Prior to PCR amplification of the variable antibody genes, B-cells from respective donors need to be isolated. In the case of viral infection and depending on when the infection occurred, the isolation of the short-lived plasmablast pool during the early antibody response or the long-lived memory B-cell and plasma cell pool may be preferred. Although the isolation of peripheral blood mononuclear cells (PBMC) from whole blood (the main source for plasmablasts) is often described for retrieving antiviral antibodies, B-cell sources such as spleen, lymph nodes (many memory B-cells), or bone marrow (the main source of plasma cells) might be considered for library construction. Good protocols for the cloning of combinatorial scFv phage display libraries including the primer sets for PCR amplification of antibody genes can be found elsewhere [17, 20–22] and are out of the scope of this chapter.

Here, we present a methodology for the recovering of potential therapeutic antibodies with unique antiviral properties from human B-cell repertoires (for workflow see **Figure 2**). This strategy has been successfully used for generating neutralizing human antibodies against HSV as a proof-of-principle [18]. The following protocol will systematically describe the procedure of generating broadly neutralizing antiviral antibodies from isolated human B-cells by a phage display technique.

2. Preliminary notes

Before starting antibody phage display, please be aware that phages are highly stable and decontamination of workspace and consumables is hard to achieve. It is best to do phage work in a special lab keeping equipment/material separated from the common bacterial workspace, especially when antibody library construction is performed. If not possible, phage work should be carried out in at least a separate workspace including a separate hood, shaker, and centrifuge. Inactivation of phage solutions can be done by incubation with diluted bleach (caution, always wear personal protection during handling) and/or sterilizing workspaces with UV light. For decontamination of tubes and Erlenmeyer flasks, bleach can be added to water-filled tubes and incubated overnight before washing, rinsing, and autoclaving. In common, single-use material is preferred for phage work. Collect phage-contaminated solutions in glass flasks and inactivate by adding bleach before dumping. Only use polypropylene (PP) tubes since phages might stick to other kinds of plastics. To prevent contamination to pipettes, always use barrier tips.

Presented protocols are intended for the selection and screening of antibody libraries based on the scFv antibody format being cloned in phagemid vectors as pIII fusion with an intrinsic amber stop codon and under the *lac* promoter (inducible by IPTG, repressible by glucose). Many current antibody phage display libraries are constructed in phagemid vectors with listed features (e.g., most derivatives of pHEN, pComb3X, pHAL, and pCANTAB), although other selection relevant features such as signal peptides, molecular tags, etc., might differ. Please check features of your antibody library used prior to selection and screening and change protocols accordingly if necessary. If using libraries based on phagemid vectors with *lac* promoter, **always add ≥2% glucose** to the media to repress scFv-pIII protein expression as long as antibody phages are not produced. Lower amounts of glucose results in background expression of pIII fusions and clones with growth advantages (e.g., truncated scFvs) might overgrow leading to a reduced library diversity. More detailed information about antibody phage display [24] and commonly used phagemid vectors can be found elsewhere [25].

Independent of the source of your antibody library, always try to package antibody libraries from primary bacteria stocks, never from secondary stocks or using phage-packaged libraries to infect bacteria. Only correctly stored (−80°C) primary glycerol bacteria stocks guarantee highest initial antibody diversity. For novel libraries or if not familiar with antibody phage display, perform test selection and subsequent screening using not relevant proteins such as bovine serum albumin.

3. Materials

A. Preparation of scFv-phages

- 2xTY medium: 16 g/l tryptone, 10 g/l yeast extract, 5 g/l NaCl, dissolved in ultrapure water, autoclaved, and stored at room temperature (RT).
- 2xYT-GA: 900 ml 2xYT medium, supplemented with 100 ml glucose stock solution and 1 ml ampicillin stock solution right before use.
- Kanamycin stock solution (2000×): 100 mg/ml kanamycin sulfate dissolved in ultrapure water, filter-sterilized, stored at −20°C.
- Ampicillin stock solution (1000×): 100 mg/ml ampicillin sodium salt dissolved in ultrapure water, filter-sterilized, stored at −20°C.
- 20% (w/v) glucose stock solution (10×): 200 g/l D-glucose dissolved in ultrapure water, filter-sterilized, stored at 4°C.
- Helper phage VCSM13 (Agilent Technologies) or M13K07 (e.g., NEB Biolabs), Kanamycin-resistant.
- Optional for oligomeric display: hyperphage M13 K07ΔpIII (Progen Biotechnik).
- 2xYT-GK agar plates (100 mm): 16 g tryptone, 10 g yeast extract, 5 g NaCl, and 15 g agar dissolved in 900 ml ultrapure water, autoclaved, cooled down to 50°C, and supplemented with 100 ml glucose stock solution and 500 μl kanamycin stock solution right before pouring, stored at 4°C.
- 1 M IPTG stock solution (20,000×): 2.38 g isopropyl β-D-1-thiogalactopyranoside dissolved in 10 ml ultrapure water, filter-sterilized, stored at −20°C.

- Induction medium 2xYT-AKI: 2xYT supplemented with 1 ml ampicillin stock solution, 500 µl kanamycin stock solution, and 50 µl IPTG stock solution (IPTG concentration depending on phagemid vector used), no glucose (!), prepared right before use.
- Polypropylene (PP) centrifugation tubes: 2 and 50 ml (single-use), 250 ml (reusable).
- PEG/NaCl solution: 200 g/l polyethylene glycol 6000, 146.1 g/l NaCl, dissolved in ultrapure water, autoclaved, stored at 4°C.
- Optional for Western blot analysis: primary murine anti-pIII monoclonal IgG (MoBiTec, diluted 1:1000 milk in phosphate-buffered saline (MPBS)) and secondary goat anti-mouse HRP-conjugated antibody (Jackson ImmunoResearch, diluted 1:10,000 in MPBS).

B. Determination of the phage titer

- TG1 bacteria strain (e.g., Lucigen).
- M9 minimal stock solution (5×): 56.4 g/l M9 minimal salt (Sigma Aldrich) dissolved in ultrapure water, autoclaved, stored at 4°C.
- 1 M $MgSO_4$ stock solution: 6.02 g $MgSO_4$ dissolved in 50 ml ultrapure water, filter-sterilized, stored at 4°C.
- Thiamine stock solution: 50 mg thiamine hydrochloride dissolved in 50 ml ultrapure water, filter-sterilized, stored at −20°C.
- M9/+Thi minimal plates (100 mm): 15 g agar dissolved in 780 ml ultrapure water, autoclaved and supplemented with 200 ml M9 minimal salt stock solution, 20 ml glucose stock solution (see A), 1 ml $MgSO_4$ solution, and 1 ml thiamine stock solution.
- 2xYT-GA agar plates (100 mm): 16 g tryptone, 10 g yeast extract, 5 g NaCl, and 15 g agar dissolved in 900 ml ultrapure water, autoclaved, cooled down to 50°C, and supplemented with 100 ml glucose stock solution and 1 ml ampicillin stock solution right before pouring, stored at 4°C.

C. Selection of antigen-specific scFv-phages

- 5 ml Nunc MaxiSorp™ immunotubes (Thermo Fisher Scientific).
- Phosphate-buffered saline (PBS): 1.42 g/l Na_2HPO_4, 0.24 g/l KH_2PO_4, 0.2 g/l KCl, 8.0 g/l NaCl, dissolved in ultrapure water, adjusted to pH 7.4, autoclaved, stored at RT.
- PBST: phosphate-buffered saline supplemented with 0.1% Tween20.
- MPBS: 2% nonfat dry milk in phosphate-buffered saline, prepared right before use.
- TG1 bacteria strain (e.g., Lucigen).
- 2xYT-GA agar plates (100 mm round, 150 mm round, or 245 mm square): see B.
- Phage elution buffer: 0.1 M glycine-HCl, 0.5 M NaCl, dissolved in ultrapure water, adjusted to pH 2.2, filter-sterilized, stored at 4°C.

- Phage neutralization buffer: 1 M Tris-HCl dissolved in ultrapure water, adjusted to pH 9.5, filter-sterilized, stored at 4°C.
- Trypsin-PBS solution: 10 μg/ml trypsin (e.g., from porcine pancreas by Sigma Aldrich) dissolved in PBS, pH 7.4, prepared right before use.

D. Polyclonal phage ELISA (ppELISA)

- PBS and PBST: see C.
- 96-well microtiter ELISA plate (e.g., Nunc Maxisorp™ by Thermo Fisher Scientific).
- Murine anti-M13 monoclonal antibody HRP-conjugate (GE Healthcare), diluted 1:5000 in MPBS.
- TMB substrate solution (e.g., Thermo Fisher Scientific).
- Stop solution (2 M H_2SO_4): concentrated sulfuric acid dissolved 1:9 in ultrapure water.

E. Screening for monoclonal binders

(I) Monoclonal phage (mpELISA) screening:

- Sterile 96-well polypropylene round-bottom microplates (e.g., Greiner Bio-One).
- Breathable sealing membrane for microplates (e.g., Sigma Aldrich).
- 96-pin microplate replicator (Boekel Scientific).
- 8-channel pipettes (20 μl and 200 μl).
- 2xYT-glycerol: 2xYT dissolved in 50% glycerol and 50% ultrapure water, autoclaved, stored at RT.
- 2xYT-GA medium, ampicillin stock solutions, glucose stock solution, kanamycin stock solution, IPTG stock solution, helper phage VCSM13 or M13K07, and induction medium 2xYT-AKI: see A.
- PBS, PBST: see C.
- Maxisorb™ ELISA plates, anti-M13 monoclonal HRP-conjugate, TMB substrate, and stop solution: see D.

(II) Soluble scFv screening:

- HB2151 bacterial strain (Nordic BioSite).
- M9/+Thi minimal plates, 2xYT-GA plates: see B.
- 2xYT medium, ampicillin stock solution, glucose stock solution: see A.
- Sterile 96-well PP round-bottom microplates, breathable sealing membrane, microplate replicator, 8-channel pipettes: see E-I.
- 1 M sucrose stock solution: 342.3 g/l dissolved in ultrapure water, filter-sterilized, stored at 4°C.

- Potassium phosphate buffer: 0.17 M KH_2PO_4, 0.72 M K_2HPO_4, adjusted to pH 7.0; filter-sterilized, stored at 4°C.
- Buffered 2xYT (pH 7.0): 900 ml 2xYT medium supplemented with 100 ml potassium phosphate buffer, filter-sterilized, stored at 4°C.
- Induction medium 2xYT-SAI: buffered 2xYT supplemented with 50 ml sucrose stock solution, 1 ml ampicillin stock solution, and 50 μl IPTG stock solution (IPTG concentration depending on phagemid vector used), prepared right before use.
- Primary scFv-tag-specific monoclonal antibody (e.g., anti-myc, anti-His): 5 μg/ml diluted in MPBS.
- Secondary anti-primary polyclonal antibody HRP conjugate (e.g., Jackson ImmunoResearch): 1:10,000 diluted in MPBS.

F. Identification of complete scFv fragments by colony PCR and sequencing

- LB high salt medium: 10 g/l tryptone, 5 g/l yeast extract, 10 g/l NaCl, dissolved in ultrapure water, autoclaved, stored at RT.
- Taq PCR Core Kit, QIAquick PCR Purification Kit, QIAprep Spin Miniprep Kit, and QIAquick Gel Extraction Kit (optional): all from Qiagen.
- Colony PCR/sequencing primers flanking the scFv insert (most pHEN phagemids):

P1 (LMB3long, forward) 5′-CAGGAAACAGCTATGACCATGATTAC-3′; and

P2 (fdseqlong, reverse) 5′-GACGTTAGTAAATGAATTTTCTGTATGAGG-3′.

- 96-well PCR plate and sealing (e.g., BRAND).
- Sterile 96-well PP round-bottom microplates (e.g., Greiner Bio-One).
- 2xYT-glycerol: see E-I

G. Small-scale expression of soluble scFvs for functional characterization

- HB2151 bacterial strain: see E-II.
- M9/+Thi minimal plates, $MgSO_4$ stock solution: see B.
- 2xYT-GA, 2xYT-GK agar plates (100 mm), IPTG stock solution: see A.
- Induction medium 2xYT-GA with 0.1% glucose: 995 ml 2xYT medium, supplemented with 5 ml glucose stock solution and 1 ml ampicillin stock solution right before use.
- Periplasmic preparation buffer: 200 g/l sucrose, 30 mM Tris-HCl, 1 mM EDTA, diluted in ultrapure water, adjusted to pH 8.0, stored at 4°C.
- PBS: see C.
- Low protein-binding sterile syringe filters (0.22 μm): e.g., Millex-GV Filter (PVDF, 4 mm diameter) by EMD Millipore.

- Dialysis: D-Tube™ Dialyzer (MWCO 12–14 kDa) by EMD Millipore or dialysis membrane (e.g., Spectra/Por 4 dialysis membrane, MWCO 12–14 kDa, by Spectrum Laboratories).
- Lysozyme solution: 50 mg/ml lysozyme, in ultrapure water, prepared right before use.
- NPI-10 buffer: 50 mM NaH_2PO_4, 300 mM NaCl, 10 mM imidazole, dissolved in ultrapure water, adjusted pH to 8.0, filter-sterilized, stored at 4°C.
- Ni-NTA Spin Columns (Qiagen).

H. Functional antibody characterization by plaque reduction neutralization test

- Complete culture medium: e.g., Vero cells, 10% heat-inactivated fetal bovine serum (FBS) (optional: supplemented with penicillin/streptomycin solution).
- Sterile cell culture plates (6-well, 12-well, and 48-well): e.g., by Greiner Bio-One.
- Carboxymethyl cellulose (CMC) medium: 2/3 volume of sterile complete culture medium and 1/3 volume of CMC solution, stored at 4°C.
- CMC solution: 20 g/l carboxymethyl cellulose sodium salt dissolved in PBS (added slowly under stirring), autoclaved, stored at RT.
- Crystal violet solution: 200 mg/l crystal violet dissolved in 1 ml ethanol, filled up to 1 l with ultrapure water, stored at RT.
- 5% formaldehyde solution: 135 ml/l formaldehyde stock solution (37%), diluted in PBS, stored at RT.

I. Production of helper phage

- Top-agar: 2xYT supplemented with 7.5 g/l agar, autoclaved.
- 2xYT-agar plates (100 mm): 16 g/l tryptone, 10/l g yeast extract, 5/l g NaCl, and 15/l g agar dissolved in ultrapure water, autoclaved, poured as thin layers, stored at 4°C.
- 2xYT medium, helper phage VCSM13 or M13K07, kanamycin stock solution, PEG/NaCl solution: see A.
- TG1 bacteria strain, M9/+Thi minimal plates: see B.

4. Protocols

A. Preparation of scFv-phages

Cloned scFv antibody libraries are stored at −80°C as bacteria glycerol stocks and has to be packed into scFv-phages for selection using target antigen or virus stock (see Protocol C). The following protocol describes the superinfection of a log phase library bacterial culture with helper phage comprising kanamycin resistance (see Section I for the production of helper phages) and PEG purification of produced scFv-phages.

A1. Inoculate prewarmed 2xYT-GA to an initial OD_{600nm} of 0.1 with freshly thawed library glycerol stock (~1 ml). Typically, we inoculate 250 ml in a 1 L baffled Erlenmeyer flask for libraries of large library size up to 10^9 independent bacteria clones. The inoculated volume depends on library diversity and might vary between 50 ml and > 2 l. For libraries cloned from virus-infected donors, an initial library size of 10^7 and inoculating 100 ml is sufficient (**Note 1**).

A2. Grow bacteria at 250 rpm at 37°C until they reach log phase (OD_{600nm} of about 0.5). This typically takes about 2½ h (**Note 2**).

A3. Infect the log phase bacteria culture by adding freshly thawed helper phage VCSM13 or M13K07 (for preparation of helper phage: see Protocol I) with a multiplicity of infection of 20:1 (phage-to-cell-ratio). Infection is best performed by swirling the flask to distribute phages, followed by 30 min standing and 30 min shaking at 250 rpm and 37°C. Exclusively in the first round of selection, infection of the antibody library can be done by hyperphage M13 K07ΔpIII for oligomeric display of scFvs on the phage surface (**Note 3**).

A4. Superinfection of bacterial culture can be monitored by plating 1 μl of the infected bacteria (diluted in 100 μl 2xYT) onto 2xYT-GK agar plates. Successful infection should result in a bacteria lawn the next day.

A5. To induce expression of scFv-pIII fusion proteins, harvest bacteria by centrifugation (4000 × *g*, 10 min, 4°C) in PP tubes (either 50 or 250 ml) and resuspend bacteria in glucose-free induction medium 2×YT-AKI (**Note 4**).

A6. Incubate culture overnight shaking at ≤30°C (**Note 5**).

A7. On the next day, pellet bacteria (4000 × *g*, 10 min, 4°C) and transfer supernatant containing the antibody phages into fresh 50 ml PP tubes (40 ml per tube).

A8. Add 8 ml of prechilled PEG/NaCl to 40 ml supernatant (1/5 volume). Mix well and incubate for at least 1 h on ice (**Note 6**).

A9. Harvest phages by centrifugation (10,000 × *g*, 20 min, 4°C). Make sure to remove PEG/NaCl completely since remaining PEG leads to losing phages in the next step. Therefore, pour away the PEG solution and remove residuals with gauze or centrifuge again and aspirate remaining solution (**Note 7**).

A10. Pure phage preparation gives white pellets. Brownish pellets indicate contamination with bacteria debris. One (*Option 1*) or two (*Option 2*) precipitation steps may be performed. Especially in the first round of selection, we recommend to precipitate twice.

Option 1: Resuspend phage pellets in 1 ml of PBS per tube transfer in 2 ml tubes and centrifuge at high speed in a microcentrifuge (3 min, 4°C). Transfer the phage-containing supernatant into a fresh tube and determine the phage titer as colony-forming units (see Protocol B).

Option 2: Resuspend the phage pellets in 40 ml of ice cold PBS and pellet the bacteria by centrifugation (4000 × *g*, 10 min, 4°C). Save the supernatant and precipitate a second time (8 ml PEG/NaCl to 40 ml supernatant) for ≥1 h on ice or overnight. Proceed as described in *Option 1*.

A11. Store the phage at 4°C and proceed as soon as possible with scFv selection. *Optional*: filter supernatant through 0.45 μm filter. Filtered phages may be stored up to 2 weeks. To prevent proteolysis of the antibody fragments, proteolysis inhibitors might be added. Although not recommended for selection since displayed antibody fragment might be denatured, long-term storage of packaged library can be done by adding sterile glycerol (15% final concentration) and freezing at −80°C (**Note 8**).

B. Determination of phage titer

Prior to selection, titer of produced scFv-phages should be determined. Phage titration can be done by different methods including counting plaque-forming units (pfu) on bacterial lawns or counting the total particle number. More easily, phage titer is determined as colony-forming units (cfu) by easy countable bacteria colonies on selection plates as described below.

B1. Streak out TG1 from frozen, uninfected bacteria stock onto minimal M9/+Thiamine plates (**Note 9**).

B2. Inoculate 5 ml of 2xYT with grown single colony of TG1 and grow overnight (250 rpm, 37°C).

B3. On the next day, inoculate 10 ml of 2xYT with 100 µl of overnight culture and grow culture until the log-phase is reached (OD_{600} of about 0.5). This will take about 2½ h. *Optional*: Check overnight TG1 cultures for infection by plating 100 µl/plate on 2xYT-GA agar and 2xYT-GK agar. No colonies should grow (**Note 10**).

B4. In parallel, prepare serial dilution for phage titration. Expect about 10^{13} to 10^{14} cfu/ml out of 1 l culture. To guarantee that all phages can infect bacteria, prepare serial dilutions of phage in PBS by diluting 10 µl into 990 µl (10^2, 10^4, and 10^6). Pipette 10 µl of the 10^6 dilution to 990 µl of the log-phase TG1 culture (10^8 dilution) and infect bacteria at 37°C (30 min standing, 30 min shaking) (**Note 11**).

B5. After infection, prepare up to five 1:10 serial dilutions (100–900 µl) of infected bacteria in 2xYT medium. Plate 100 µl of infected bacteria and dilutions onto 2xYT-GA plates. Additionally, plate 100 µl of TG1 culture as negative controls on 2xTY-GA and 2xYT-GK plates. Incubate plates overnight at 30°C. Alternatively, spot 10 µl/dilution in triplicates onto 2xYT-GA plates and dry before overnight incubation.

B6. The next day, count colonies on countable plates and calculate phage titer as colony-forming units (cfu/ml). If colonies are too small to count, increase temperature to 37°C. No colonies should be visible on control plates.

C. Selection of antigen-specific scFv-phages

The following protocol describes the selection of target-specific scFv-phages using recombinant viral protein or virions immobilized on immunotubes. Usually ≥3 selection rounds are performed to enrich specific binding scFv-phages.

C1. For the first round of selection, coat an immunotube with 10–50 µg protein dissolved in 1 ml PBS and incubate the parafilm-sealed tube overnight at 4°C. For subsequent rounds, decrease the protein concentration for more stringent conditions (1–5 µg/ml). If oligopeptides are used for the selection procedure, coat 2–5 µg/ml for all rounds. Alternatively, immunotubes might be coated with a virus stock if the target antigen is unknown (**Note 12**).

C2. On the same day, prepare uninfected TG1 overnight culture as described (see B1–B3).

C3. The next day, wash tube three times with PBS by filling the tube with PBS using a wash bottle and removing the liquid immediately by pouring.

C4. Block the remaining binding sites by filling the empty immunotube completely with MPBS to the brim and incubate for about 2 h at RT.

C5. In parallel, preincubate packaged library (10^{12} to 10^{13} cfu) or phages from subsequent rounds (10^{11} to 10^{12} cfu) in MPBS (2–4% final milk concentration) for at least 1 h by slow overhead rotation in PP tubes (volume depends on volume used for coating immunotubes). Especially in the first round of selection, use 100-fold excess of scFv-phages compared with final library size to increase capturing promising binders (**Note 13**).

C6. Inoculate 20 ml of 2xYT with 200 µl of overnight culture and grow culture until the log-phase is reached (OD_{600} of about 0.5). This will take about 2½ h. Log phase TG1 can be stored on ice until infection with eluted phage. *Optional*: Check for infection of overnight TG1 culture by plating 100 µl on 2xYT-GA and 2xYT-GK plates.

C7. Empty the immunotube, add the preblocked phage solution, seal it with parafilm, and incubate for 90 min gently shaking followed by 30 min standing at the bench.

C8. In the last 30 min of incubation, start washing the immunotubes. In the first selection round, wash 10× (5× with PBST and 5× with PBS). In the following rounds, increase stringency of washing by adding more wash cycles (second round: 20× cycles, third round: 30× cycles, etc.).

C9. Elution of antigen-bound scFv-phages can be done by different methods. We prefer either acid elution (*Option 1*) or protease elution (*Option 2*).

Option 1 (*acid elution*): completely remove remaining buffer, add 1 ml acid elution buffer (pH 2.2) and incubate for about 8 min (longer incubation can destroy the phage). Rotate sealed tubes in an overhead rotator if using >1 ml for coating. Pipette eluted phage to about 100 µl neutralization buffer in a novel PP tube (**Note 14**).

Option 2 (*protease elution*): many common phagemid vectors possess a trypsin cleavage site between the scFv and pIII protein (e.g., all phagemids containing the myc or FLAG tag) that can be used for elution. Add 1 ml freshly prepared trypsin-PBS to the tubes and incubate for 10 min standing (1 ml coated tubes) or overhead rotation (>1 ml coated tubes) (**Note 15**).

C10. Per selection, inoculate 14 ml of log-phase TG1 culture with the eluted phage solution in fresh 50 ml tubes. Infect at 37°C by 30 min standing and 30 min shaking. *Optional*: fill the empty immunotube with 5 ml of log-phase TG1 and perform infection at 37°C as described above. After infection, combine both cultures for following steps.

C11. To monitor the success of an antibody selection, the eluted phage titer can be determined after each selection round. Therefore, make serial dilutions of the TG1 culture after infection (e.g., by plating 100 µl of undiluted culture, 10^2, 10^4, and 10^6 dilutions onto 2xYT-GA plates). Incubate plates at 30°C overnight and count colonies to determine the eluted phage titer after each round. Typically for successful enrichment of specific binders, the eluted phage titer should increase from about 10^4–10^6 in the first round up to the total number used for bacterial infection in subsequent rounds (~10^{10}).

C12. Centrifuge the remaining TG1 culture (3500 × *g*, 10 min, RT), resuspend pellets in about 1 ml 2xYT, and plate onto either one large square plate (245 × 245 mm) or 3 round 15 cm plates containing 2xYT-GA agar.

C13. Grow plates overnight at 30°C and harvest bacteria by adding sterile-filtered 15% glycerol in 2xYT (about 10 ml totally). Harvest cells with flamed glass spreader. Mix very well and freeze bacteria glycerol stock at −80°C.

C14. Perform subsequent selection rounds. Resolve 100–400 μl of the glycerol stock from the previous round in 100 ml 2xYT-GA to start OD_{600nm} of 0.1 and perform selection following the Protocols A, B, and C (**Note 16**).

D. Polyclonal phage ELISA (ppELISA)

After performing repeated rounds of selection, the scFv-phage preparations from the different rounds should be analyzed by ppELISA to identify if target-specific scFv-phage were successfully enriched.

D1. Coat a 96-well ELISA plate with the target antigen (or virus stock: usually 1×10^5–1×10^7 pfu/ml) and control proteins at 2–10 μg/ml (100 μl/well) in PBS, seal plate with parafilm, and incubate overnight at 4°C. In total, coat two wells of target and control proteins plus two wells as blank for each selection round (R0, R1, R2, R3, etc.).

D2. The next day, remove coating solution and block entire plate with MPBS (400 μl/well) for 2 h at RT.

D3. Dilute phages from the different selection rounds to 10^{12} cfu/ml in MPBS, pipette 100 μl/well, and incubate for 1 h at RT.

D4. Wash plate 3× with PBST and 3× with PBS. **Note 17**

D5. Add 100 μl/well of HRP-conjugated anti-M13 antibody diluted 1:5000 in MPBS and incubate for 1 h at RT.

D6. Wash plate 3× with PBST and 3× with PBS.

D7. Add 100 μl/well of TMB substrate solution and incubate until blue color has developed (up to 30 min). Stop reaction by adding 50 μl/well of stop solution. Read absorbance at 450 nm in a microplate reader (**Note 18**).

E. Screening for monoclonal binders

After successful antibody selection (see Protocols A–D), you will end up with an enriched pool of target-specific scFv-phages that must be screened for single binding antibodies ("monoclonals"). Screening can be done differently, using scFv-phages, scFv-pIII fusion proteins, or soluble scFv fragments. For beginners, we recommend screening as monoclonal phages by mpELISA (see Protocol E-I) since scFv-phages can be easily produced and detected by anti-phage HRP conjugates. Sometimes, screening as soluble fragments (see Protocol E-II) is preferred since screening as scFv-phages might result in false positive binders; meaning binding is dependent on the entire antibody-pIII fusions/phage. However, soluble screening requires switching the bacteria strain to a nonamber suppressor strain (e.g., HB2151).

E-I. Monoclonal phage (mpELISA) screening

E1. Plate TG1 glycerol stocks from target-enriched selection rounds as confirmed in ppELISA (see Protocol D) on 2xYT-GA selection plates to obtain single colonies. Alternatively, use the plates that have been prepared for the determination of the phage titer (see Protocol B).

E2. Fill a sterile 96-well round-bottom plate with 100 μl/well of 2xYT-GA.

E3. Pick (single!) TG1 colonies from selection plates that are positively enriched rounds using sterile toothpicks or pipette tips and inoculate one well/colony. Keep wells H6 and H12 free as blank. Seal plate with breathable membrane (**Note 19**).

E4. Incubate plate at 37°C overnight while shaking. This will be your master plate (**Note 20**).

E5. On the next day, transfer an aliquot of the culture to a new plate containing 100 μl/well 2xYT-GA. Pipette either about 5 μl/well from the master plate using a multichannel pipette to the new induction plate or use a 96-well induction device with sterile metal pins for induction.

E6. Add 50 μl/well 2xYT containing 50% glycerol to the masterplate and freeze sealed plate at −20°C.

E7. Incubate induction plate for about 2½ h in the phage orbital shaker until bacteria reach log-phase (37°C, 200 rpm).

E8. Infect bacteria 1:20 with helper phage, i.e., 10 μl/well of a 10^{11} cfu/ml dilution (100 μl log-phase bacteria containing 5×10^7 bacteria and should be infected by 10^9 phages). Infect for 30 min standing and 30 min shaking at 37°C.

E9. Centrifuge plate (10 min, 3000 × *g*, 4°C), discard supernatant, and resuspend bacteria pellets in 180 μl/well of induction medium 2xYT-AKI. No glucose!

E10. Seal plate with a breathable membrane and incubate the induction plate overnight at 37°C.

E11. Coat two ELISA Maxisorb™ plates per induction plate by pipetting 100 μl/well of antigen/virus stock to the first half (columns 1–6) and control protein to the second-half (columns 7–12) of the plates. Use 2–10 μg/ml antigen/control protein diluted in PBS for coating. Seal plates and incubate overnight at 4°C.

E12. The next day, block ELISA plates with MPBS for 2 h at RT.

E13. Remove blocking solution and add 50 μl/well 4% MPBS.

E14. Centrifuge the induction plate for 10 min at 3000 × *g* and 4°C. The supernatant can be transferred to a new PP microplate and stored at 4°C.

E15. Pipette 50 μl/well of the supernatant from the induction plate to one antigen-coated column and one control protein-coated column (e.g., column 1 of the induction plate to columns 1 and 7 of the ELISA plate, column 2 to columns 2 and 8) and incubate for 1 h at RT.

E16. Wash plate 3× with PBST and 3× with PBS.

E17. Add 100 μl/well of HRP-conjugated anti-M13 antibody diluted 1:5000 in MPBS and incubate for 1 h at RT.

E18. Wash plate 3× with PBST and 3× with PBS.

E19. Add 100 µl/well of TMB substrate solution and incubate until blue color has developed (up to 30 min). Stop reaction by adding 50 µl/well of stop solution. Read absorbance at 450 nm in a microplate reader (**Note 21**).

E-II. Soluble scFv screening

E20. Grow bacteria strain HB2151 on M9/+Thi minimal plates and prepare log phase-HB2151 culture (OD_{600nm} of 0.5) as described before (see B1–B3).

E21. Take 10 µl of eluted phages from the different positively enriched selection rounds and infect 1 ml of log-phase HB2151 at 37°C (30 min standing, 30 min shaking).

E22. Prepare different dilutions of the phage-infected HB2151 culture in 2xYT (e.g., 10^2, 10^4, 10^6), plate 100 µl of the dilutions on 2xYT-GA plates, and grow overnight at 30°C. Alternatively, spot 10 µl/dilution on 2xYT-GA plates in triplicates.

E23. The next day, prepare a masterplate as described above (see E2–E4) by picking single HB2151 colonies.

E24. Inoculate an induction plate (see E5) and freeze the masterplate after adding 50% 2xYT/glycerol (see E6).

E25. Grow induction plate for around 3 h until OD_{600nm} of about 1 is reached.

E26. Centrifuge the induction plate (10 min, 3000 × *g*, 4°C) and completely remove the supernatant by carefully pipetting without disturbing the bacteria pellet.

E27. Resuspend the bacteria pellets in 180 µl/well of buffered 2xYT-SAI medium. No glucose! Seal the plate with breathable membrane and incubate the induction plate overnight at 30°C while shaking (**Note 22**).

E28. Perform ELISA as described in E11 to E19. However, soluble scFvs must be detected by a tag-specific antibody (e.g., anti-myc and anti-His) followed by washing and incubation with anti-primary HRP conjugated antibody. Alternatively, when using scFv libraries entirely based on the kappa light chain, detection can be performed with protein A-HRP or protein L-HRP using 3% BSA for blocking (lower backgrounds).

F. Identification of complete scFv fragments by colony PCR and sequencing

After screening for monoclonal binders (scFv-phages or soluble scFv fragments), hits should be analyzed for the presence of the full-length scFv insert (VH and VL) prior to sequencing. Selection of bacterial clones with incomplete inserts is a common issue observed with antibody phage display. Bacteria encoding for incomplete fragments with lower affinities often show growth advantages compared with those encoding for full-length scFvs and might be predominantly enriched during selection. To retrieve complete scFvs, we recommend analysis of colonies after screening by colony PCR as described below prior to sequencing. The following protocol allows PCR amplification of scFv inserts for size analysis and fast sequencing. Moreover, prepared plasmid DNA and glycerol stocks are useful for sequencing, cloning, electroporation in HB2151, or direct expression of soluble scFv (Protocol G) that can be used for subsequent functional analysis (see Protocol H).

F1. Streak out the masterplate glycerol stocks from wells that have been identified as antigen-specific binders by screening (see Protocol E) on 2xYT-GA plates and grow overnight at 30°C.

F2. Fill sterile 96-well plate with 100 μl/well LB medium.

F3. Prepare PCR master mix using Taq PCR Core Kit according to manufacturer's recommendations preparing 50 μl/reaction and using scFv insert flanking primers, e.g., P1 (LMB3long) and P2 (fdseqlong) if using pHEN derivatives.

F4. Distribute 50 μl/well of PCR master mix into a 96-well PCR plate.

F5. Use sterile pipette tips to pick single colonies and inoculate one well of the PCR plate and afterward the corresponding well of the medium-filled masterplate.

F6. Run PCR according to manufacturer's recommendations using an annealing temperature of 53°C and 30 cycles.

F7. Analyze 25 μl/sample on a 1% agarose gel containing ethidium bromide. Complete scFv inserts run at about 1 kb when using pHEN phagemids and primer P1 and P2.

F8. Purify remaining 25 μl PCR product of full-length scFvs by QIAquick PCR Purification Kit according to manufacturer's recommendations by eluting DNA in ultrapure water (**Note 23**).

F9. Sequence inserts using a primer designed to either bind downstream or upstream of the forward (P1) or reverse primer (P2) used for colony PCR. Although colony PCR primer (or shorter versions thereof) might be used as well, sequencing primer binding within the amplified scFv insert might increase sequence quality.

F10. Use 100 μl of infected medium from positive binders for inoculation of 6 ml LB high-salt medium supplemented with 100 μg/ml ampicillin and grow culture overnight at 37°C.

F11. The next day, use 1 ml of grown culture to prepare bacterial stock by adding 0.5 ml 50% 2xYT/glycerol and freeze at −20°C. Use remaining culture to prepare plasmid DNA using QIAprep Spin Miniprep Kit according to manufacturer's recommendations by eluting DNA in ultrapure water (**Note 24**).

F12. Analyze obtained scFv sequences for sequence inaccuracies using molecular cloning software (e.g., SnapGene). VH and VL genes can be analyzed by the Fab Analysis online tool by aligning the scFv sequences to the VBASE2 database [26] to identify closest antibody germline sequences as well as to identify the CDR regions of the scFvs.

Preliminary notes prior to antibody fragment production and functional characterization

Antigen/virus-specific scFvs needs to be further characterized for virus neutralization. This step is challenging since the neutralization capacity of antibodies often depends on the antibody valency as observed for HSV, varicella-zoster virus, HIV, and rabies [27, 28]. In these cases, bivalent antibodies (IgG) or antibody fragments (F(ab)$_2$) neutralized the virus with an exceptional efficiency, while monovalent Fab or scFv fragments did not or only when used at very high concentrations (e.g., 300 times higher than IgG). Although the production of soluble scFvs from phagemid libraries for functional characterization is a simple procedure (see Protocol G), it allows only the production of monovalent fragments that might be insufficient for virus neutralization in some cases. Therefore, the cloning of the VH and VL genes of virus-specific scFvs into other bivalent antibody formats (e.g., scFv-Fc, diabody, minibody) using a high-throughput, recombinant protein expression systems should be considered to increase the likelihood of isolating potent antiviral antibodies (e.g., transient HEK 293 expression platform from National Research Council Canada). The screening of virus-specific antibodies for virus neutralization can be performed either with bivalent or monovalent antibodies. The choice of the method (e.g., reporter virus and cell line) strongly depends on the virus itself. You need the suitable cell culture system to test neutralizing effects of antibodies on the viral replication. In this chapter, we demonstrate the identification of an HSV-neutralizing scFvs as an example for the isolation of neutralizing antibodies from phage display libraries. As mentioned above, this procedure can be modified for the screening of bivalent antibodies and for other viruses.

G. Small-scale expression of soluble scFvs for functional characterization

After the identification of scFvs with a unique sequence, soluble scFv can be produced in small scale to analyze their biological function, e.g., for their neutralizing capacity in case of antiviral antibodies. The protocol below describes the soluble expression of scFvs in the periplasm of nonamber suppressor strain HB2151 that allows the correct formation of disulfide bonds. ScFvs are recovered by periplasmic extraction followed by one-step purification using Immobilized metal ion affinity chromatography (IMAC) for His-tagged scFvs. Please adapt the protocol when using other tags for purification or upscale if higher quantities of scFvs are needed.

G1. Streak out HB2151 glycerol stock of unique scFv clones on 2xYT-GA agar plates to obtain single colonies (**Note 25**).

G2. Inoculate 5 ml 2xYT-GA with single picked colony and grow overnight at 37°C while shaking.

G3. The next day, inoculate 200 ml 2xYT-GA containing reduced concentration of 0.1% glucose with 2 ml of overnight culture and grow culture at 37°C until OD_{600nm} of 1 is reached.

G4. Add 0.2 ml IPTG stock solution (i.e., 1 mM final concentration) to the cultures and grow culture overnight at RT (**Note 26**).

G5. Harvest bacteria by centrifugation (6000 × *g*, 15 min, 4°C) and resuspend the pellets in 5 ml periplasmic preparation buffer supplemented with 1 ml/l of freshly prepared lysozyme stock solution.

G6. Incubate preparation on ice for 30 min and stabilize spheroblasts by adding 50 µl 1 M $MgSO_4$ (i.e., 10 mM final concentration).

G7. Centrifuge preparations (12,000 × *g*, 30 min, 4°C) to clarify periplasmic fractions.

G8. Dialyze scFvs using D-Tube™ Dialyzer (MWCO 12–14 kDa) overnight at 4°C against NPI-10 buffer (**Note 27**).

G9. Purify scFvs by IMAC employing Ni-NTA spin columns following the manufacturer's protocol and loading columns several times with the scFv preparations.

G10. Analyze samples by reduced SDS-PAGE and Coomassie stain (and/or Western blot) to check for purity.

G11. Dialyze scFvs against PBS buffer, filter-sterilize using low-protein-binding filter (0.22 μm) and measure protein concentration (e.g., by Nanodrop using calculated extinction coefficient and molecular mass).

G12. Store scFvs at 4°C and proceed as soon as possible to characterization. ScFv stability can differ dramatically depending on the sequence from few days to several years. Do not freeze scFvs since many tend to aggregate after thawing. Oligomeric state of scFv can be analyzed by gel filtration chromatography.

H. Functional antibody characterization by plaque reduction neutralization test

In the case of screening antiviral antibodies, scFvs can be screened in neutralization and/or protection assays that detect antiviral activities of antibodies *in vitro* or *in vivo* [29]. As the "gold standard" assay for screening and neutralizing capacity of antibodies, plaque reduction neutralization test (PRNT) can be performed where the $PRNT_{50}$ value is used to describe the neutralization activity. The protocol below describes a PRNT-based assay to screen for best neutralizing scFvs and was optimized for HSV-specific and neutralizing scFvs.

H1. Cultivate cell line suitable to form plaques when infected with virus of interest (e.g., Vero cells for HSV, dengue virus) according to supply recommendations. Most virus sustainable cell lines are recommended to be propagated and stored in low passage levels to guarantee susceptibility for plaque formation.

H2. Seed cells in 6-well cell culture plates with 5×10^5 cells/well and grow in 5 ml/well complete culture medium in a humidified cell incubator at 37°C and 5% CO_2 for one to three days and until a confluency of at least 90% is reached (**Note 28**).

H3. To screen for the best neutralizing antibody, dilute all scFvs to a constant concentration (e.g., 4 μM) in appropriate culture medium supplemented with penicillin/streptomycin solution. For some viruses, reduction of the FBS concentration is recommended. If the $PRNT_{50}$ should be determined, prepare twofold serial dilution of scFvs (at least five steps) that is the amount of antibody required to neutralize 50% of the infectious virus particles (**Note 29**).

H4. Freshly thaw cryostock with a known titer of plaque-forming units (pfu) at RT and dilute to 600 pfu/ml (same medium as in H3).

H5. Pipette 300 μl of diluted scFvs (or PBS as negative control) to 300 μl of the virus preparation in a sterile plate and incubate the scFv-virus mixtures at 37°C for 1 h.

H6. Carefully aspirate old medium from cell plates and wash with 2 ml PBS. Always pipette to the wall of the wells to not destroy the cell monolayer.

H7. Add 500 μl/well of the scFv-virus mixtures to each well and tilt plates as described above. Include virus only to every plate. ScFvs should be tested in at least duplicates.

H8. Incubate plates at 37°C for about 1 h (time can vary between 30 and 90 min depending on the cell/virus). During incubation, carefully tilt all the plates 10–15 min.

H9. Remove inoculum and wash cells with 3 ml/well PBS.

H10. Add 3 ml/well CMC medium and incubate plates in the humidified incubator (37°C, 5% CO_2) for three days.

H11. Fixate the cells with formaldehyde solution (3 ml/well for 5 min) and stain with crystal violet solution (800 μl/well) for 2 min.

H12. Wash wells once with PBS and twice with ultrapure water (2 ml/well).

H13. Count plaques and calculate percentage of neutralization as follows:

% of neutralization = 100 – [(no. of plaques: virus + antibody)/no. of plaques: virus only) × 100].

When analyzing serial dilutions of scFvs, percentage of neutralization can be plotted against scFvs concentration to determine the $PRNT_{50}$ values.

After functional characterization, produced scFvs should be characterized for specificity and affinity in binding to recombinant antigen and, more importantly, to intact virions. The specificity of scFvs to recombinant proteins can be easily analyzed by ELISA using recombinant virus antigens (or virus lysates). While scFv affinities has to be determined by kinetic measurements (e.g., by surface plasmon resonance or biolayer interferometry), estimation of apparent scFv affinities can be quickly performed by ELISA. Therefore, recombinant antigen is coated on ELISA plates and 1:2 serial dilutions of purified scFvs (e.g., 1 μM start concentration) are incubated in triplicates followed by detection via tag-specific IgGs and anti-IgG HRP conjugate. The half-maximal effective concentration (EC_{50}) of saturated binding corresponds to the KD value and can be used for affinity ranking of scFvs. However, immobilization of antigens/virions on plastic can alter conformation of coated proteins leading to antibodies recognizing epitopes that are not found on intact virions. Alternatively, binding affinity of antibody fragments can also be estimated by flow cytometry using antigen overexpressing cell lines [30], e.g., by using Vero cell being infected with HSV [18, 28].

In conclusion, broadly neutralizing human monoclonal antibodies represent an excellent opportunity for the prevention and therapy of viral infections and are a potent tool to identify neutralizing epitopes on viral proteins for vaccine approaches. Phage display technology became a potent tool to isolate human neutralizing antibodies and should be considered as a validated technique for future approaches.

I. Production of helper phage

Larger preparation of helper phage (VCSM13 or M13K07) being used for superinfection to prepare scFv-phages for selection (Protocol A) and screening (Protocol E-I) can be obtained following the protocol below. Hyperphage cannot be produced without recombinant *E. coli* strain and must be purchased.

http://dx.doi.org/10.5772/intechopen.70139

I1. Thaw primary phage stock and prepare 10^2 dilutions (100 μl) in 2xYT medium.

I2. Mix helper phage dilution with equal volume of log-phase TG1 culture prepared as described above (see B1–B3) to infect bacteria at 37°C (30 min standing and 30 min shaking).

I3. Melt top agar in a microwave, aliquot in glass tubes while hot, and cool down tubes to 42°C in a prewarmed water bath.

I4. Pipette infected bacteria to top agar tubes, mix quickly, and immediately cast top agar onto prewarmed (37°C) 2xYT plates. Grow plates overnight at 30°C (**Note 30).**

I5. The next day, pick a single small plaque from grown bacteria lawns and transfer into 3 ml 2xYT that was inoculated with 100 μl of TG1 overnight culture right before.

I6. Incubate culture for 3 h at 37°C while shaking and use grown culture to inoculate 500 ml of 2xYT.

I7. After one further hour of growing, add 200 μl kanamycin stock solution and grow overnight at 37°C while shaking.

I8. The next day, pellet bacteria (4000 × *g*, 10 min, 4°C), transfer 40 ml of supernatant into 50 ml PP tubes and precipitate phage as described in Protocols A8–A10 (**Note 31**).

I9. To inactivate the remaining bacteria, either heat helper phage preparation for 15 min at 65°C (recommended) or filter through low protein binding 0.45 μm filter (**Note 32**).

I10. Aliquot the phage preparation into 2 ml PP tubes and snap freeze the tubes in liquid nitrogen prior to storage at ≤−20°C.

I11. Determine phage titer as plaque-forming unit (pfu/ml) as described above (see I1–I4) using 1:10 serial phage dilutions from 10^8 to 10^{13} for infecting 100 μl log phage TG1 and counting plaques on countable plates (**Note 33).**

5. Notes

Note 1: To minimize loss of diversity, very large libraries (>10^9 independent clones) should always be stored as sublibraries that can be separately packed and combined prior to selection. Antibody selection should be only performed with freshly packaged (sub-)libraries that have been kept at 4°C for short as possible. Due to loss of diversity, we do not recommend selection with frozen phage preparations or phage antibodies that have been packaged from secondary library stocks. Importantly, minimize freeze and thaw steps of your primary library and keep it frozen at −80°C until needed.

Note 2: Correct growing temperature is crucial for phage display. Too low a temperature (<34°C) might result in ineffective formation of pili that are necessary for successful infection by phage.

Note 3: Oligomeric display of scFvs in the first round of selection by infection with hyperphage can greatly improve selection efficacy and can reduce loss of interesting binders during the initial selection step improving the average display from 0.01 up to 5 antibody fragments per phage. Please note that hyperphage infection results in scFv-phages without wild-type pIII proteins that are necessary for successful infection. To restore the wild-type infectivity, hyperphage-packed libraries should be eluted by a protease cutting between the antibody fragment and the pIII protein (e.g., trypsin works well for pSEX and most pHEN derivatives). To check for suitable proteases for your phagemid, you might analyze your vector on PeptideCutter (ExPASy database) and perform Western blot analysis of digested antibody phages using an anti-pIII antibody for detection (see Note 8).

Note 4: Expression of scFv-pIII fusion proteins with *lac* promoter-based phagemid vectors can be performed by using glucose-free media without or a low concentration of IPTG (about 5 μM to 500 μM final concentration depending on used phagemid). However, strong induction of the *lac* promotor by too high concentration of IPTG might reduce the expression of complete scFv-pIII fusion proteins. Induction conditions should be optimized and antibody presentation on phages can be analyzed by SDS PAGE and Western blot using primary anti-pIII detection system (see Note 8).

Note 5: Reducing temperature to 30°C or lower guarantees better expression and folding of complete antibody fusions that otherwise might be overgrown by incomplete fusions. Moreover, lower temperature helps to reduce degradation/cleavage of antibody fragments on the phage surface.

Note 6: Longer incubation on ice or 4°C might result in better precipitation of antibody phage and higher yields.

Note 7: To save time, we perform phage pelletation in Beckman centrifuges, equipped with fixed angel rotors such as JA 16.250 that allows higher speed centrifugation in 250 ml reusable or 50 ml disposable PP tubes if using adapters. If not available, centrifugation with swinging buckets and lower speed can be performed, but centrifugation time should be increased accordingly.

Note 8: Helper phage/hyperphage packaged libraries can be analyzed by SDS-PAGE and Western blot. Run reduced phage samples on 10% SDS PAGE and incubate membrane with primary anti-pIII monoclonal antibody and secondary anti-mouse polyclonal serum HRP conjugate, using ECL substrate for detection. Although wild-type pIII has a calculated molecular weight of about 45 kDa, it runs at about 60 kDa in SDS-PAGE. Accordingly, complete scFv-pIII constructs can be detected at about 90 kDa.

Note 9. TG1 is an amber suppressor *E. coli* strain most widely used for antibody phage display. Growing TG1 on proline-deficient M9 minimal plates guarantees maintenance of the F′ episome important for production of pili necessary for phage infection. For growing of TG1, M9 plates must be additionally supplemented with thiamine due to a chromosomal mutation in the thiamine biosynthesis.

Note 10: OD_{600} of culture is critical. Do not overgrow or grow below 34°C. Bacteria can be kept on ice for a while (30 min up to a few hours), but cells might start losing pili after longer incubations.

Note 11: One ml of log phase TG1 (OD_{600nm} of 0.5) corresponds to about 5×10^8 bacteria. Always infect with at least 1:10 phage-to-cell ratio for titration, i.e., do not use more than 5×10^7 phages for 1 ml log-phase TG1.

Note 12: If enough antigen is available, increase volume of coating solution up to 5 ml, especially in the first round of selection. Only use highly pure (>90%), freshly prepared protein from sources you can trust. Do not use proteins that have been stored at 4°C for prolonged periods. If using oligopeptides or virions for selection, immobilization condition should be optimized due to lower coating efficacies and/or reduced accessibility of epitopes. Test different buffer/pH/additives for immobilization on MaxiSorp™ plates (e.g., 50 mM carbonate buffer pH 9.6) using tag-specific antibody enzyme conjugates for detection in ELISA. Alternatively, antigens might be biotinylated and immobilized on streptavidin-coated tubes/plates or be captured in solution using streptavidin dynabeads [31].

Note 13: If using proteins with large tags/fusions (e.g., Fc region, GST tag) for antibody selection, supplement the preincubation solution with respective proteins to reduce enrichment of binders against those parts. If using biotinylated oligopeptides immobilized on streptavidin-coated immunotubes, preincubate phages with streptavidin to deplete streptavidin-specific binders.

Note 14: To check pH of final solution, perform microtitration using pH indicator strips to determine volume of neutralization buffer required to get a final pH of 7.2–7.4.

Note 15: Always elute hyperphage-packaged libraries by protease elution to guarantee highest infectivity of eluted phages.

Note 16: We usually perform three rounds of selection, but this might be increased up to five or more. However, performing additional rounds might lead to loss of diversity and enrichment of binders having growth advantages that might occur (e.g., truncated scFvs).

Note 17: Washing can be done by hand using a small plastic box filled with buffer. Remove all liquid by inverting the plates and hitting it onto paper towels. Change buffer and towels frequently. For better reproducibility and when screening larger amounts of plates, wash plates using a microplate washer (e.g., BioTek Instruments, Tecan).

Note 18: Successful enrichment of specific binding scFv-phages should be seen as increasing of target-specific signals compared to control antigens. For a typical result see [18], Figure 4A.

Note 19: Try to pick single colonies. Sometimes picking of double colonies or a spillover from well to well might occur. Secondary screen of positive well (hit-picking) can be performed. If performing high-throughput screening on a regular basis, automation of the picking process by colony pickers (e.g., Molecular Devices) might be considered.

Note 20: Most universal orbital shakers for bacterial culture possess an orbit diameter of about one inch that works very well for Erlenmeyer flasks (25 ml up to 2 l) and shaking at about 200 to 250 rpm. However, growing bacterial culture in microtiter plates can be more challenging due to evaporation, contamination, and oxygen transfer. To prevent contamination, shaking at a lower speed (about 180 rpm) can be performed although oxygen supply is reduced as well. Alternatively, PP deep well plates can be used for screening. To prevent evaporation, plates can be tape-fixed in an additional plastic bag or use PBS-filled plates at the bottom and top when using microplate holders. The highest yield of soluble scFvs can be obtained with special temperature-controlled shakers with a small orbital diameter (0.12 inch) and shaking at high speed (1000 rpm).

Note 21: Usually, antigen-specific binding is defined as signals at least five times higher than the background. For a typical result, see [18], Figure 4B and C.

Note 22: The 2% glucose guarantees repression of antibody expression within the first 3 h of growing. To induce antibody expression, medium must be replaced by induction medium without glucose and optimized concentration of IPTG. Many scFvs show very low yield in the supernatant after expression in *E. coli* and periplasmic extraction is highly recommend prior to ELISA, e.g., by resuspending bacteria pellets in 180 μl/well periplasmic preparation buffer (see Protocol G) for 30 min on ice. However, as shown by Hust et al. [32], buffered 2xYT-SAI and growing cultures overnight at 30°C can improve production in *E. coli* for some scFvs even without performing periplasmic extraction.

Note 23. Adjusting PCR conditions to obtain single scFvs bands on agarose gel is important for successful sequencing of PCR fragments, e.g., by increasing annealing temperature. Alternatively, scFv bands can be recovered by QIAquick Gel Extraction Kit or sequencing can be done using plasmid DNA (see F10).

Note 24: Plasmid DNA can be used for electroporation into self-made electrocompetent HB2151 if scFv-phage screening with TG1 bacteria was performed beforehand. If already in HB2151 after soluble screening, the glycerol stock can be used to obtain single colonies on 2xYT-GA plates for small-scale production of soluble scFvs (see Protocol G). Alternatively, plasmid DNA can be used for subcloning into bacterial expression vectors without pIII gene.

Note 25. For time reasons, we recommend soluble expression of scFvs in nonamber suppressor strain such as HB2151 when using phagemid with the amber stop codon between the scFv and the pIII protein. Otherwise, scFvs can also be subcloned into expression vector without the pIII gene. If clones are still in TG1 after phage screening, phagemid DNA can be transformed into self-made competent HB2151. Use standard protocol for generation of chemically or electrocompetent HB2151. Alternatively use commercially available competent nonamber suppressor strains for soluble production (e.g., SS320 by Lucigen, or Express I^q by NEB).

Note 26. Reducing the temperature for soluble scFv expression is important for proper folding and stability of produced scFvs.

Note 27: As a cheaper option for dialysis in small scale, we recommend using 2 ml PP tubes without lids, filled with scFv preparations, and sealed with square cut dialysis membrane fixed with rubber band and parafilm. If using other tags for purification, dialyze in recommended buffer prior purification.

Note 28: Determine best number/growing conditions for your cell line. Gently tilt plate about five times horizontally after seeding to guarantee that uniform monolayers of cells are formed. PRNT assay can be adapted to plates with higher well number (e.g., 12–24 well/plates) by reducing pfu and volumes used. Presented protocol was optimized for PRNT with HSV and Vero cells. Cell line and optimal conditions are different for each virus and should be optimized for best results (e.g., scFv-virus incubation time, absorption time on cells, percentage of CMC for overlay, working virus dilution and volume, incubation time after infection).

Note 29: Since performing of the PRNT is laborious and time-consuming, using a single concentration of scFvs for neutralization usually allows a good head-to-head comparison to identify best neutralizing scFvs. In a second step, most promising scFvs can be cloned into other (bivalent) Ab formats (e.g., scFv-Fc) and tested in more detail by analyzing $PRNT_{50}$ (or more precisely even $PRNT_{70}$ or $PRNT_{90}$).

Note 30: The temperature of melted top agar should be exactly at 42°C before casting. Higher temperatures might kill *E. coli* bacteria, while at lower temperatures, the top agar might solidify too fast before pouring nice layers on plates.

Note 31: Although helper phage supernatant can be directly used after heat treatment, we recommend purifying and concentrating by one or two steps of PEG/NaCl precipitation.

Note 32: Using 0.22 μm filter for phage filtration is not recommended due to loss of filamentous phages. If clogging of 0.45 μm filter occurs, centrifuge phage preparation at high g-force at 4°C prior to filtration.

Note 33: Using 10^8 phage dilution guarantees an at least tenfold excess of helper phage to bacteria for infection. Avoid additional freeze-and-thaw cycles of helper phage preparations. Titer of frozen helper phage might drop over time during storage and titration should be repeated after several months. Sterile glycerol up to a final concentration of 50% prior to snap freezing can be added to prolong storage time. Review Ref. [33] for more information about correct storage of phages.

Acknowledgements

We thank Buck Rogers and Cedric Mpoy for discussions and corrections on the manuscript.

Author details

Philipp Diebolder[1] and Adalbert Krawczyk[2]*

*Address all correspondence to: adalbert.krawczyk@uni-due.de

1 Department of Radiation Oncology, Washington University School of Medicine, St. Louis, USA

2 Institute for Virology, University Hospital Essen, University of Duisburg-Essen, Essen, Germany

References

[1] Casadevall A, Scharff MD. Return to the past: The case for antibody-based therapies in infectious diseases. Clinical Infectious Diseases. 1995;**21**:150-161

[2] Marasco WA, Sui J. The growth and potential of human antiviral monoclonal antibody therapeutics. Nature Biotechnology. 2007;**25**:1421-1434

[3] Hemming VG. Use of intravenous immunoglobulins for prophylaxis or treatment of infectious diseases. Clinical and Diagnostic Laboratory Immunology. 2001;**8**:859-863

[4] Kohler G, Milstein C. Continuous cultures of fused cells secreting antibody of predefined specificity. Nature. 1975;**256**:495-497

[5] Ecker DM, Jones SD, Levine HL. The therapeutic monoclonal antibody market. MAbs. 2015;**7**:9-14

[6] Gresl T, Storz U, Sandercock C. An update on obtaining and enforcing therapeutic antibody patent claims. Nature Biotechnology. 2016;**34**:1242-1244

[7] Pelegrin M, Naranjo-Gomez M, Piechaczyk M. Antiviral monoclonal antibodies: Can they be more than simple neutralizing agents? Trends in Microbiology. 2015;**23**:653-665

[8] Kwong PD, Mascola JR, Nabel GJ. Broadly neutralizing antibodies and the search for an HIV-1 vaccine: The end of the beginning. Nature Reviews Immunology. 2013;**13**:693-701

[9] Bornholdt ZA, Turner HL, Murin CD, Li W, Sok D, et al. Isolation of potent neutralizing antibodies from a survivor of the 2014 Ebola virus outbreak. Science. 2016;**351**:1078-1083

[10] Caskey M, Klein F, Nussenzweig MC. Broadly neutralizing antibodies for HIV-1 prevention or immunotherapy. The New England Journal of Medicine. 2016;**375**:2019-2021

[11] Corti D, Lanzavecchia A. Broadly neutralizing antiviral antibodies. Annual Review of Immunology. 2013;**31**:705-742

[12] Krawczyk A, Arndt MA, Grosse-Hovest L, Weichert W, Giebel B, et al. Overcoming drug-resistant herpes simplex virus (HSV) infection by a humanized antibody. Proceedings of the National Academy of Sciences of the United States of America. 2013;**110**:6760-6765

[13] Sattentau Q. Avoiding the void: Cell-to-cell spread of human viruses. Nature Reviews Microbiology. 2008;**6**:815-826

[14] Traggiai E, Becker S, Subbarao K, Kolesnikova L, Uematsu Y, et al. An efficient method to make human monoclonal antibodies from memory B cells: Potent neutralization of SARS coronavirus. Nature Medicine. 2004;**10**:871-875

[15] Wilson PC, Andrews SF. Tools to therapeutically harness the human antibody response. Nature Reviews Immunology. 2012;**12**:709-719

[16] Frenzel A, Schirrmann T, Hust M. Phage display-derived human antibodies in clinical development and therapy. MAbs. 2016;**8**:1177-1194

[17] Diebolder P. Generation of "LYmph Node Derived Antibody Libraries" (LYNDAL): A concept for recovering human monoclonal antibodies with therapeutic potential [Dissertation]. University of Stuttgart; 2014. XIV, 164 p. DOI: 10.18419/opus-9017

[18] Diebolder P, Keller A, Haase S, Schlegelmilch A, Kiefer JD, et al. Generation of "LYmph Node Derived Antibody Libraries" (LYNDAL) for selecting fully human antibody fragments with therapeutic potential. MAbs. 2014;**6**:130-142

[19] Vaughan TJ, Williams AJ, Pritchard K, Osbourn JK, Pope AR, et al. Human antibodies with sub-nanomolar affinities isolated from a large non-immunized phage display library. Nature Biotechnology. 1996;**14**:309-314

[20] Frenzel A, Kugler J, Wilke S, Schirrmann T, Hust M. Construction of human antibody gene libraries and selection of antibodies by phage display. Methods in Molecular Biology. 2014;**1060**:215-243

[21] Little M, Welschof M, Braunagel M, Hermes I, Christ C, et al. Generation of a large complex antibody library from multiple donors. Journal of Immunological Methods. 1999;**231**:3-9

[22] Welschof M, Christ C, Hermes I, Keller A, Kleist C, et al. Generation and screening of a modular human scFv expression library from multiple donors. Methods in Molecular Biology. 2003;**207**:103-121

[23] de Haard HJ, van Neer N, Reurs A, Hufton SE, Roovers RC, et al. A large non-immunized human Fab fragment phage library that permits rapid isolation and kinetic analysis of high affinity antibodies. The Journal of Biological Chemistry. 1999;**274**:18218-18230

[24] Kuhn P, Fuhner V, Unkauf T, Moreira GM, Frenzel A, et al. Recombinant antibodies for diagnostics and therapy against pathogens and toxins generated by phage display. Proteomics Clinical Applications. 2016;**10**:922-948

[25] Qi H, Lu H, Qiu HJ, Petrenko V, Liu A. Phagemid vectors for phage display: Properties, characteristics and construction. Journal of Molecular Biology. 2012;**417**:129-143

[26] Mollova S, Retter I, Hust M, Dübel S, Müller W. Analysis of single chain antibody sequences using the VBASE2 Fab analysis tool. In: Kontermann R, Dübel S, editors. Antibody Engineering. Berlin, Heidelberg: Springer Berlin Heidelberg; 2010. pp. 3-10

[27] Both L, Banyard AC, van Dolleweerd C, Wright E, Ma JK, et al. Monoclonal antibodies for prophylactic and therapeutic use against viral infections. Vaccine. 2013;**31**:1553-1559

[28] Krawczyk A, Krauss J, Eis-Hubinger AM, Daumer MP, Schwarzenbacher R, et al. Impact of valency of a glycoprotein B-specific monoclonal antibody on neutralization of herpes simplex virus. Journal of Virology. 2011;**85**:1793-1803

[29] Hangartner L, Zinkernagel RM, Hengartner H. Antiviral antibody responses: The two extremes of a wide spectrum. Nature Review Immunology. 2006;**6**:231-243

[30] Benedict CA, MacKrell AJ, Anderson WF. Determination of the binding affinity of an anti-CD34 single-chain antibody using a novel, flow cytometry based assay. Journal of Immunological Methods. 1997;**201**:223-231

[31] Chames P, Baty D. Phage display and selections on biotinylated antigens. In: Kontermann R, Dübel S, editors. Antibody Engineering. Berlin, Heidelberg: Springer Berlin Heidelberg; 2010. pp. 151-164

[32] Hust M, Steinwand M, Al-Halabi L, Helmsing S, Schirrmann T, et al. Improved microtitre plate production of single chain Fv fragments in *Escherichia coli*. New Biotechnology. 2009;**25**:424-428

[33] Fortier LC, Moineau S. Phage production and maintenance of stocks, including expected stock lifetimes. Methods in Molecular Biology. 2009;**501**:203-219

Chapter 5

Colony Assay for Antibody Library Screening: Outlook and Comparison to Display Screening

Mieko Kato and Yoshiro Hanyu

Additional information is available at the end of the chapter

http://dx.doi.org/10.5772/intechopen.72149

Abstract

Recombinant monoclonal antibodies are established by screening the antibody libraries. To obtain antibodies with a high specificity and affinity, an efficient screening process with a highly diverse library including low background signals is necessary. One of the most extensively used methods is the phage display method. Although phage display screening is a powerful tool for enriching clones from vast libraries, it is not easy to identify single clones with an antigen recognition function only through several rounds of biopanning. The application of colony assays for screening antibody libraries can identify clones with a high reliability by a direct observation of the antibody-antigen binding during the screening process; however, the size of the library that can be dealt with is limited. This chapter describes the colony assay as a current screening technology used in recombinant monoclonal antibody production, the possible problems in this method, and discusses the outlook for this technology.

Keywords: colony assay, screening, antibody library, scFv, *E. coli*, phage display

1. Introduction

The use of recombinant technology for antibody selection offers several advantages over conventional antibody selection strategies, such as the selection of antibodies against toxic or non-immunogenic antigens unattainable using conventional methods [1, 2], the ability to select positive clones from vast libraries [3], the realization of in vitro screening [4], and the bypass of animal usage [5]. The selection and production of recombinant monoclonal antibodies require the creation of highly diverse libraries [6] and the subsequent identification of positive clones using a screening technology with low background signals [7]. In particular, the variable domains of the antibody heavy and light chain (V_H and V_L) are isolated

INTECH
open science | open minds

© 2018 The Author(s). Licensee InTech. This chapter is distributed under the terms of the Creative Commons Attribution License (http://creativecommons.org/licenses/by/3.0), which permits unrestricted use, distribution, and reproduction in any medium, provided the original work is properly cited. (cc) BY

from the lymph tissue of immunized animals and linked together for creating a single-chain variable fragment (scFv) library, and Fab libraries are constructed too. In general, the antibody fragments used for screening are the scFvs. Currently, entirely synthetic libraries [8–11] and naïve libraries [12] are being used. These antibody gene libraries are incorporated into a phagemid or plasmid and expressed in phage or *Escherichia coli* (*E. coli*). Further, panning [13] or colony assays [14] are performed to isolate scFvs possessing affinity to the antigen, thereby establishing monoclonal antibodies. This step, the screening of antibody libraries, is critical for establishing monoclonal antibody fragments with a high affinity and specificity against the antigen. One of the most extensively used methods is the phage display method [15, 16]. The display of the antibody repertoires on the surface of bacteriophages and their selection through panning enables the isolation of monoclonal antibodies [17]. Phage display is also widely used for affinity maturation [18, 19], in which mutations are introduced into the variable domains of an antibody gene mainly into CDRs to produce antibodies with a higher affinity as the original clone [20]. In addition, cell surface panning techniques [1, 21, 22] are being developed to establish antibodies recognizing membrane proteins on living cells that are difficult to produce using the conventional methods. Technologies that enable liquid panning rather than immobilizing the antigens to a solid phase have also been proposed for phage display to establish antibodies that recognize protein conformation [23]. Screening with a colony assay induces the actual expression of the scFvs themselves and involves a direct confirmation of the antigen-antibody binding, lending it the advantage of a low false-positive rate. In addition, the method can be easily used to screen libraries in the order of magnitude larger than those that can be screened with the hybridoma technology. However, this method poses several problems: it requires extensive and complex manipulation of assay steps, the expression of antibody fragments could be at times nonexistent or very low, and the extensive manipulation during the assay can lead to contamination and death of the *E. coli* cells, potentially preventing gene retrieval. Although this technique is not complete and not widely applied, further development and improvement can render it highly beneficial.

2. Antibody library screening

A critical step in the establishment of antigen-specific monoclonal antibody fragment clones is the screening of the recombinant-antibody libraries [6, 7]. Methods for screening the antibody libraries can be largely divided into two strategies [24]: the display and repertoire cloning strategies (**Figure 1**).

2.1. Display strategies for antibody library screening

In the display strategy [25], the antibody fragment and its gene, i.e., the antigen recognition function and information, are joined, and antibody fragments with an affinity against the antigen are screened. Phage display systems in which an scFv joined to the filamentous phage coat protein, g3p, is displayed on the phage are extensively used [15, 16]. Other display systems include yeast display systems in which scFvs are displayed on the surface of yeast [26]; mRNA display [27]; ribosome display in which a ribosome, mRNA, and an scFv are

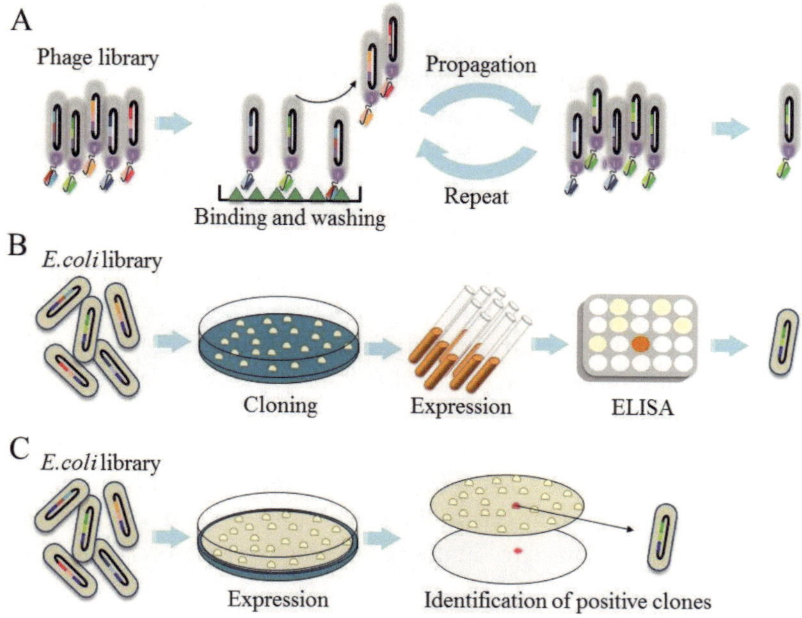

Figure 1. Strategies for antibody library screening. (A) Display strategy: scheme of the phage display panning process. (B) Repertoire cloning strategy: scheme of the cloning and assay process. (C) Detection of antigen-specific antibody fragments released from a bacterial colony by a colony assay.

integrated [28]; bacterial surface display [29]; and mammalian cell surface display [30, 31] for human antibody discovery. In these display systems, panning is applied for screening [13]. The antigen is immobilized on the surface of a microtiter plate, and the scFv library can be screened with phage display and with ribosome/mRNA display. Weakly bound clones are removed by washing, retaining the specific clones bound to the antigen (**Figure 1A**). This panning method is characterized by repeated selection, proliferation, and the enrichment of positive clones for enabling the processing of large libraries. For yeast, bacterial and mammalian cell surface display FACS with the cells displaying the recombinant antibody fragments using labeled antigen is applied.

2.2. Repertoire cloning strategies for antibody library screening

In contrast, in repertoire cloning strategies, the antibody library is transformed into *E. coli*; the scFvs are expressed and secreted from a single clone, and scFvs are screened by ELISA (**Figure 1B**). Clones are selected based on assays, using scFv characteristics such as the affinity; thereby, this method offers advantages such as low false-positive rates and the ability to reliably identify clones with a high affinity. However, an assay must be performed for each individual *E. coli* clone, and only the positive clones are selected. There is no enrichment process in the screening method, and only limited libraries can be used for antibody selection.

Particularly, antibody repertoires from immunized animals with a clone number of approximately 10^6 are suitable for the repertoire cloning but not naïve and synthetic antibody repertoires with high clone numbers (10^9–10^{12} clones). During the assay, a clone from an *E. coli* library is cultured, and its expression is induced. The reactivity of the expressed scFv against the antigen is measured. Clones exhibiting high reactivity are selected as the positive clones. In this method, only a few thousands of clones can be examined simultaneously, even if a multi-well microtiter plate is used. Although this number is higher than the clones obtained by the hybridoma technique, positive clones cannot be efficiently obtained, when the positive ratio is low.

Colony assay in which periplasmic expression and *E. coli* colony formation lifted onto filters are used provides a method for handling large libraries (**Figure 1C**). In colony assay, the clones do not need to be picked up individually before screening; all the colonies on the plate can be assayed simultaneously. Thus, numerous clones can be assayed from a single plate. Antibody fragments released by bacteria were detected by a phage plaque assay in earlier experiments [32, 33]. Libraries of the antibody fragments were expressed in *E. coli* using phage λ vectors [34, 35]. Then, the active fragments secreted from the viable *E. coli* colonies were detected by colony-lift immunoassay [36]. With the colony assay, considerably larger libraries can be dealt with because the number of colonies screened can be easily increased.

2.3. Screening with a phage display

In a phage display system, panning is used to isolate phages that display the antibody fragments exhibiting affinity to the antigen (**Figure 1A**). Positive clones are established by selecting only the phages that displays antibody fragments (primarily scFvs) fused to the g3p coat proteins on the surface of the filamentous phage, which have affinity to the antigen. This method has the advantage of processing large libraries (~10^{11}) [3, 37]. The antigen is immobilized, and the recombinant phage bound to the antigen is left intact; weakly bound recombinant phages are washed away. The remaining recombinant phages, which possess a binding capacity are detached from the antigen by acid treatment and infected into *E. coli*. Further, *E. coli* cells are cultured to propagate positive clones. The *E. coli* clones expressing the phagemids are then infected with a helper phage, and the phages displaying scFvs with binding capacities are collected. Panning is performed repeatedly for the selected group of phages. The repeated selection and propagation of positive clones enrich clones with antibodies comprising binding capacities to the antigen. Then, single clones are isolated at the final step with high binding capacities [38]. This method renders it possible to handle large libraries.

One limitation of this method is that the high background during panning selection often results in false-positive clones. A specific antigen-binding activity is typically not the only driving force exploited during the panning process [39, 40]. Multiple rounds of panning have been documented to frequently cause a strong bias for antibodies directed against immunodominant epitopes and abundant proteins [41], resulting in the loss of the library's diversity and of valuable antibody clones. Several factors influence the selection of the antigen-specific clones and produce undesired effects; these factors include a high efficiency of expression and folding despite poor antigen-binding activity, the nonspecific hydrophobic binding properties of the phage particle itself, and a superior compatibility with the host cells, not related to the antibody fragment affinity.

However, as several antibody fragments are themselves toxic to *E. coli*, these clones will be lost during panning, even if they possess a high affinity. Conversely, repeated panning may result in the relatively preferential propagation of clones with reduced *E. coli* toxicity, even if the clones do not possess a high binding capacity. Toxicity to *E. coli* can increase the background, resulting in several false-positive clones being obtained. This situation renders panning extremely difficult; it is not easy to establish single positive clones only through several rounds of panning [14]. Although the phage display is a powerful tool for establishing monoclonal antibodies, it is used less frequently than expected [39].

3. Colony assay for antibody library screening

As an alternative antibody-screening tool, the colony assay can be used which is sometimes superior to the phage display method [42]. The advantage of this method is that the antibody-antigen binding can be directly observed during the screening process, reducing the selection of false-negative clones [24]. Thus, the colony assay presents notable advantages over the phage display and biopanning method.

3.1. Principle of the colony assay

In the colony assay (**Figure 2**), antibody libraries are expressed in *E. coli* for the selection of clones with a favorable affinity to the antigen. An scFv library is transformed into *E. coli* cells, and afterward transformed *E. coli* cells are plated on appropriate agar plates. After growing of the colonies, they are lifted onto a filter. Further, an expression-inducing reagent such as isopropyl-β-$_{D}$-thiogalactopyranoside (IPTG) is applied, inducing the expression and secretion of scFvs from the *E. coli* cells (**Figure 2A**). scFvs with the desired affinity will diffuse out and bind the antigen coated on the membrane beneath the colonies. However, scFvs without affinity will not bind the antigen (**Figure 2B**), and the unbound scFvs are washed away. Then, the bound scFvs with an affinity against the antigen are detected using an enzymatic method. The His-tags attached to the scFvs are detected with anti-His antibodies (**Figure 2C**). Positive clones are identified as the colonies corresponding to positive signals (**Figure 2D**).

3.2. Filter-sandwich assay

Dreher et al. [43, 44] improved the colony assay by developing the filter-sandwich colony-screening assay (hereafter, the filter-sandwich assay) for selecting positive clones; *E. coli* colonies are grown directly on a hydrophilic filter, which is then transferred to an antigen-coated membrane soaked with IPTG solution and placed on an agar plate containing IPTG to induce antibody fragment production. The antibody fragments produced by the colonies diffuse out and bind to the antigen on the membrane. The presence of antibody fragments bound to the membrane is then detected, and the spot is superimposed on the colony. This method circumvents the difficult technique of lifting the colony [14, 36]. In addition, the filter-sandwich assay was further optimized. The procedure can now be performed by a single step [45] under tightly controlled IPTG concentration for expression of the scFvs.

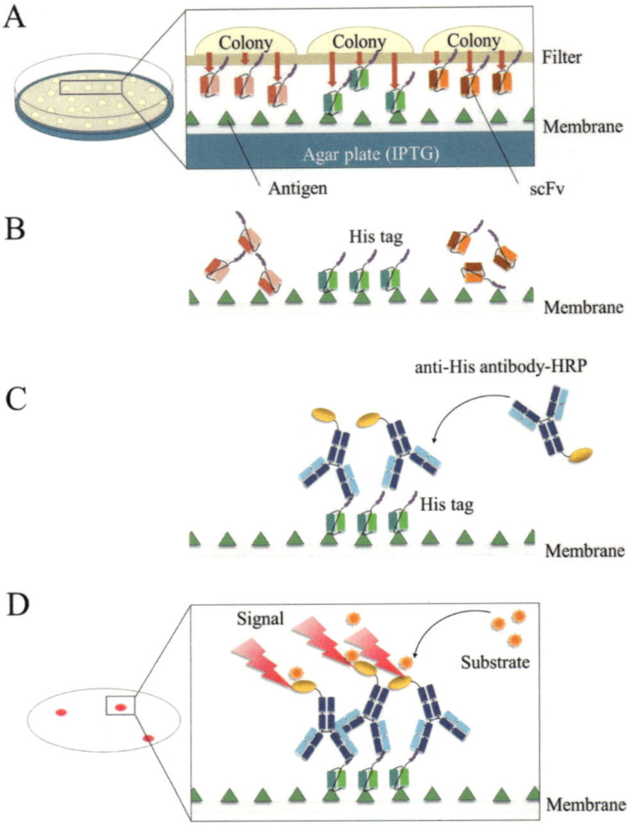

Figure 2. Scheme of the colony assay principle. (A) scFvs are expressed and secreted from *E. coli*. (B) scFvs with the desired affinity bind the antigen beneath the colonies. (C) Bound scFvs with an affinity against the antigen are detected using an enzymatic method. (D) Positive clones are identified as the colonies corresponding to positive signals.

3.3. Procedure for filter-sandwich assay

The procedure used in the filter-sandwich colony assay is depicted schematically in **Figure 3**.

In particular, the RNAs are isolated from the lymph tissue of immunized animals, and the corresponding cDNA is synthesized; this cDNA is used as the template for the polymerase chain reaction (PCR) amplification of the V_L and V_H domains. Further, the variable domains are assembled to an scFv and cloned into an expression vector to create the scFv libraries [46]. As expression vector, for example, pET22b (+), containing a *pelB* signal sequence for periplasm expression and a His-tag sequence for the detection of the scFv expression driven by the T7 promoter, is used. The antibody repertoire is transformed into *E. coli*, and the filter sandwich assay is performed as described in **Figure 3**.

The hydrophilic PVDF filter is placed on an agar plate. Transformed *E. coli* with the scFv libraries is spread onto the filter and incubated. After the formation of the bacterial colonies on the filter surface, the filter harboring the colonies is transferred to an antigen-coated nitrocellulose membrane on the agar plate containing IPTG and incubated to induce scFv expression.

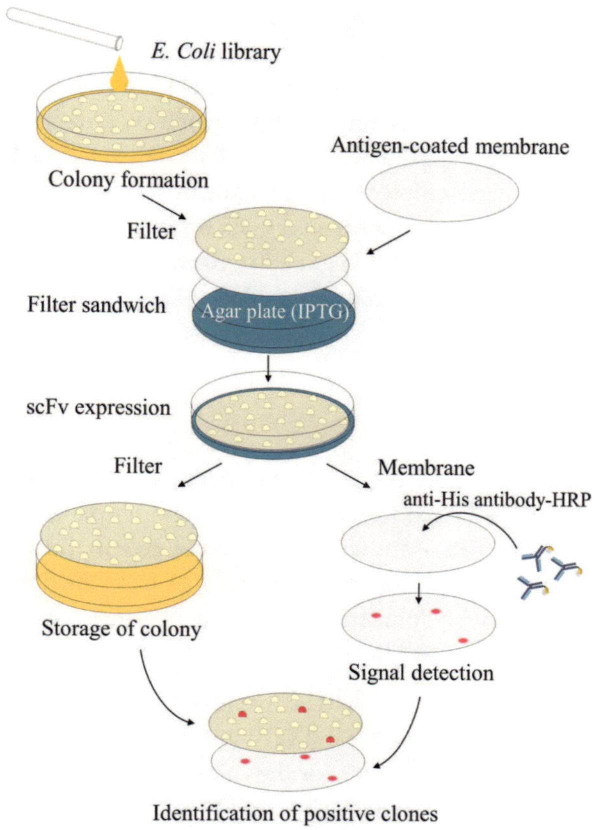

Figure 3. Procedure for filter-sandwich colony assay.

Then, the filter harboring the colonies is removed, placed on a fresh plate, and stored for the later recovery of the bacteria. Subsequently, antigen-bound scFvs on the nitrocellulose membrane are detected with chemiluminescence from a horseradish peroxidase (HRP)-conjugated anti-His antibody. The filter harboring the colonies and the image presenting the chemiluminescence data are superimposed, and positive colonies corresponding to the chemiluminescence signals are identified. These positive clones are transferred to a medium and incubated. The plasmid encoding the scFv gene with an affinity against the antigen is purified, and the antibody coding sequence is determined.

3.4. Establishing monoclonal antibody fragments by colony assay

A colony assay is used for screening the antibody fragments against a variety of antigens, with optimizations for each specific purpose. The recombinant antibody fragments against EspA and the intimin of *E. coli* O157:H7 were established by colony filter screening [47]. Colony-lift assay was combined with phage display, using cell-coated filters to screen the phage libraries for cell-binding clones [48]. Robert et al. developed subtractive colony filter screening to select scFvs that recognize atherosclerotic but not the normal aorta [49]. Giovannoni et al.

isolated antiangiogenesis antibodies from combinatorial libraries by iterative colony filter screening: colonies located around the positive signals were selected, and the screening step was repeated; monoclonal scFvs were established after several rounds of the assay [50]. Neumann-Schaal et al. developed a colony-screening method in which *E. coli* colonies producing the required scFv were selected in the presence of ampicillin conjugated to the antigen of interest; this method relies on the neutralization of the conjugate by the produced scFv. The scFvs were identified against biotin by the growth of the scFv library-expressing *E. coli* in the presence of a biotin-ampicillin conjugate [51]. Kumada et al. improved the sensitivity of the colony assay utilizing antibody-coupled liposome encapsulating HRP [52].

4. Summary

It is possible to screen 3–5 × 10^3 clones on a 10-cm diameter plate in a filter-sandwich assay, whereas in the hybridoma method, dozens of 96-well microtiter plates are required for screening these clones. Further, the filter-sandwich assay can be readily upscaled by increasing the number of plates. Therefore, the number of positive clones from the filter-sandwich assay can be higher than that from the hybridoma method. This would increase the chance of obtaining monoclonal antibody fragments with the desired affinity, specificity, and function.

However, the filter-sandwich assay needs to be improved further for the selection of positive clones, particularly with respect to the reliability of the antibody fragment expression and the handling of the colonies during the assay. For the colony assay, the control of the expression level is critical. Because the scFv expression by itself is considerably toxic to *E. coli*, an excess induction of expression, namely, exposure to an excess of the expression-inducing reagent (IPTG), leads to cell death and prevents the selection of antigen-specific scFvs. Conversely, exposure to insufficient IPTG induces inadequate antibody expression for the detection of signals from positive clones. In the filter-sandwich assay, expression induction is not stringently controlled because the concentration of the IPTG added to the cells cannot be precisely controlled. IPTG reaches the colonies by diffusing through the filter from the antigen-coated membrane and the agar plate. Quantitative control of the expression level is required for superior screening. This uncertainty in the IPTG concentration in the filter-sandwich assay also causes a problem in the induction timing. For appropriate induction, the colony size is a critical factor [14, 44]; however, the colony continues to grow during the assay. Hence, the timing of the expression induction is crucial for proper expression. If the ITPG diffusion is delayed, an initially small colony would grow too large for proper induction to occur; however, if the colonies are too small, the signal from each colony is inadequate for detecting the antigen binding. The induction strength cannot be accurately determined, particularly during the step, when the filter is transferred to the IPTG-containing plate to initiate the induction of expression. These induction-related uncertainties in the filter-sandwich assay lead to unstable expression and failure in isolating the antibody-encoding genes. Stringent control of the expression level is critical. Various factors related to the expression vector, such as the promoter, strength of the ribosomal binding site, fusion tags, and the copy number, must be optimized [53–57]. The incubation temperature is also an important factor in controlling the expression strength [58]. For inducing expression, additional methods such as the cold-shock system [59] should be examined. Expression-inducing reagents that are less toxic than IPTG to *E. coli*, such as rhamnose [60], should also be tested.

In the filter-sandwich assay, before the induction of antibody expression, the filter harboring the colonies must be transferred without disturbance. This transfer requires delicate manipulation of the filter and frequently produces unwanted stress on the filter, occasionally disturbing the colonies themselves. A method that does not require the transfer of the filter should be developed for more efficient antibody establishment. Recently, a single-step colony assay was established by us using a tightly controlled IPTG concentration for scFv expression [45]. One advantage is also that no transfer of the filter on which the colonies are grown to the antigen-coated membrane is necessary.

The establishment of a high-quality antibody library and efficient screening are the most important factors for successful recombinant antibody selection and production. Improvements in the screening technology are critical for quickly and reliably establishment of high-performance antibodies. Phage display screening is a powerful tool for this purpose; however, it has certain disadvantages such as the frequent selection of false-positive clones, but it can easily deal with a vast library. On the other hand, screening with a colony assay could identify the positive clones reliably; however, it cannot deal with a large complex library. Thus, screening methods using a display panning system and a colony assay have certain advantages and disadvantages, respectively. They should be utilized cooperatively, depending on the purpose of the experiments. Hence, condensing the library by phage display and then cloning the positive clones by colony assay would be advantageous. To efficiently establish high-quality antibodies, the adequate choice of these technologies and their combination would be crucial.

Author details

Mieko Kato[1] and Yoshiro Hanyu[2*]

*Address all correspondence to: y.hanyu@aist.go.jp

1 Bio-Peak Co., Ltd., Takasaki, Japan

2 Structural Physiology Research Group, Biomedical Research Institute, National Institute of Advanced Industrial Science and Technology (AIST), Tsukuba, Japan

References

[1] Jones ML, Alfaleh MA, Kumble S, Zhang S, Osborne GW, Yeh M, et al. Targeting membrane proteins for antibody discovery using phage display. Scientific Reports. [Internet]. May 18, 2016;**6**:26240. Available from: http://www.nature.com/articles/srep26240 [Accessed: Jan 28, 2017]

[2] Griffiths AD, Williams SC, Hartley O, Tomlinson IM, Waterhouse P, Crosby WL, et al. Isolation of high affinity human antibodies directly from large synthetic repertoires. EMBO Journal. [Internet]. Jul 15, 1994;**13**(14):3245-3260. Available from: http://www.pubmedcentral.nih.gov/articlerender.fcgi?artid=395221&tool=pmcentrez&rendertype=abstract [Accessed: Sep 28, 2015]

[3] Bradbury A, Sblattero D. Exploiting recombination in single bacteria to make large phage antibody libraries. Nature Biotechnology. [Internet]. Jan 1, 2000;**18**(1):75-80. Available from: http://www.ncbi.nlm.nih.gov/pubmed/10625396 [Accessed: Jan 8, 2017]

[4] Geyer CR, McCafferty J, Dübel S, Bradbury ARM, Sidhu SS. Recombinant antibodies and in vitro selection technologies. Methods in Molecular Biology. [Internet]. Jan 2012;**901**:11-32. Available from: http://www.ncbi.nlm.nih.gov/pubmed/22723092 [Accessed: Sep 10, 2015]

[5] Marks JD, Hoogenboom HR, Bonnert TP, McCafferty J, Griffiths AD, Winter G. By-passing immunization. Human antibodies from V-gene libraries displayed on phage. Journal of Molecular Biology. [Internet]. Dec 5, 1991;**222**(3):581-597. Available from: http://www.ncbi.nlm.nih.gov/pubmed/1748994 [Accessed: Jan 29, 2017]

[6] Hust M, Frenzel A, Schirrmann T, Dübel S. Selection of recombinant antibodies from antibody gene libraries. Methods in Molecular Biology. [Internet]. Jan 2014;**1101**:305-320. Available from: http://www.ncbi.nlm.nih.gov/pubmed/24233787 [Accessed: Sep 3, 2015]

[7] Hoogenboom HR. Selecting and screening recombinant antibody libraries. Nature Biotechnology. [Internet]. Sep 2005;**23**(9):1105-1116. Available from: http://www.ncbi.nlm.nih.gov/pubmed/16151404 [Accessed: Mar 9, 2015]

[8] Rothe C, Urlinger S, Löhning C, Prassler J, Stark Y, Jäger U, et al. The human combinatorial antibody library HuCAL GOLD combines diversification of all six CDRs according to the natural immune system with a novel display method for efficient selection of high-affinity antibodies. Journal of Molecular Biology. [Internet]. Feb 29, 2008;**376**(4):1182-1200. Available from: http://www.ncbi.nlm.nih.gov/pubmed/18191144 [Accessed: Sep 28, 2015]

[9] Chen G, Sidhu SS. Design and generation of synthetic antibody libraries for phage display. Methods in Molecular Biology. [Internet]. Jan 2014;**1131**:113-131. Available from: http://www.ncbi.nlm.nih.gov/pubmed/24515463 [Accessed: Sep 15, 2015]

[10] Lerner RA. Combinatorial antibody libraries: New advances, new immunological insights. Nature Reviews Immunology. [Internet]. Jul 4, 2016;**16**(8):498-508. Available from: http://www.nature.com/doifinder/10.1038/nri.2016.67 [Accessed: Jan 28 2017]

[11] Prassler J, Thiel S, Pracht C, Polzer A, Peters S, Bauer M, et al. HuCAL PLATINUM, a synthetic fab library optimized for sequence diversity and superior performance in mammalian expression systems. Journal of Molecular Biology. [Internet]. Oct 14, 2011;**413**(1):261-278. Available from: http://www.ncbi.nlm.nih.gov/pubmed/21856311 [Accessed: Sep 28, 2015]

[12] Hust M, Frenzel A, Meyer T, Schirrmann T, Dübel S. Construction of human naive antibody gene libraries. Methods in Molecular Biology (Clifton, NJ). [Internet]. 2012;**907**:85-107. Available from: http://www.ncbi.nlm.nih.gov/pubmed/22907347 [Accessed: Apr 5, 2017]

[13] Parmley SF, Smith GP. Antibody-selectable filamentous fd phage vectors: affinity purification of target genes. Gene. [Internet]. Dec 20, 1988;**73**(2):305-318. Available from: http://www.ncbi.nlm.nih.gov/pubmed/3149606 [Accessed: Sep 28, 2015]

[14] Rauth S, Schlapschy M, Skerra A. Selection of antibody fragments by means of the filter-sandwich Colony screening assay. In: Kontermann R, Dübel S, editors. Antibody Engineering. Berlin Heidelberg: Springer; 2010. pp. 255-266

[15] McCafferty J, Griffiths AD, Winter G, Chiswell DJ. Phage antibodies: Filamentous phage displaying antibody variable domains. Nature. [Internet]. Dec 6, 1990;**348**(6301):552-554. Available from: http://www.ncbi.nlm.nih.gov/pubmed/2247164 [Accessed: Jul 22, 2015]

[16] Hoogenboom HR, de Bruïne AP, Hufton SE, Hoet RM, Arends JW, Roovers RC. Antibody phage display technology and its applications. Immunotechnology. [Internet]. Jun 1998;**4**(1):1-20. Available from: http://www.ncbi.nlm.nih.gov/pubmed/9661810 [Accessed: Jan 6, 2017]

[17] Boldicke T, Tesar M, Griesel C, Rohde M, Grone HJ, Waltenberger J, et al. Anti-VEGFR-2 scFvs for cell isolation. Single-chain antibodies recognizing the human vascular endothelial growth factor receptor-2 (VEGFR-2/flk-1) on the surface of primary endothelial cells and preselected CD34+ cells from cord blood. Stem Cells. 2001;**19**(1):24-36

[18] Steinwand M, Droste P, Frenzel A, Hust M, Dübel S, Schirrmann T. The influence of antibody fragment format on phage display based affinity maturation of IgG. MAbs Journal. [Internet]. 2014;**6**(1):204-218. Available from: http://www.pubmedcentral.nih.gov/articlerender.fcgi?artid=3929444&tool=pmcentrez&rendertype=abstract [Accessed: Nov 25, 2014]

[19] Thie H, Voedisch B, Dübel S, Hust M, Schirrmann T. Affinity maturation by phage display. Methods in Molecular Biology [Internet]. Jan 2009;**525**:309-322. xv. Available from: http://www.ncbi.nlm.nih.gov/pubmed/19252854 [Accessed: Sep 28, 2015]

[20] Prassler J, Steidl S, Urlinger S. In vitro affinity maturation of HuCAL antibodies: Complementarity determining region exchange and RapMAT technology. Immunotherapy [Internet]. 2009 Jul;**1**(4):571-583. Available from: http://www.ncbi.nlm.nih.gov/pubmed/20635988 [Accessed: Sep 28, 2015]

[21] Giordano RJ, Cardó-Vila M, Lahdenranta J, Pasqualini R, Arap W. Biopanning and rapid analysis of selective interactive ligands. Nature Medicine. [Internet]. Nov 2001; **7**(11):1249-1253. Available from: http://www.ncbi.nlm.nih.gov/pubmed/11689892 [Accessed: Sep 29, 2015]

[22] Akahori Y, Kurosawa G, Sumitomo M, Morita M, Muramatsu C, Eguchi K, et al. Isolation of antigen/antibody complexes through organic solvent (ICOS) method. Biochemical and

Biophysical Research Communications. [Internet]. Jan 23, 2009;**378**(4):832-835. Available from: http://www.ncbi.nlm.nih.gov/pubmed/19071089 [Accessed: Sep 29, 2015]

[23] Haque A, Tonks NK. The use of phage display to generate conformation-sensor recombinant antibodies. Nature Protocols. [Internet]. Dec 2012;**7**(12):2127-2143. Available from: http://www.pubmedcentral.nih.gov/articlerender.fcgi?artid=3712638&tool=pmcentrez&rendertype=abstract [Accessed: Sep 29, 2015]

[24] Kato M, Hanyu Y. Screening technologies for recombinant antibody libraries. Archives of Medical Research. 2015;**2**(7):12-18

[25] Grönwall C, Ståhl S. Engineered affinity proteins – Generation and applications. Journal of Biotechnology [Internet]. 2009;**140**(3):254-269. Available from: http://www.sciencedirect.com/science/article/pii/S0168165609000340 [Accessed: Apr 5, 2017]

[26] Feldhaus MJ, Siegel RW. Yeast display of antibody fragments: A discovery and characterization platform. Journal of Immunological Methods [Internet]. Jul 2004;**290**(1-2):69-80. Available from: http://www.ncbi.nlm.nih.gov/pubmed/15261572 [Accessed: Sep 28, 2015]

[27] Fukuda I, Kojoh K, Tabata N, Doi N, Takashima H, Miyamoto-Sato E, et al. In vitro evolution of single-chain antibodies using mRNA display. Nucleic Acids Research. [Internet]. 2006;**34**(19):e127. Available from: http://www.ncbi.nlm.nih.gov/pubmed/17012279 [Accessed: Apr 5, 2017]

[28] Schaffitzel C, Hanes J, Jermutus L, Plückthun A. Ribosome display: An in vitro method for selection and evolution of antibodies from libraries. Journal of Immunological Methods [Internet]. Dec 10, 1999;**231**(1-2):119-135. Available from: http://www.ncbi.nlm.nih.gov/pubmed/10648932 [Accessed: 2015 Sep 28]

[29] Daugherty PS, Chen G, Olsen MJ, Iverson BL, Georgiou G. Antibody affinity maturation using bacterial surface display. Protein Engineering. [Internet]. 1998;**11**(9):825-832. Available from: https://chemengr.ucsb.edu/~ceweb/faculty/daugherty/pdfs/04.pdf [Accessed: Apr 5, 2017]

[30] King DJ, Bowers PM, Kehry MR, Horlick RA. Mammalian cell display and somatic hypermutation in vitro for human antibody discovery. Current Drug Discovery Technologies [Internet]. Mar 2014;**11**(1):56-64. Available from: http://www.ncbi.nlm.nih.gov/pubmed/23978037 [Accessed: Jan 28, 2017]

[31] Bowers PM, Horlick RA, Kehry MR, Neben TY, Tomlinson GL, Altobell L, et al. Mammalian cell display for the discovery and optimization of antibody therapeutics. Methods. [Internet]. Jan 1, 2014;**65**(1):44-56. Available from: http://www.ncbi.nlm.nih.gov/pubmed/23792919 [Accessed: Jan 29, 2017]

[32] Huse WD, Sastry L, Iverson SA, Kang AS, Alting-Mees M, Burton DR, et al. Generation of a large combinatorial library of the immunoglobulin repertoire in phage lambda. Science [Internet]. Dec 8, 1989;**246**(4935):1275-1281. Available from: http://www.ncbi.nlm.nih.gov/pubmed/2531466 [Accessed: Jan 6, 2017]

[33] Caton AJ, Koprowski H. Influenza virus hemagglutinin-specific antibodies isolated from a combinatorial expression library are closely related to the immune response of the donor. Proceedings of the National Academy of Sciences of the United States of America. [Internet]. Aug 1990;**87**(16):6450-6454. Available from: http://www.ncbi.nlm.nih.gov/pubmed/1696733 [Accessed: Jan 6, 2017]

[34] Mullinax RL, Gross EA, Amberg JR, Hayt BN, Hogrefe HH, Kubitz MM, et al. Identification of human antibody fragment clones specific for tetanus toxoid in a bacteriophage lambda immunoexpression library. Proceedings of the National Academy of Sciences of the United States of America. 1990;**87**(October):8095-8099

[35] Persson MA, Caothien RH, Burton DR. Generation of diverse high-affinity human monoclonal antibodies by repertoire cloning. Proceedings of the National Academy of Sciences of the United States of America. [Internet]. Mar 15, 1991;**88**(6):2432-2436. Available from: http://www.pubmedcentral.nih.gov/articlerender.fcgi?artid=51246&tool=pmcentrez&rendertype=abstract [Accessed: Sep 28, 2015]

[36] Rodenburg CM, Mernaugh R, Bilbao G, Khazaeli MB. Production of a single chain anti-CEA antibody from the hybridoma cell line T84.66 using a modified colony-lift selection procedure to detect antigen-positive ScFv bacterial clones. Hybridoma [Internet]. 1998 Feb;**17**(1):1-8. Available from: http://www.ncbi.nlm.nih.gov/pubmed/9523232 [Accessed: Jan 8, 2017]

[37] Hust M, Steinwand M, Al-Halabi L, Helmsing S, Schirrmann T, Dübel S. Improved microtitre plate production of single chain Fv fragments in *Escherichia coli*. New Biotechnology. [Internet]. Sep 2009;**25**(6):424-428. Available from: http://www.ncbi.nlm.nih.gov/pubmed/19552889 [Accessed: Sep 3, 2015]

[38] Schaefer JV, Honegger A, Plückthun A. Construction of scFv fragments from hybridoma or spleen cells by PCR assembly. In: Kontermann R, Dübel S, editors. Antibody Engineering. Berlin Heidelberg: Springer; 2010. pp. 21-44

[39] Nelson AL. Antibody fragments: Hope and hype. MAbs Journal. 2010;**2**:77-83

[40] Hammers CM, Stanley JR. Antibody phage display: Technique and applications. Journal of Investigative Dermatology. [Internet]. Feb 2014;**134**(2):e17. Available from: http://www.ncbi.nlm.nih.gov/pubmed/24424458 [Accessed: Jan 28, 2017]

[41] De Wildt RM, Mundy CR, Gorick BD, Tomlinson IM. Antibody arrays for high-throughput screening of antibody-antigen interactions. Nature Biotechnology. [Internet]. 2000;**18**(9):989-994. Available from: http://www.ncbi.nlm.nih.gov/pubmed/10973222

[42] Pini A, Ricci C, Bracci L. Phage display and colony filter screening for high-throughput selection of antibody libraries. Combinatorial Chemistry & High Throughput Screening. [Internet]. Nov 1, 2002;**5**(7):503-510. Available from: http://www.eurekaselect.com/openurl/content.php?genre=article&issn=1386-2073&volume=5&issue=7&spage=503 [Accessed: Jun 18, 2016]

[43] Dreher ML, Gherardi E, Skerra A, Milstein C. Colony assays for antibody fragments expressed in bacteria. Journal of Immunological Methods [Internet]. Jun 3, 1991;**139**(2):197-205. Available from: http://www.ncbi.nlm.nih.gov/pubmed/2045660 [Accessed: Sep 28, 2015]

[44] Skerra A, Dreher ML, Winter G. Filter screening of antibody Fab fragments secreted from individual bacterial colonies: Specific detection of antigen binding with a two-membrane system. Analytical Biochemistry. [Internet]. Jul 1991;**196**(1):151-155. Available from: http://www.ncbi.nlm.nih.gov/pubmed/1888028 [Accessed: Sep 28, 2015]

[45] Kato M, Hanyu Y. Single-step colony assay for screening antibody libraries. Journal of Biotechnology. [Internet]. Aug 10, 2017;**255**:1-8. Available from: http://www.ncbi.nlm.nih.gov/pubmed/28641985 [Accessed: Aug 24, 2017]

[46] Kato M, Hanyu Y. Construction of an scFv library by enzymatic assembly of VL and VH genes. Journal of Immunological Methods. 2013;**396**(1-2):15-22

[47] Kühne SA, Hawes WS, La Ragione RM, Woodward MJ, Whitelam GC, Gough KC. Isolation of recombinant antibodies against EspA and intimin of *Escherichia coli* O157:H7. Journal of Clinical Microbiology. [Internet]. Jul 1, 2004;**42**(7):2966-2976. Available from: http://jcm.asm.org/cgi/doi/10.1128/JCM.42.7.2966-2976.2004 [Accessed: Jan 6, 2017]

[48] Radosević K, Voerman JSA, Hemmes A, Muskens F, Speleman L, de Weers M, et al. Colony lift assay using cell-coated filters: a fast and efficient method to screen phage libraries for cell-binding clones. Journal of Immunological Methods. [Internet]. Jan 15, 2003;**272**(1-2):219-233. Available from: http://www.ncbi.nlm.nih.gov/pubmed/12505726 [Accessed: Jan 6, 2017]

[49] Robert R, Jacobin-Valat MJ, Daret D, Miraux S, Nurden AT, Franconi JM, et al. Identification of human scFvs targeting atherosclerotic lesions: Selection by single round in vivo phage display. The Journal of Biological Chemistry. 2006;**281**(52):40135-40143

[50] Giovannoni L, Viti F, Zardi L, Neri D. Isolation of anti-angiogenesis antibodies from a large combinatorial repertoire by colony filter screening. Nucleic Acids Research. [Internet]. Mar 1, 2001;**29**(5):E27. Available from: http://www.pubmedcentral.nih.gov/articlerender.fcgi?artid=29740&tool=pmcentrez&rendertype=abstract [Accessed: Sep 28, 2015]

[51] Neumann-Schaal M, Messerschmidt K, Grenz N, Heilmann K. Use of antibody gene library for the isolation of specific single chain antibodies by ampicillin–antigen conjugates. Immunology Letters. [Internet]. Mar 2013;**151**(1-2):39-43. Available from: http://www.ncbi.nlm.nih.gov/pubmed/23453960 [Accessed: Jan 6, 2017]

[52] Kumada Y, Maehara M, Minami N, Nogami M, Katoh S. Colony lift immunoassay utilizing antibody-coupled liposomes encapsulating HRP. Biochemical Engineering Journal. 2006;**29**(1-2):98-102

[53] Rosano GL, Ceccarelli EA. Recombinant protein expression in *Escherichia coli*: Advances and challenges. Frontiers in Microbiology. 2014;**5**:1-17

[54] Sharma SK, Suresh MR, Wuest FR. Improved soluble expression of a single-chain antibody fragment in *E. coli* for targeting CA125 in epithelial ovarian cancer. Protein Expression and Purification. [Internet]. Oct 2014;**102**:27-37. Available from: http://linkinghub.elsevier.com/retrieve/pii/S104659281400165X [Accessed: Jan 29, 2017]

[55] Esposito D, Chatterjee DK. Enhancement of soluble protein expression through the use of fusion tags. Current Opinion in Biotechnology. [Internet]. Aug 2006;**17**(4):353-358. Available from: http://www.ncbi.nlm.nih.gov/pubmed/16781139 [Accessed: Apr 26, 2015]

[56] Kato M, Hanyu Y. Fusion of Zif268 to the C-terminus of Scfvs promotes expression of the active form in the cytoplasm of *Escherichia coli* abstract. Biochemistry & Molecular Biology Journal. 2016;**2**(1):1-7

[57] Islam MM, Khan MA, Kuroda Y. Analysis of amino acid contributions to protein solubility using short peptide tags fused to a simplified BPTI variant. Biochimica et Biophysica Acta (BBA) – Proteins and Proteomics [Internet]. Oct 2012;**1824**(10):1144-1150. Available from: http://www.ncbi.nlm.nih.gov/pubmed/22728531 [Accessed: Jan 29, 2017]

[58] Schaefer JV, Plückthun A. Improving expression of scFv fragments by co-expression of periplasmic chaperones. In: Kontermann R, Dübel S, editors. Antibody Engineering [Internet]. Berlin, Heidelberg: Springer Berlin Heidelberg; 2010. pp. 345-361. Available from: http://link.springer.com/10.1007/978-3-642-01147-4 [Accessed: Aug 27, 2015]

[59] Hu X, O'Hara L, White S, Magner E, Kane M, Wall JG. Optimisation of production of a domoic acid-binding scFv antibody fragment in *Escherichia coli* using molecular chaperones and functional immobilisation on a mesoporous silicate support. Protein Expression and Purification. [Internet]. Mar 2007;**52**(1):194-201. Available from: http://linkinghub.elsevier.com/retrieve/pii/S1046592806002580 [Accessed: 2017 Jan 29]

[60] Giacalone MJ, Gentile AM, Lovitt BT, Berkley NL, Gunderson CW, Surber MW. Toxic protein expression in *Escherichia coli* using a rhamnose-based tightly regulated and tunable promoter system. BioTechniques. 2006;**40**(3):355-364

Construction and Characteristics of a Recombinant Single-Chain Antibody Fragment against Bacterial Type III Secretion

Teiji Sawa, Atsushi Kainuma, Kiyoshi Moriyama and
Yoshifumi Naito

Additional information is available at the end of the chapter

http://dx.doi.org/10.5772/intechopen.70316

Abstract

Pseudomonas aeruginosa, a Gram-negative pathogen, causes life-threatening infections. Lung injury and the development of sepsis depend largely on expression of the virulence genes associated with the type III secretion system of this bacterium. The type III secretion system functions as a molecular syringe to deliver type III secretory toxins directly into the cytosol of eukaryotic cells and also acts to inhibit innate immune mechanisms, thereby preventing bacterial clearance. Antibodies against PcrV, the cap structure in the translocational needle of type III secretory apparatus of *P. aeruginosa,* block toxin translocation of the type III secretion system. We have been investigating the therapeutic use of a recombinant anti-PcrV single-chain antibody. In this chapter, as a preliminary step toward an antibody-based immunotherapy against bacterial infections, we summarize our experience of constructing a recombinant single-chain antibody (called scFv166), in which the heavy (V_H) and light chain (V_L) variable regions of the anti-PcrV monoclonal IgG are joined by a flexible peptide linker. The practical methodologies used to make recombinant scFv166 against a bacterial protein component are described in detail.

Keywords: single-chain antibody, PcrV, *Pseudomonas aeruginosa,* type III secretion system

1. Introduction

Bacterial infections still frequently cause life-threatening diseases in humans. New pathogens have emerged, old pathogens have reemerged, and the prevalence of multidrug resistant microorganisms has increased despite the introduction of various new antibiotics since antibacterial agents were first developed in the early twentieth century. The difficulties

INTECH
open science | open minds

© 2018 The Author(s). Licensee InTech. This chapter is distributed under the terms of the Creative Commons Attribution License (http://creativecommons.org/licenses/by/3.0), which permits unrestricted use, distribution, and reproduction in any medium, provided the original work is properly cited. (cc) BY

associated with treating infections in immunocompromised patients have increased the need for new adjunctive immunotherapies. During the last 20 years, major advances in the techniques used to generate human antibodies and humanize murine monoclonal antibodies have seen antibody-based therapies to arrive as potential candidates for adjuvant therapies for infectious diseases. However, today, antibody therapy for bacterial infections is still indicated in relatively few situations, although more attention should be focused on it because of the increased levels of bacterial drug resistance and higher numbers of immunocompromised patients.

We have been investigating the therapeutic use of recombinant antibodies against the Gram-negative pathogen, *P. aeruginosa*. *P. aeruginosa* is an opportunistic pathogen responsible for a variety of acute infections in immunocompromised patients, and chronic infections in those with cystic fibrosis [1, 2]. *P. aeruginosa* is also highly resistant to various antibiotics and causes nosocomial pneumonia with an associated high mortality rate despite aggressive treatment with antimicrobial drugs [3, 4]. We have been studying the pathogenesis of acute infections caused by *P. aeruginosa* to identify a therapeutic target in this pathogen, and have reported that its ability to cause epithelial injury, to disseminate into the circulation, and to avoid host innate immune responses is highly associated with its type III secretion system (TTSS) [5–9]. The TTSS of Gram-negative bacteria mediates the translocation of toxins from the bacterial cytoplasm directly into the cytosol of host eukaryotic cells [10, 11]. Once inside the eukaryotic cell, these translocated bacterial toxins interfere with signal transduction. TTSSs with homology to *P. aeruginosa* have been described in most Gram-negative bacterial pathogens (e.g., *Yersinia, Shigella, Salmonella,* and *Escherichia coli*), and all of them are associated with pathogenicity [12].

Here, as a preliminary step toward antibody-based immunotherapy against bacterial infections, we summarize our trial to block the TTSS-associated virulence of *P. aeruginosa* using recombinant antibody technologies. Especially, cloning of the variable domains of the light and heavy chain from a hybridoma cell and assembling the cloned V_H and V_L domains to recombinant single-chain antibody (scFv) to confirm the binding to the target antigen are required steps to humanize murine antibody. In addition to a brief explanation of the *P. aeruginosa* TTSS and the concept of a virulence blockade, the advantage of a recombinant single-chain antibody (scFv), the detailed methods to clone the variable domains from hybridoma cells and construction of scFv166, in which the heavy (V_H) and light chain (V_L) variable regions of the anti-PcrV monoclonal IgG molecule are joined by a flexible peptide linker, will be described.

2. Antibody-based blockade of *P. aeruginosa* type III secretion

P. aeruginosa translocates its virulent TTS toxins (ExoS, ExoT, ExoU, and ExoY) directly into eukaryotic cells to disrupt their normal cellular processes [12, 13]. The translocation of ExoS and ExoT proteins, which both have ADP-ribosyltransferase and GTPase activities, inhibits the phagocytic activities of macrophages [14, 15]. The translocation of ExoU, which has patatin-like phospholipase A_2 activity, is correlated with acute cytotoxicity *in vitro* and lung damage, sepsis, and mortality in animal models [7, 16–20]. The translocation of ExoY, which possesses adenylate cyclase activity, causes an increase of cytosolic cyclic AMP in eukaryotic cells and affects cell morphology [21]. In our past clinical study, we discovered an association between patients infected with TTSS-expressing *P. aeruginosa* strains and mortality [22], and other reports from various countries have supported the association of TTSS with severe clinical outcomes in patients infected with this bacterium [19].

In the TTSS, the translocated toxins are not exposed extracellularly and evade direct recognition by the host immune system. Therefore, targeting the protein factors involved in the "*secretion*" or the "*translocation*" process of the TTSS seems a rational approach for blocking TTS virulence. To target the TTSS of *P. aeruginosa,* we have been developing neutralizing antibodies capable of blocking the translocation process of the TTSS [23]. An obvious candidate for a protective antigen was PcrV as it shares relatively high homology with the protective antigen from *Yersinia* sp., LcrV [6, 24-33]. Using genetic analyses, we demonstrated that PopD and PcrV were required for the delivery of *P. aeruginosa*-encoded TTS toxins [23]. In addition, recombinant TTS proteins, such as ExoU, PcrV, and PopD, were produced, purified, and tested for their protective capacities in a model of acute lung infection in mice. Only PcrV was protective in these experiments. Antibodies to PcrV protected against type III intoxication as shown by the inhibition of translocation of ExoY and by the inhibition of macrophage cytotoxicity mediated by ExoU. Passive protection with anti-PcrV reduced the inflammatory response, minimized bacteremia, and prevented septic shock [23]. Moreover, the protective capacity of the antibody was Fc-independent because $F(ab')_2$ fragments of polyclonal anti-PcrV were also effective [34–36].

In our previous study, the Mab166 murine monoclonal antibody, which has neutralizing effects on virulence of the *P. aeruginosa* TTSS, was developed [35]. Also, the Fab fragments of the Mab166 had comparable therapeutic effects to the whole IgG of Mab166 in preventing *P. aeruginosa*-induced acute lung injury, and the Fc-dependent opsonization of the bacteria does not seem critical for the efficacy of the Mab166 [36]. These results implicate that the blockade of type III secretion-associated virulence can be attained by the effective Fab fragment of IgG molecules. Because the Fc-portion of IgG may induce unfavorable inflammatory responses such as complement fixation, activation of macrophages, the administration of the whole IgG may cause some inflammatory side effects. If the Fab fragment had the same therapeutic potency as the whole IgG, the therapeutic administration of either Fab fragments or scFv might overcome the disadvantages of the intratracheal administration of whole IgG. Therefore, the *E. coli*-derived recombinant scFv against PcrV is attractive to be an effective therapeutic agent against *P. aeruginosa* pneumonia.

In the next chapter, we describe the methods used to clone the variable antibody domains V_H and V_L from hybridoma cells and assembly of a single-chain antibody as an *E. coli*-derived recombinant protein. Previously, the engineered recombinant Fab fragment against PcrV was humanized to allow it to be considered for adjunctive therapy in patients [37–39].

3. Methods for construction of a single-chain antibody

3.1. Cloning the variable V_H and V_L domains from hybridoma cells

3.1.1. Poly A⁺ RNA extraction

The anti-PcrV IgG Mab166 hybridoma cell line [35] was cultured in a standard culture medium. After the cells had reached confluence in a 75 cm^2 flask, they were harvested by centrifugation at 600 rpm for 5 min. The cell pellet was homogenized in 2 mL of TRIzol™ reagent (Thermo Fisher Scientific, Waltham, MA, USA), and total RNA extracted after chloroform fractionation, isopropanol precipitation, and washing with 70% ethanol. Poly A^+ RNA was extracted with an oligotex mRNA spin-column (Qiagen, Valencia, CA).

3.1.2. RNA oligo-capping

To clone the variable V_H and V_L domains from the total RNA, the oligo-capping method reported by Maruyama and Sugano [40] using a GeneRacer™ kit (Thermo Fisher Scientific) was used. mRNA (250 ng) was incubated with calf intestinal phosphatase at 50 °C for 1 h to dephosphorylate non-mRNA or truncated mRNA species. After the reaction, phenol-chloroform extraction and ethanol precipitation were performed, and the dephosphorylated RNA was incubated with tobacco acid pyrophosphatase at 37°C for 1 h to remove the 5′-cap structure from the full-length mRNA. After phenol-chloroform extraction and ethanol precipitation, the synthetic RNA oligo (GeneRacer™ RNA Oligo, Thermo Fisher Scientific) was ligated to the decapped RNA with T4 RNA ligase at 37°C for 1 h. After phenol-chloroform extraction and ethanol precipitation, the RNA was suspended in diethylpyrocarbonate-treated water.

3.1.3. Reverse transcription of mRNA

The RNA-oligo ligated, full-length mRNA was reverse transcribed using a 54 base-pair primer containing an 18 nucleotide dT tail (GeneRacer™ Oligo-dT, Thermo Fisher Scientific) and avian myeloblastosis virus reverse transcriptase at 42°C for 1 h. After the reaction, the sample was diluted four times with sterile water.

3.1.4. Construction of a single-chain antibody gene

The cDNAs encoding V regions of the heavy and light (kappa) chains were PCR-amplified using a set of primers (V_H forward: 5'-TGA GGA GAC GGT GAC TGA GGT TCC-3', V_H reverse : 5'-CAG GTG CAG CTG AAG CAG TCA GG-3', V_{k2} forward: 5'-CCG TTT TAT TTC CAG CTT GGT CCC-3', V_k reverse : 5'-GAC ATC CAG ATG ACT CAG TCT CCA-3'). PCRs were run over 30 cycles (94°C for 30 sec, 60°C for 40 sec, and 72°C for 40 sec). V_H and V_L fragment-amplified PCR products were purified separately by agarose gel electrophoresis. The PCR products derived from the murine immunoglobulin V_H and V_L domain of Mab166 were subcloned into a pCR2.1 vector (TOPO cloning™, Thermo Fisher Scientific) and submitted to a DNA sequencing service for DNA sequence acquisition and analysis. Sequencing of the immunoglobulin variable genes for Mab166 was analyzed by The International imMunoGeneTics Database IMGT (http://www.imgt.org).

The purified V_H and V_L cDNAs were each assembled into a single gene using a DNA linker fragment-encoding a glycine-serine $(Gly_4Ser)_3$ linker peptide, thereby connecting the two cDNAs in the correct reading frame. Assembly PCR was run with a set of primers to multiply V_H-linker-V_L. The assembled fragment was amplified using two oligonucleotide primers with either an *Nco*I or *Xba*I restriction enzyme site at the 5′ end to facilitate cloning of the PCR product into a pBAD/gene III plasmid (Thermo Fisher Scientific) (**Figure 1**). The ligation mixture was used to transform *E. coli* TOP10 cells (Thermo Fisher Scientific), and subsequently to transform *E. coli* LMG194.

3.2. Expression and purification of recombinant single-chain antibody fragments

3.2.1. Expression and purification of scFv166

scFv166 protein expression was induced in the *E. coli* plasmid-harboring transformants by adding L-arabinose to a final concentration of 0.004%. After 24 h culture at 26°C with agitation at 200 rpm, the cells were collected by centrifugation at 5000× g for 20 min and then incubated in phosphate-buffered saline (PBS) with 1 mM ethylenediaminetetraacetic acid for 10 min on ice to obtain the periplasmic fraction. The osmotically shocked lysate was centrifuged at 15,000× g for 20 min, passed through a 0.4-μm-pore-size filter and dialyzed overnight against

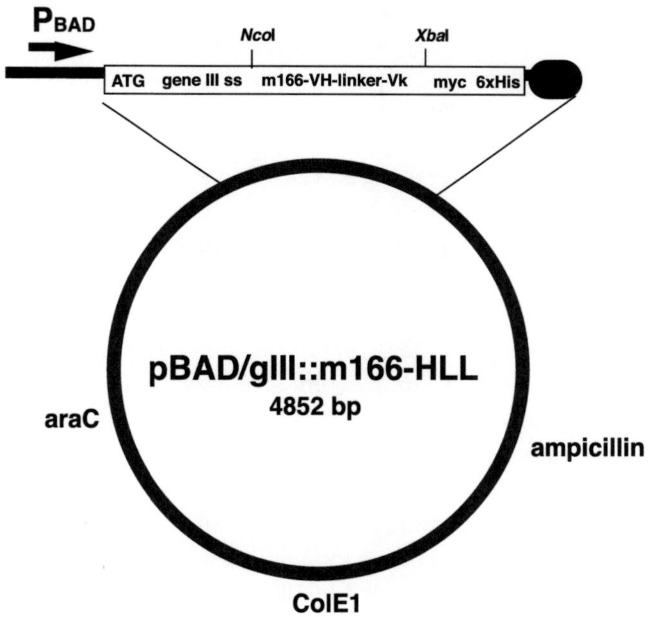

Figure 1. Expression vector pBAD/gIII::m166-HLL. The assembled scFv166 gene was subcloned into the pBAD/Gene III *E. coli* expression vector, downstream of, and in frame with, the gene III secretory leader sequence using *NcoI* and *XbaI* restriction sites.

lysis buffer (50 mM NaH_2PO_4, 300 mM NaCl, 10 mM imidazole, 0.05% Tween 20, pH 8.0). The lysate was mixed with nitrilotriacetic acid (Ni-NTA) agarose (Qiagen) for 30 min at 4°C with gentle shaking. After the Ni-NTA agarose was collected by centrifugation (4000× g), it was resuspended in lysis buffer and packed onto the chromatography column.

The column was washed twice with washing buffer (50 mM NaH_2PO_4, 300 mM NaCl, 20 mM imidazole, 0.05% Tween 20, pH 8.0), and the bound scFv166 antibodies were eluted with elution buffer (50 mM NaH_2PO_4, 300 mM NaCl, 250 mM imidazole, 0.05% Tween 20, pH 8.0). The eluate was dialyzed against PBS overnight and applied to an endotoxin removal column (Detoxi-Gel, Thermo Fisher Scientific) to get rid of the contaminating endotoxin. The purified antibodies were stored at −80°C until use.

In this study, we assembled the variable regions of the heavy and light chains of the anti-PcrV monoclonal IgG together with a glycine-serine linker in a single-chain antibody format. First, we assembled scFv166 in two different formats: one with V_H-linker-V_k positioned between the two variable segments (**Figure 2**), the other with V_k-linker-V_H positioned between two variable segments. The assembled scFv166 gene was subcloned into the *E. coli* pBAD/gene III expression vector, downstream of, and in frame with, the gene III secretory leader sequence. Expression of recombinant scFv166 was induced in *E. coli* by arabinose, after which it was purified via its C-terminal hexahistidine tag using Ni-NTA resin and conventional affinity column techniques. However, scFv-V_L-linker-V_H was highly insoluble, despite the expressed protein being detected in the whole lysates from *E. coli* cells after arabinose induction. Because scFv166 with its associated V_H-linker-V_L fragment was easier to purify as a soluble protein, we decided to focus on purifying it in that format. The purified scFv166 recognized the PcrV antigen in ELISAs and western immunoblots, as described in the next section.

3.3. Protein gels and immunoblot analyses

The purity of scFv166 was evaluated using sodium dodecyl sulfate polyacrylamide gel electrophoresis (SDS-PAGE) and Coomassie Blue staining (**Figure 3**). Briefly, samples of *E. coli* lysate were loaded onto a 4–15% Tris-HCl gel (BioRad Laboratories Inc., Hercules, CA, USA) and, after electrophoresis, the gel was stained with Coomassie Blue. For the immunoblot analysis, after SDS-PAGE, the protein was transferred to a nitrocellulose membrane and immunostained with a horseradish peroxidase-conjugated anti-c-myc IgG antibody, after which the blot was developed with a chemiluminescent substrate (ECL, GE Healthcare Bioscience, Piscataway, NJ). Immunoblots of scFv166 and precipitated *P. aeruginosa* proteins were also performed (**Figure 4**). *P. aeruginosa* PA103 was cultured in tryptic soy broth deferrated with nitrilotriacetic acid for 24 h at 31°C and, after centrifugation at 5000× g for 20 min, the supernatant was harvested. Saturated ammonium sulfate solution was added (final concentration, 55%), and the solution was incubated on ice for 1 h, and then centrifuged (20,000 × g, 30 min). The precipitated proteins were resuspended in 100 μL of PBS. After adding 100 μL of SDS-PAGE sample buffer and boiling for 5 min, the sample was analyzed by SDS-PAGE. After electrophoresis, the proteins were blotted onto a nitrocellulose membrane, and then immunostained with scFv166 and a horseradish peroxidase-conjugated anti-c-myc IgG secondary antibody, and the blot was developed with ECL.

```
Gene III signal sequence
ATG AAA AAA CTG CTG TTC GCG ATT CCG CTG GTG GTG CCG TTC TAT AGC CAT AGC ACC ATG
 M   K   K   L   L   F   A   I   P   L   V   V   P   F   Y   S   H   S   T   M

GAG CTC GAG CGG CAG GTG CAG CTG AAG CAG TCA GGA CCT GGC CTA GTG CGG CCC TCA CAG
 E   L   E   R   Q   V   Q   L   K   Q   S   G   P   G   L   V   R   P   S   Q
                                  VH-CDR1
AGC CTG TCC ATC ACC TGC ACA GTC TCT GGT TTC TCA TTA ACT AGC TAT GGT GTA CAC TGG
 S   L   S   I   T   C   T   V   S   G   F   S   L   T   S   Y   G   V   H   W
                                                VH-CDR2
GTT CGT CAG TCT CCA GGA AAG GGT CTG GAG TGG CTG GGA GTG ATA TGG AGT GGT GGA GAC
 V   R   Q   S   P   G   K   G   L   E   W   L   G   V   I   W   S   G   G   D     VH

ACA GAC TAT AAT GCA GCT TTC ATA TCC AGA CTG AGC ATC AGC AAG GAC AAT TCC AAG AGC
 T   D   Y   N   A   A   F   I   S   R   L   S   I   S   K   D   N   S   K   S

CAA CTC TTC TTT AAA ATG AAC AGT CTG CGA GCT ACT GAC ACA GCC ATA TAT TAC TGT GCC
 Q   L   F   F   K   M   N   S   L   R   A   T   D   T   A   I   Y   Y   C   A
VH-CDR3
AGA AAT AGA GGG GAT ATT TAC TAT GAT TTC ACT TAT GCC ATG GAC TAC TGG GGT CAA GGA
 R   N   R   G   D   I   Y   Y   D   F   T   Y   A   M   D   Y   W   G   Q   G
                            (G4S)3-linker
ACC TCA GTC ACC GTC TCC TCA GGT GGA GGC GGC TCA GGC GGA GGT GGC TCT GGC GGT GGC
 T   S   V   T   V   S   S   G   G   G   G   S   G   G   G   G   S   G   G   G

GGA TCG GAC ATC CAG ATG ACT CAG TCT CCA GCC TCC CTA TCT GCA TCT GTG GGA GAA ACT
 G   S   D   I   Q   M   T   Q   S   P   A   S   L   S   A   S   V   G   E   T
                                  Vk-CDR1
GTC ACC ATC ACA TGT CGA GCA AGT GGG AAT ATT CAA AAT TAT TTA GCA TGG TAT CAG CAG
 V   T   I   T   C   R   A   S   G   N   I   Q   N   Y   L   A   W   Y   Q   Q
                                            Vk-CDR2
ACA CAG GGA AAA TCT CCT CAG CTC CTG GTC TAT TCT GCA AAA ACC TTA GCA GAT GGT GTG
 T   Q   G   K   S   P   Q   L   L   V   Y   S   A   K   T   L   A   D   G   V     Vk

CCA TCA AGG TTC AGT GGC AGT GGA TCA GGA ACA CAA TAT TCT CTC AAG ATC AAC AGC CTG
 P   S   R   F   S   G   S   G   S   G   T   Q   Y   S   L   K   I   N   S   L
                                      Vk-CDR3
CAG CCT GAA GAT TTT GGG AGT TAT TAC TGT CAA CAT TTT TGG AGT ACT CCG TAC ACG TTC
 Q   P   E   D   F   G   S   Y   Y   C   Q   H   F   W   S   T   P   Y   T   F
                                              cMyc-tag
GGA GGG GGG ACC AAG CTG GAA ATA AAA CGG GCT CTA GAA CAA AAA CTC ATC TCA GAA GAG
 G   G   G   T   K   L   E   I   K   R   A   L   E   Q   K   L   I   S   E   E
                           6xHis-tag
GAT CTG AAT AGC GCC GTC GAC CAT CAT CAT CAT CAT CAT TGA
 D   L   N   S   A   V   D   H   H   H   H   H   H   *
```

Figure 2. scFv166 nucleotide sequence. After the gene III signal sequence (18 aa) and the short joint region (6 aa), the V_H region (123 aa) is followed by the glycine-serine linker (15 aa), the V_L region (108 aa), a cMyc-tag, and a hexahistidine-tag.

3.4. Affinity determination of scFv166

The affinity of scFv166 for its cognate antigen was determined by competition ELISA, and the result was compared with that of the hybridoma-derived parental Mab166, as described previously [41], **Figure 5**. Briefly, in the first step, the total antibody concentration range in which the absorbance correlates proportionately with the free antibody concentration was

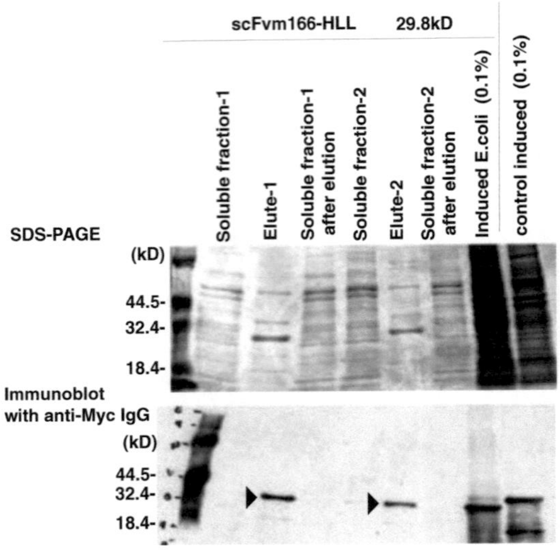

Figure 3. Expression and purification of scFv166. *E. coli* lysates were loaded onto a 4–15% gradient Tris-HCl gel and, after electrophoresis, the gel was stained with Coomassie Blue. For the immunoblot analysis, after polyacrylamide gel electrophoresis, the protein was blotted onto a nitrocellulose membrane and immunostained with a horseradish peroxidase-conjugated anti-c-Myc IgG antibody, and the blot was developed with a chemiluminescent substrate. The secreted scFv166 (298 amino acids) was detected as a 29.7 kD-band in the elute-1 and elute-2, designated by arrows. Soluble fraction: the osmotically shocked lysate; elute: the eluted solution from an Ni-NTA agarose column; soluble fraction after elution: the solution passed through an Ni-NTA agarose column (two sets of the lysate and the column elute were analyzed and labeled "–1" and "–2", respectively).

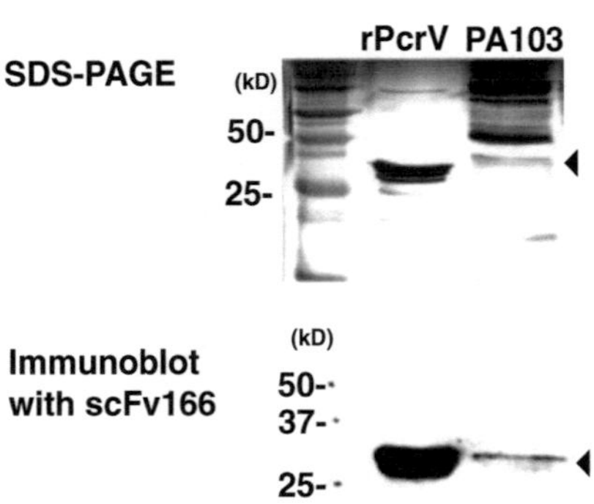

Figure 4. Immunoblot of *P. aeruginosa* proteins reacted with scFv166. Precipitated *P. aeruginosa* PA103 proteins were resuspended in 100 μL of PBS. After adding 100 μL of SDS-PAGE sample buffer and boiling for 5 min, the proteins in the sample were separated by SDS-PAGE with *E. coli*-derived recombinant PcrV (rPcrV) as a reference. After electrophoresis, the proteins were transferred to a nitrocellulose membrane, and immunostained with scFv166 and a horseradish peroxidase-conjugated secondary anti-c-Myc IgG antibody and the blot was developed with a chemiluminescent substrate. The bindings of scFv166 to both native PA103 PcrV (294 amino aicds, 32.4 kD) and recombinant PcrV (rPcrV, 306 amino acids, 33.8 kD) were detected as shown in arrows.

measured by indirect ELISA with the PcrV antigen coated at 1 μg/mL. In the second step, K_d, the dissociation constant, was measured using binding equilibrium studies (competition ELISA) to determine the concentration that gives 50% inhibition of maximum binding.

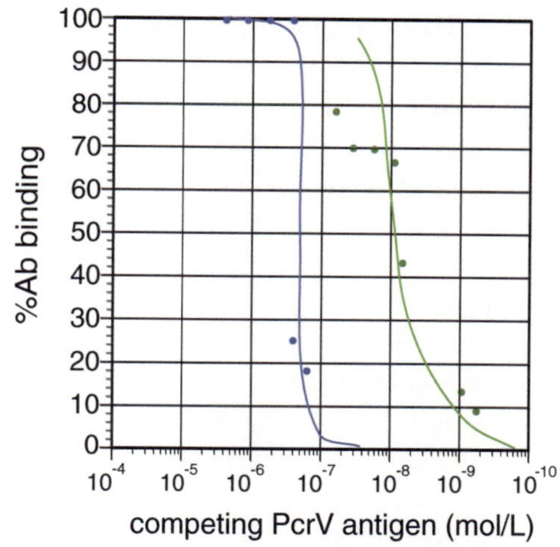

Figure 5. Binding affinities of Mab166 and scFv166 in competition ELISA. Binding affinities (K_d) of Mab166 and scFv166 to immobilized PcrV were evaluated in a competition ELISA.

4. Results

4.1. Aminoacid sequence of V_H, V_L of scFv166

The sequence of the Mab166 heavy chain region is shown in **Figure 2**. The DNA sequence of the 5′-untranslational region and a V-region segment in the heavy chain-containing complementarity determining regions (CDRs) 1 and 2 is identical (except two amino acids in the frame 3 region) to germline Musmus IGHV2S2 (IGHV subgroup 2, V_H#101, Accession #J00502). The V-region sequence also shows the same level of homology as that reported for pseudogene, IGHV2S5 (Accession #M21165). Transcription starts 24 nucleotides downstream of the TATA box of germline IGHV2S2. Nucleotides differ from the germline sequence at 10 positions, and these cause the following amino acid changes: position #61 in CDR2 S->D, #87 in FR3 V->L, #95 Q->R, and #96 S->A, #97 N->T. The first 15 nucleotides in the D-region encode the first 5 unique amino acids in CDR3, and the region consists of 16 amino acids in total. The J-region DNA sequence is identical to the IGHJ4 germline sequence (Accession #V00770). The unique CDR3 sequence includes the Arg-Gly-Asp (RGD) sequence, which functions as a recognition sequence for adhesion receptors in many adhesive proteins including fibrinogen, fibronectin, von Willebrand factor, and vitronectin.

The nucleotide sequence of the variable region of the kappa light chain, along with its predicted amino acid sequence, is shown in **Figure 2**. The CDRs are underlined, and the amino acids are numbered according to a convention. This kappa variable chain is a class II mouse kappa variable region. Although its sequence is not identical to any germline variable regions present in the data bank (The International ImMunoGeneTics Database IMGT), the DNA sequence of the 5′-untranslational region, and V-region of the kappa light chain shows the highest homology to germline Musumus IGKV12-41*01F (IGKV subgroup 12, Accession #AJ235953). Transcription starts from nine nucleotides downstream of the TATA box. Nucleotides differ from the germline sequence at four positions (+#192, C->A), (+#218, A->C), (+#250, A->T, +#251, A->C), and they cause amino acid changes at the following positions: #30 in CDR1 H->Q, #45 in FR2 K->T, and #56 in CDR2 N->S. The DNA sequence in the J-region is identical to germline IGKJ2 (Accession #V00777).

4.2. Evaluation of the expressed scFv166

Immunoblot to the anti-cMyc tag visualized the secreted scFv166 (298 amino acids) as a predicted 29.8 kD-band in the eluted solution from Ni-NTA agarose as shown in **Figure 3**. The bindings of scFv166 to both native PA103 PcrV (294 amino acids, 32.4 kD) and recombinant PcrV(rPcrV, 306 amino acids, 33.8 kD) were confirmed as shown in **Figure 4**. The binding affinity of Mab166 was 1×10^{-8} M, while that of scFv166 was 5×10^{-6} M (**Figure 5**).

4.3. Humanization and affinity maturation

The next step, for human use, after testing the binding affinity of scFv166 to a target molecule, together with the affinity maturation steps, is the elimination of the human-specific antigenic mouse amino acid sequence. In fact, Mab166 has already been humanized by antibody affinity engineering by serial epitope-guided complementarity replacement (SECR) which is a licensed humanization/affinity maturation technique of KaloBios Pharmaceutical Inc (Brisbane, California, USA) [33, 37] (**Figure 6**). In brief, SECR provides for a method for obtaining human idiologs for any nonhuman antibody to any target by epitope-guided replacement of variable regions using competitive cell-based methods in which the competitor can be either the reference antibody or a ligand that binds to the same epitope on the target as the reference antibody [37]. Fab 1A8 of humanized Mab166 by SECR bound to PcrV with approximately a twofold-higher affinity than the original murine Mab166 Fab [37]. Therefore, a further modification of scFv166 can be done by referring to the existing information available for the modified amino acid sequences in Fab 1A8 [33].

heavy chain IgG2b CDR3	murine (Mab166) humanized (1A8)	NRGDIYYDFTYAMDY NRGDIYYDFTYAXDZ (X D M/F, Z D I/S/Q)
light chain κ CDR3	murine (Mab166) humanized (1A8)	QHFWSTPYT QQFWXTPYT (X D S/G)
FR4	murine (Mab166) humanized (1A8)	FGGGTKLEIKR FGGGTKLTVLR

Figure 6. Amino acid sequence differences between murine Mab166 and humanized Fab 1A8. CDR3 in the heavy chain, CDR3 and FR4 in the light chain (*k*) of humanized Fab 1A8 have sequence modifications following humanization and affinity maturation compared to corresponding sequences of Mab166.

http://dx.doi.org/10.5772/intechopen.70316

5. Conclusion

We have shown in an *in vivo* study that instillation of a single dose of Fab into the lungs of mice protected them against a lethal pulmonary challenge with *P. aeruginosa* [36]. The ability to use a recombinant Fab fragment for the treatment of *P. aeruginosa* infection in patients with ventilator-associated pneumonia or chronically infected cystic fibrosis patients has potential to minimize acute lung injury and mortality associated with TTS virulence of *P. aeruginosa*. Further optimization, such as the affinity maturation and PEGylation, will be the next step to achieve clinical application in humans. An engineered single-chain antibody that binds to the *P. aeruginosa* PcrV protein with high affinity has strong potential to be an effective new therapeutic reagent for infections caused by *P. aeruginosa*.

Acknowledgements

This work was supported by the Japan Society for the Promotion of Science, Grant-in-Aid for Scientific Research (KAKENHI No. 24390403, 26670791, and 15H05008) and by The Ministry of Education, Culture, Sports, Science and Technology, Japan to Teiji Sawa. The research studies associated with this chapter were carried out in the University of California San Francisco (UCSF) when Teiji Sawa was an Anesthesia/UCSF faculty member, under the generous support of Dara W. Frank, Department of Microbiology and Molecular Genetics, Medical College of Wisconsin, and Jeanine P. Wiener-Kronish, Department of Anesthesia, Critical Care and Pain Medicine, Massachusetts General Hospital.

Abbreviations

CDR	complementarity determining region
P. aeruginosa	*Pseudomonas aeruginosa*
SECR	serial epitope-guided complementarity replacement
TTS	type III secretory
TTSS	type III secretion system

Author details

Teiji Sawa[1]*, Atsushi Kainuma[1], Kiyoshi Moriyama[2] and Yoshifumi Naito[1]

*Address all correspondence to: anesth@koto.kpu-m.ac.jp

1 Department of Anesthesiology, Kyoto Prefectural University of Medicine, Kyoto, Japan

2 Department of Anesthesiology, School of Medicine, Korin University, Mitaka, Japan

References

[1] Salyers AA, Whitt DD. *Pseudomonas aeruginosa*. In: Salyers AA, White DD, editors. Bacterial Pathogenesis: A Molecular Approach. Washington, DC: American Society for Microbiology Press; 1994. pp. 260-270

[2] Govan JR, Deretic V. Microbial pathogenesis in cystic fibrosis: Mucoid *Pseudomonas aeruginosa* and *Burkholderia cepacia*. Microbiological Reviews. 1996;**60**:539-574

[3] Ramirez-Estrada S, Borgatta B, Rello J. *Pseudomonas aeruginosa* ventilator-associated pneumonia management. Infection and Drug Resistance. 2016;**9**:7-18. DOI: 10.2147/IDR.S50669

[4] Grgurich PE, Hudcova J, Lei Y, et al. Management and prevention of ventilator-associated pneumonia caused by multidrug-resistant pathogens. Expert Review of Respiratory Medicine. 2012;**6**:533-555. DOI: 10.1586/ers.12.45

[5] Kudoh I, Wiener-Kronish JP, Hashimoto S, et al. Exoproduct secretions of *Pseudomonas aeruginosa* strains influence severity of alveolar epithelial injury. American Journal of Physiology. 1994;**267**:L551-L556

[6] Yahr TL, Mende-Mueller LM, Friese MB, et al. Identification of type III secreted products of the *Pseudomonas aeruginosa* exoenzyme S regulon. Journal of Bacteriology. 1997;**179**:7165-7168

[7] Finck-Barbançon V, Goranson J, Zhu L, et al. ExoU expression by *Pseudomonas aeruginosa* correlates with acute cytotoxicity and epithelial injury. Molecular Microbiology. 1997;**25**:547-557

[8] Sawa T, Ohara M, Kurahashi K, et al. In vitro cellular toxicity predicts *Pseudomonas aeruginosa* virulence in lung infections. Infection and Immunity. 1998;**66**:3242-3249

[9] Kurahashi K, Kajikawa O, Sawa T, Ohara M, Gropper MA, Frank DW, Martin TR, Wiener-Kronish JP. Pathogenesis of septic shock in *Pseudomonas aeruginosa* pneumonia. Journal of Clinical Investigation. 1999;**104**:743-750

[10] Hueck CJ. Type III protein secretion systems in bacterial pathogens of animals and plants. Microbiology and Molecular Biology Reviews. 1998;**62**:379-433

[11] Galan JE, Collmer A. Type III secretion machines: Bacterial devices for protein delivery into host cells. Science. 1999;**284**:1322-1328

[12] Yahr TL, Goranson J, Frank DW. Exoenzyme S of *Pseudomonas aeruginosa* is secreted by a type III pathway. Molecular Microbiology. 1996;**22**:991-1003

[13] Frank DW. The exoenzyme S regulon of *Pseudomonas aeruginosa*. Molecular Microbiology. 1997;**26**:621-629

[14] Goranson J, Frank DW. Genetic analysis of exoenzyme S expression by *Pseudomonas aeruginosa*. FEMS Microbiology Letters. 1996;**135**:149-155

[15] Sawa T. The molecular mechanism of acute lung injury caused by *Pseudomonas aeruginosa*: From bacterial pathogenesis to host response. Journal of Intensive Care Medicine. 2014;**2**:10. DOI: 10.1186/2052-0492-2-10

[16] Sato H, Frank DW, Hillard CJ, et al. The mechanism of action of the *Pseudomonas aeruginosa*-encoded type III cytotoxin, ExoU. EMBO Journal. 2003;**22**:2959-2969. DOI: 10.1093/emboj/cdg290

[17] Tamura M, Ajayi T, Allmond LR, et al. Lysophospholipase A activity of *Pseudomonas aeruginosa* type III secretory toxin ExoU. Biochemical and Biophysical Research Communications. 2004;**316**:323-331. DOI: 10.1016/j.bbrc.2004.02.050

[18] Pankhaniya RR, Tamura M, Allmond LR, et al. *Pseudomonas aeruginosa* causes acute lung injury via the catalytic activity of the patatin-like phospholipase domain of ExoU. Critical Care Medicine. 2004;**32**:2293-2299

[19] Sawa T, Shimizu M, Moriyama K, et al. Association between *Pseudomonas aeruginosa* type III secretion, antibiotic resistance, and clinical outcome: A review. Critical Care. 2014;**18**:668. DOI: 10.1186/s13054-014-0668-9

[20] Sawa T, Hamaoka S, Kinoshita M, et al. *Pseudomonas aeruginosa* type III secretory toxin ExoU and its predicted homologs. Toxins. 2016;**8**:307. DOI: 10.3390/toxins8110307

[21] Yahr TL, Vallis AJ, Hancock MK, et al. ExoY, an adenylate cyclase secreted by the *Pseudomonas aeruginosa* type III system. Proceedings of the National Academy of Sciences of the United States of America. 1998;**95**:13899-13904

[22] Roy-Burman A, Savel R, Racine S, et al. Type-III protein secretion is associated with death in lower respiratory and systemic *Pseudomonas aeruginosa* infections. Journal of Infectious Diseases. 2001;**183**:1767-1774

[23] Sawa T, Yahr TL, Ohara M, et al. Active and passive immunization with the *Pseudomonas* V antigen protects against type III intoxication and lung injury. Nature Medicine. 1999; **5**:392-398

[24] Burrows TW, Bacon GA. The basis of virulence in *Pasteurella pestis*: Antigen determining virulence. British Journal of Experimental Pathology. 1956;**37**:481-493

[25] Burrows TW, Bacon GA. The effects of loss of different virulence determinants on the virulence and immunogenicity of strains of *Pasteurella pestis*. British Journal of Experimental Pathology. 1958;**39**:278-291

[26] Lawton WD, Erdman RI, Surgalla MJ. Biosynthesis and purification of V and W antigens in *Pasteurella pestis*. Journal of Immunology. 1963;**91**:179-184

[27] Une T, Brubaker RR. Role of V antigen in promoting virulence and immunity in *Yersiniae*. Journal of Immunology. 1984;**133**:2226-2230

[28] Motin VL, Nakajima R, Smirnov GB, et al. Passive immunity to *Yersiniae* mediated by anti-recombinant V-antigen and protein A-V antigen fusion peptide. Infection and Immunity. 1994;**62**:4192-4201

[29] Hill J, Leary SEC, Griffin K, et al. Regions of *Yersinia pestis* V antigen that contribute to protection against plague identified by passive and active immunization. Infection and Immunity. 1997;**65**:4476-4482

[30] Leary SEC, Williamson ED, Griffin KF, et al. Active immunization with recombinant V antigen from *Yersinia pestis* protects mice against plague. Infection and Immunity. 1995;**63**:2854-2858

[31] Anderson Jr. GW, Leary SEC, Williamson ED, et al. Recombinant V antigen protects mice against pneumonic and bubonic plague caused by F1-capsule-positive and -negative strains of *Yersinia pestis*. Infection and Immunity. 1996;**64**:4580-4585

[32] Sawa T, Wiener-Kronish JP. A therapeutic strategy against the shared virulence mechanism utilized by both *Yersinia pestis* and *Pseudomonas aeruginosa*. Anesthesiology Clinics of North America. 2004;**22**:591-606

[33] Sawa T, Ito E, Nguyen VH, et al. Anti-PcrV antibody strategies against virulent *Pseudomonas aeruginosa*. Human Vaccines & Immunotherapeutics. 2014;**10**:2843-2852. DOI: 10.4161/21645515.2014.971641

[34] Shime N, Sawa T, Fujimoto J, et al. Therapeutic administration of anti-PcrV $F(ab')_2$ in sepsis associated with *Pseudomonas aeruginosa*. Journal of Immunology. 2001;**167**:5880-5886

[35] Frank DW, Vallis A, Wiener-Kronish JP, et al. Generation and characterization of a protective monoclonal antibody to *Pseudomonas aeruginosa* PcrV. Journal of Infectious Diseases. 2002;**186**:64-73

[36] Faure K, Fujimoto J, Shimabukuro DW, et al. Effects of monoclonal anti-PcrV antibody on *Pseudomonas aeruginosa*-induced acute lung injury in a rat model. Journal of Immune Based Therapies and Vaccines. 2003;**1**:2

[37] Baer M, Sawa T, Flynn P, et al. An engineered human antibody fab fragment specific for *Pseudomonas aeruginosa* PcrV antigen has potent antibacterial activity. Infection and Immunity 2009;**77**:1083-1090. DOI: 10.1128/IAI.00815-08

[38] Francois B, Luyt CE, Dugard A, et al. Safety and pharmacokinetics of an anti-PcrV PEGylated monoclonal antibody fragment in mechanically ventilated patients colonized with *Pseudomonas aeruginosa*: A randomized, double-blind, placebo-controlled trial. Critical Care Medicine. 2012;**40**:2320-2326. DOI: 10.1097/CCM.0b013e31825334f6

[39] Milla CE, Chmiel JF, Accurso FJ, et al. Anti-PcrV antibody in cystic fibrosis: A novel approach targeting *Pseudomonas aeruginosa* airway infection. Pediatric Pulmonology. 2013;**49**:650-658. DOI: 10.1002/ppul.22890

[40] Maruyama K, Sugano S. Oligo-capping: A simple method to replace the cap structure of eukaryotic mRNAs with oligobonucleotides. Gene. 2002;**138**:171-174

[41] Djavadi-Ohaniance L, Goldberg ME, Friguet B. Measuring antibody affinity in solution. In: McCafferty J, Hoogenboom HR, Chiswell DJ, editors. Antibody Engineering. New York: Oxford University Press Inc.; 1996. pp. 77-97

Chapter 7

Separation of Monoclonal Antibodies by Analytical Size Exclusion Chromatography

Atis Chakrabarti

Additional information is available at the end of the chapter

http://dx.doi.org/10.5772/intechopen.73321

Abstract

Size exclusion chromatography (SEC) is a powerful tool for the separation of biotherapeutics such as monoclonal antibodies (mAb) and others such as antibody drug conjugates (ADCs), biosimilars, and bi-specific mAbs as well as other therapeutic proteins. Detection of purified protein heterogeneity is essential. Heterogenic impurities cause immunogenic response. More than 99% purity is needed for the medicinal purpose. Size exclusion chromatography (SEC) is used to monitor this purity level in the quality control (QC) process of the biopharmaceutical industry. With the increased use of ultra-high-performance liquid chromatography (UHPLC) instruments in QC laboratories today, instead of the conventional HPLC, it is important to have a size exclusion chromatography (SEC) column which is compatible with both UHPLC and conventional HPLC instruments. Orthogonal and complimentary modes such as reversed phase chromatography (RPC), hydrophobic interaction chromatography (HIC), and ion exchange chromatography (IEC) can also be used along with SEC. SEC columns are generally modified with diol groups on the surface to prevent a secondary interaction. Surface and pore characteristics of the SEC columns are critical for the separation. Pore characteristics need to be optimized to have high resolution of mAb monomer from dimer and higher order aggregates as well as from fragments. Shallow calibration curve is necessary for the best resolution. Overall, the separation of monoclonal antibodies from the impurities by analytical size exclusion chromatography column is primarily discussed in this chapter. The evaluation of the different peak parameters such as retention time, peak asymmetry, column efficiency, peak resolution, run time, and loading capacity is also briefly discussed. Finally, the tips and tricks for the best separation and maintaining the column health are also discussed.

Keywords: mAb, monoclonal antibody, heterogeneity, aggregate, SEC, size exclusion, ADC, bi-specific antibody, mass spectroscopy

INTECH
open science | open minds

© 2018 The Author(s). Licensee InTech. This chapter is distributed under the terms of the Creative Commons Attribution License (http://creativecommons.org/licenses/by/3.0), which permits unrestricted use, distribution, and reproduction in any medium, provided the original work is properly cited.

1. Introduction

Antibodies belong to a family of globular proteins called immunoglobulins [1]. Immunoglobulin G (IgG) is the most common. Eighty percent of all the antibodies present in the blood are IgG [2]. IgG is a relatively large molecule (approx. 150 kDa). It has four subclasses, which are IgG1, IgG2, IgG3, and IgG4 [3]. Monoclonal antibodies are antibodies derived from one unique B cell clone [4]. They have single antigenic determinant specificities [5]. Monoclonal antibodies are screened and isolated by special procedures, expressed, and purified [6]. Monoclonal antibodies, particularly IgG1, have tremendous application in biotherapeutics. Other subclasses such as IgG2 and IgG4 are also used as biotherapeutic, and interest in these two antibody classes is also increasing. As for today, IgG1 comprise most of the mAb biotherapeutic drugs in the market. Twenty-nine new mAbs are presently undergoing late-stage clinical trials, including human and humanized IgG1, IgG2, and IgG4 molecules [7]. Few IgG2 and IgG4 drugs are already available such as OKT3 (Muronomab-CD3), a murine IgG2a drug from Johnson & Johnson (1986), Bexxar (Tositumomab-I-131), and a murine IgG2a drug radiolabeled with I-131 from Corixa/GSK (2003). IgG4 antibodies are evolving as an important class of cancer immunotherapies [8].

Size exclusion chromatography (SEC) is a powerful analytical tool for the separation of monoclonal antibodies and other proteins [9]. SEC, as a strategy for the isolation and purification of antibodies, is not new; in 1989, high-resolution Superose 6 HR 10/30 fast protein liquid chromatography (FPLC) columns were used. [10]. Since then, many researchers used SEC for the purification of antibodies. The literature search for the number of "publications on the purification of monoclonal antibodies by size exclusion chromatography" [11] shows that between 1983 and 2003, there was a surge of research in this regard (**Figure 1**).

For the large-scale purification of monoclonal antibody biotherapeutics, Protein A is commonly used as the primary capture step. Following the use of Protein A chromatography, SEC is used to characterize the Protein A purified fractions. Size exclusion chromatography (SEC) is primarily used for the separation in analytical HPLC and for routine quality control

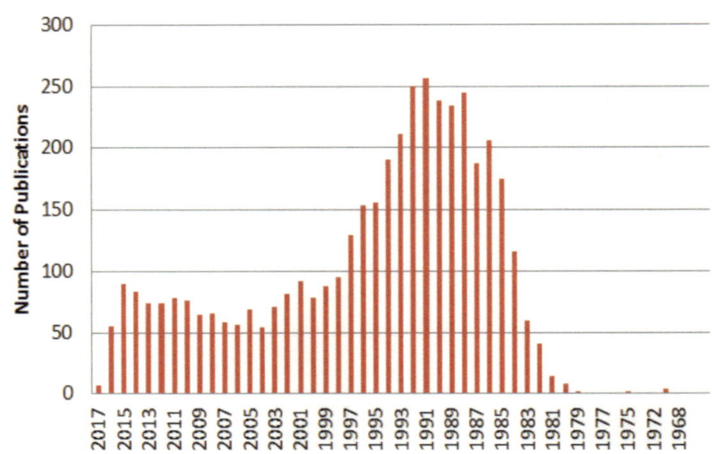

Figure 1. Number of publications dealing with size exclusion chromatography over the years.

analysis of the mAb. Detection wavelength of 280 nm is commonly used. SEC combined with multi-angle light scattering is one method for the characterization of the molar mass distribution of mAb, ADC, and other biomolecules [12].

In this chapter, certain aspects of size exclusion chromatography and its use in the analytical purification or separation of monoclonal antibodies are discussed. Secondary interactions, effects of particle size and pore size on the SEC separation, particularly in resolving monomer peak from dimer and fragment peaks with a better resolution are also discussed. Selection of the right SEC column is critical to achieve the goal of separation. The calibration curve has a very important role in this regard. Since there are different kinds of proteins differing in structure and shape, many vendors provide calibration curves using globular protein standards, branched standards, and linear standards, so that the separation range can ideally be interpreted under the chromatographic conditions.

Reproducible separation of a monomer from its dimer and other high molecular weight (HMW) impurities, fragments, and other low molecular weight (LMW) impurities is needed during the purification of the mAb biotherapeutic. Optimized particle chemistry and packing of SEC column help in this regard. mAb analysis using a mobile phase containing an appropriate amount of selected organic solvents such as isopropyl alcohol (IPA) may be needed to prevent alteration of peak retention time, poor peak shape, or resolution. Few examples are shown to elaborate this. Digestion with papain or pepsin is commonly applied to obtain antibody fragments without the loss of activity—this is discussed in the context of selecting right SEC columns from a variety of particle sizes, pore sizes, and dimensions. Forced degradation studies are needed to assess the stability of the protein, to understand the mechanism of degradation by oxidation, heat, light, or hydrolysis. Forced degradation study by SEC is separately discussed in Section 2.7. Interest in the accurate molecular weight analysis of intact monoclonal antibody IgG1 by SEC using MS-friendly mobile phases is increasing, and it is discussed in Section 4. Section 5 focuses mostly on the use of chromatographic methods which are orthogonal or complimentary size exclusion and useful to detect the protein heterogeneity. The use of ultra HPLC is needed for fast separation, and many methods already developed in HPLC need to be easily transferred to UHPLC. Section 6 briefly discusses the usefulness of a SEC column compatible to both HPLC and UHPLC instruments by easy method transfer. Section 7 is about desalting of mAb or any biopolymer solution, not by dialysis membrane or spin column but by using an analytical SEC HPLC column. The use of SEC column in hydrophilic liquid chromatography (HILIC) mode is interesting and can separate the nucleobases (Section 8). This chapter ends with few remarks about the tips and tricks for size exclusion chromatography.

2. Size exclusion chromatography and purification of monoclonal antibodies

2.1. Size exclusion chromatography

Size exclusion chromatography uses a molecular sieving retention mechanism [13], based on differences in the hydrodynamic radii or differences in size of analytes such as proteins. Large sample molecules cannot penetrate or only partially penetrate the pores of the stationary phase. So, the larger molecules elute first and smaller molecules elute later, the order of elution being a function of the size.

SEC is the only mode of chromatography where theoretically there is no interaction of the analyte with a stationary phase. The whole process of partitioning or separating the different molecular species is due to the entropy factor and not due to adsorption, ΔH being equal to zero. Pure Silica particles are most commonly used as base material in this type of chromatography of biomolecules. Since the separation of the biomolecule by SEC will depend on its hydrodynamic radii, two proteins of the same molecular weight (such as 70 kDa) may elute at two different retention times, if there is a difference in their hydrodynamic radii (**Figure 2**). So, any factor at any stage of purification, affecting the shape of the protein, will affect the elution volume or retention time.

Unless otherwise mentioned, SEC analyses discussed in this chapter were carried out using the mobile phase 100 mM KH_2PO_4/Na_2HPO_4, pH 6.7, 100 mM Na_2SO_4, 0.05% NaN_3. Agilent 1100, Agilent 1200 HPLC and Thermo Ultimate 3000 UHPLC systems and associated software were used for integration and peak analysis. Sodium azide (NaN_3) was used as an antibacterial agent to prevent fouling of the phosphate buffer. Detection wavelength was 280 nm unless otherwise mentioned. Flow rates and injection volume of the sample are varied as needed. Reproducibility for calculation of % relative standard deviation (RSD) was based on 10 consecutive injections. Linearity of both monomer and dimer during loading study was calculated based on peak areas versus total material loaded during injection. Please refer to individual chromatograms for the respective chromatographic conditions.

2.2. SEC and secondary interaction

As mentioned earlier, among all modes of chromatography, it is only during the size exclusion chromatography where the analyst does not demonstrate any kind of interaction with the stationary phase. During all other chromatographic modes, an analyst demonstrates some kind of interaction between the protein and the stationary phase, followed by the elution using

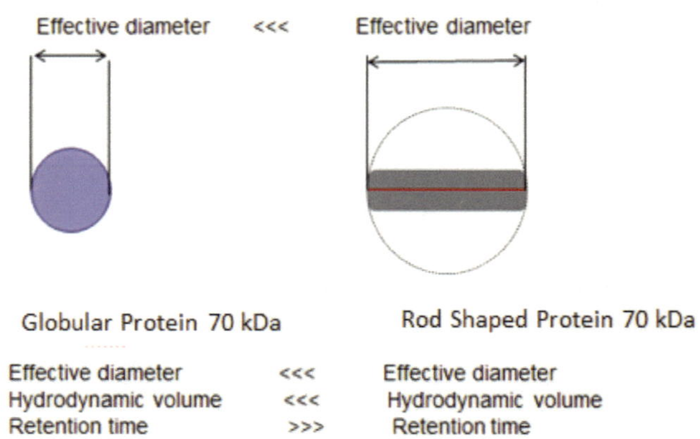

Figure 2. Comparison of globular and rod-shaped proteins.

a stronger solvent. This is because SEC is purely a separation technique based on the permeability of the protein through the pores. Any factor which will prevent the free passage through the pores will result into a nonideal SEC condition. These interactions between proteins and the stationary phases are called secondary interactions. The secondary interactions are based on charge-related interactions or hydrophobicity-related interactions. The secondary interaction coming from the free silanol groups present on the silica surface of the stationary phase is often protected by a diol-bonded coating on the stationary phase which shields the silica surface from such action [14].

In a real-world situation, any secondary interaction between the stationary phase and the proteins including monoclonal antibodies needs to be taken care of by selecting the right column where the stationary phase is effectively coated, and free silanol groups are inaccessible to proteins. Further method development by optimizing the chromatographic conditions may be needed to get the best separation. Ionic and hydrophobic interactions between the sample and the column packing material can be avoided by controlling the ionic strength. A general rule of thumb is that low ionic strength (<0.1 M) may induce charge-related secondary interactions and high ionic strength (>1.0 M) may lead to hydrophobicity-related secondary interactions, while the concept of low or high concentration may vary from mAb to mAb depending on the nature of the individual one. For each protein sample, there will be an optimal buffer type and salt concentration for the best separation that results in the highest resolution and recovery. This can be found out by trial and error approach only. If a sticky protein comes into contact with the stationary phase (dotted line in the figure below), it may undergo a conformational change; the binding constant of the conformationally changed protein can be so strong that it would not elute out of the column (**Figure 3**). The use of additives may be needed. Arginine prevents binding to the surface [15]. Similarly, a number of other additives may also be used to minimize the secondary interactions. The use of isopropyl alcohol (IPA) as another additive to avoid nonspecific interaction and the reproducibility of the analysis is somewhat discussed in the Section 2.5.

There is no universal protocol for working with additives to avoid nonspecific interactions for all proteins. Chromatographic conditions preventing secondary interactions need to be found out by trial-and-error type of experiments with a variety of additives.

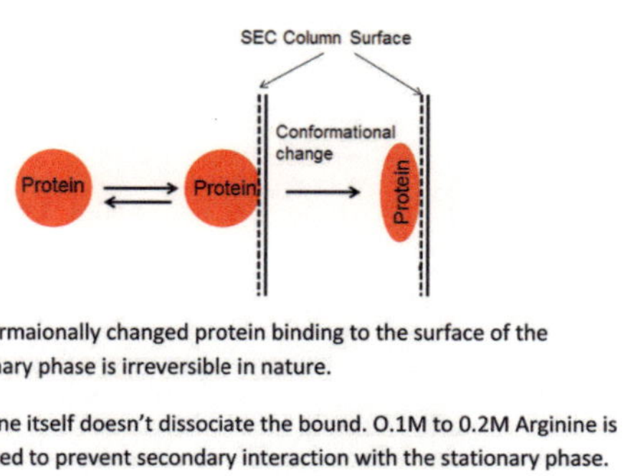

Figure 3. Binding of a protein to the stationary phase and the influence of arginine.

2.3. Effect of particle size and pore size of the stationary phase on SEC separation

Particle size and pore size are important factors for better peak shape, peak sensitivity, and resolution. SEC columns with smaller particle size yield better separation and resolution but with higher back pressure as expected from the basic chromatography theory.

Pore characteristics need to be optimized for SEC separation of biomolecules. To have the high resolution of a mAb monomer from dimer and higher order aggregates as well as from fragments, permeability through the pores of the SEC stationary phases is needed. This is similar to accessibility of the pore needed in reverse phase chromatography (RPC) for better mass transfer kinetics. The larger pore size helps in more efficient permeation of the biomolecules inside the pores, resulting in better size-based separation (**Figure 4**); 8–14 nm pores are not suitable for the separation of large intact biomolecules and its aggregates since they are too large to enter into the pores. SEC columns with 25 nm pore size are widely available and popular for SEC separation of biomolecules. In the last few years, even larger pore size, such as 30 nm SEC columns, became available in the market, which enables increased permeability of the higher order aggregates of large biomolecules.

Increase in the pore volume of the packing material results into a shallower slope in the calibration curve and increases the spread in elution time between compounds with different molecular masses and improves resolution. But there is a limit to what extent the pore of a particle of definite size can be stretched to its maximum. This is because as the pore volume of a packing material increases, the strength of the packing material generally decreases, making the material more fragile. **Figure 5** [16] illustrates the relation between the particle and pore characteristics to the resolution and other peak parameters.

It is important to compromise between the particle sizes and pore volume in order to get the desired separation. Pore characteristics of the SEC column need to be optimized to have a high resolution of a mAb monomer from a dimer and higher order aggregates, as well as from fragments. For large biomolecules, such as therapeutic proteins and monoclonal antibodies (mAbs), a larger exclusion limit will yield better separation particularly of the dimer and higher order aggregates from the monomer.

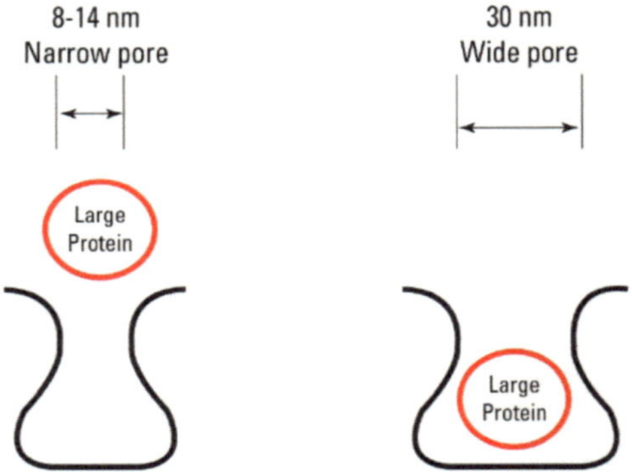

Figure 4. Permeation of large molecules into pores depends on the pore size.

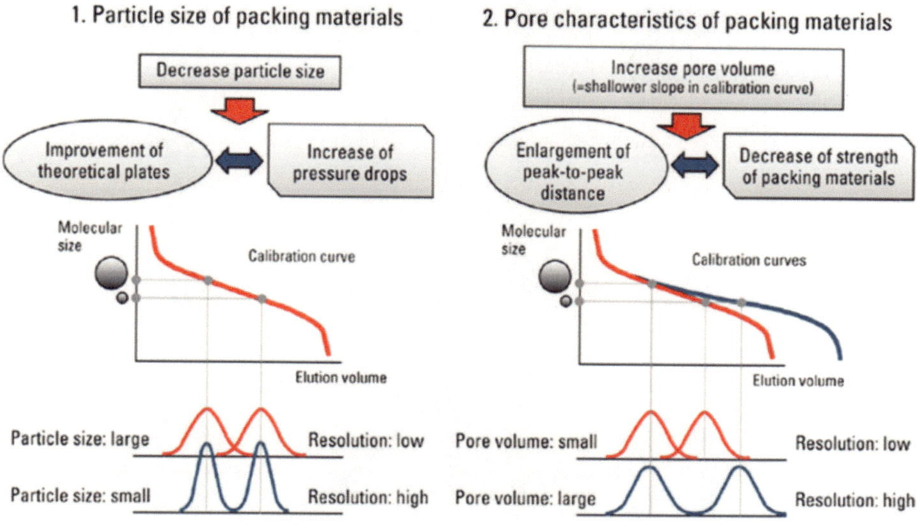

Figure 5. Relation between the particle and pore characteristics to the resolution and other peak parameters.

2.4. SEC column selection and calibration curve

In the absence of any secondary or non-SEC retention mechanism, the calibration yields an S-shaped curve containing a linear portion in between the total exclusion and total inclusion limits. In **Figure 6** [17], the calibration curve was generated using three different types of standards (globular, branched, and linear).

The red line in **Figure 6** represents the average molecular weight of the monoclonal antibody (mAb) IgG (150 kDa). If we follow the calibration curve generated by globular proteins (•), mAb is eluting very close to the total exclusion limit of TSKgel G2000SW, while it is eluting very close to the total inclusion limit of TSKgel G4000SW, resulting into poor separation of the monomer from its impurities in both the cases. But in the middle panel, as seen in the case of TSKgel G3000W, the monomer is eluting around in the middle of the linear range of the calibration curve, so the monomer peak can clearly be separated from its dimer and higher order aggregates and fragment impurities way better than with the other two columns. It is the pore volume between total exclusion and total inclusion volume which is important. The greater the pore volume per unit column volume, the better the separation. In other words, the shallower the calibration curve, the better the separation. All SEC columns with the same dimension, particle size, and pore size from different vendors otherwise may look identical, but the pore volume per unit column volume may not be the same. An analyst can gain advantage by selecting a column with larger pore volume per unit column volume.

Different SEC columns obtained from different vendors, having the same dimensions and particle size as labeled on the individual columns, may apparently look alike. The difference is in the pore volume per unit column volume due to the differences in particle size and pore size distributions, packing quality, and so on. In general, the better the pore volume per unit

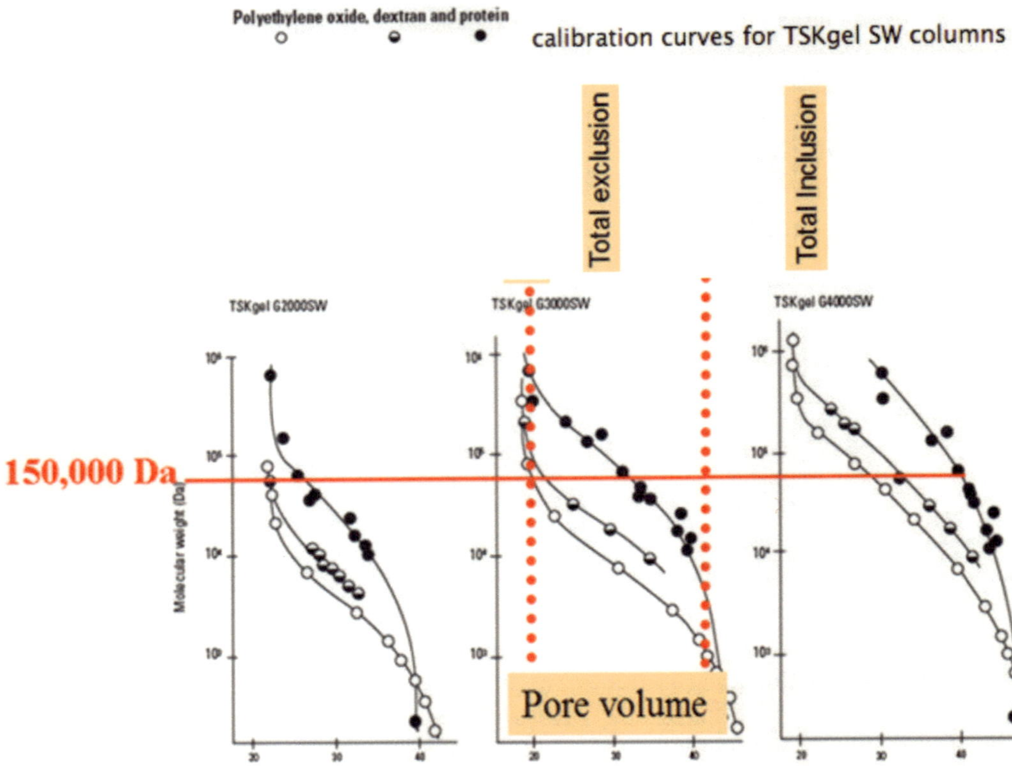

Figure 6. Elution profile of mAb IgG obtained with TSKgel G2000SW, TSKgelG3000W, or TSKgel G4000SW columns.

column volume, the better the separation and resolution of proteins from a SEC column. This is a very critical criterion when selecting a SEC column for better separation.

2.5. Separation of HMW and LMW species by SEC and reproducibility

A chromatographer uses SEC primarily to separate monoclonal antibodies from its impurities or heterogeneities. The monomer IgG1 peak (150 kDa) needs to be purified from its dimer, trimer, or higher order aggregates popularly known as high molecular weight (HMW) species and the fragments which are known as the low molecular weight (LMW) species. SEC is widely accepted as a work horse for routine quality control with its purpose to monitor these HMW and LMW impurities from a mAb monomer. Protein aggregation of biotherapeutics is a common issue. Even a very small amount of aggregates may cause an immunogenic response in the human body and needs to be removed from the monoclonal antibody monomer. More than 99% purity is needed for medicinal purpose [17]. The formulation containing the pure monomer monoclonal antibody needs to be monitored for its stability. The purified protein in the formulation may also undergo aggregation over time. Protein aggregation can happen at any stage during expression and purification. Temperature, pH, ionic strength, concentration and many other factors can give rise to protein instability, leading to aggregation. Effect of ions on protein agitation and temperature-induced aggregation of mAbs has been reported in the literature [18]. Specific racemization of Heavy-Chain Cysteine-220 in the hinge region is identified as a possible cause of degradation during storage. Increased hydrophobicity can increase the likelihood of aggregate formation during manufacturing and storage [19]. Freeze-thaw cycles too can cause an aggregation of an already purified protein [20]. Formation of aggregates may be induced by light as well [21]. That is the reason why all registration applications for new molecular entities and associated drug products require photo-stability data [22]. Increased resolution between the monomer peak and other HMW and LMW impurities is the key for the purification of monoclonal antibodies. SEC can monitor the stability during storage. The removal of HMW and LMW impurities is equally important for application of newly emerging biotherapeutics such as ADCs, bi-specific antibodies, biosimilars, and bio betters as well. As an example from the recent literature report, aggregate and fragment levels were determined by SEC-HPLC for the characterization of bi-specific antibodies [23]. A single chain variable fragment (scFv), composed of the variable regions of the heavy chain (V_H) and the light chain (V_L), is gaining interest too as it retains the specificity of the original IgG. The scFv format is often used, but one problem that cannot be easily solved by purification is the fact that hybridomas can secrete different monoclonal antibodies [24]. Literature reports a few interesting articles about the concept of mAbs being a perfectly defined entity to researchers. The following is an excerpt from the commentary as shown here [25]. "most researchers consider monoclonal antibodies to be perfectly defined reagents with single specificities" but "Hybridomas frequently secrete more than one light and/or heavy chain." So "the problem is probably best summarized thus: antibodies sold as different are often identical, while antibodies sold as identical are often different (thanks to Natalie de Souza (editor Nature Methods) for this pithy insightful observation), and the customer does not know which is which." In another interesting article, the authors have discussed that "two kappa immunoglobulin light chains are secreted by an anti-DNA hybridoma" and its implications for isotypic exclusion are discussed [26]. Biotherapeutic scientist needs to be aware of these facts while analyzing mAb. The separation of scFvs from dimers and aggregates is also important; most of the affinity purified scFv fractions are monitored by SEC.

Different mAbs may have different amount of impurities under native conditions. Representative chromatograms of the separation of four different monoclonal antibodies (IgG1) at 0.75 mL/min using a 4 μm; 4.6 mm ID × 15 cm TSKgel SuperSW mAb HTP column are shown in **Figure 7** [27]. This analysis clearly showed that under native conditions different monoclonal IgG1 antibodies had different extent of HMW and LMW species based on the individual % peak area analysis (data not shown here). The monomer peak eluted as fast as in 2 min.

A chromatographer needs to choose a suitable column based on the separation criteria the chromatographer is looking for. Comparison of the analysis of mAb aggregates using 15 and 30 cm long TSKgel UP-SW3000, 2 μm columns using the same mobile phase and flow rate is shown below [28].

Fast separation of the HMW and LMW species is important. The effect of the column length should be taken into account when selecting a column in this regard. The results indicate that the TSKgel UP-SW3000 column with a shorter length yielded a similar profile to the 30-cm

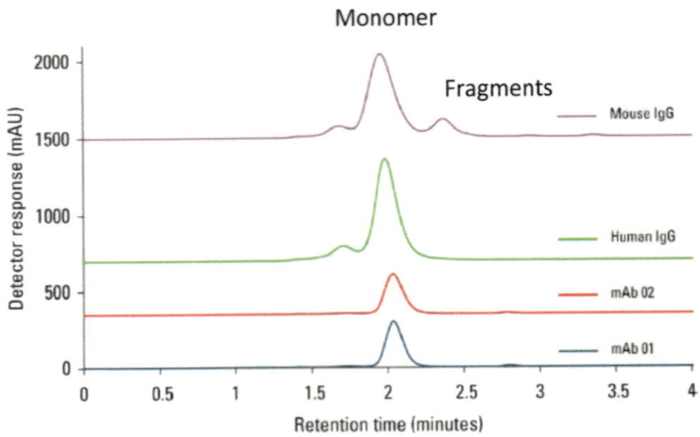

Figure 7. Separation of four different mAbs on a 4 μm; 4.6 mm ID × 15 cm TSKgel SuperSW mAb HTP column.

column with 50% less run time and 50% lower backpressure at a typical flow rate of 0.35 mL/min (**Figure 8**). The resolution between dimer and monomer is still maintained within the acceptable range. Thus, a shorter column could be successfully used for the separation of the dimer and monomer, reducing the overall runtime by half but the resolution of the fragment on the LMW side of the monomer slightly decreased. The longer column yielded a better resolution. As long as the resolution is 1.5 and above yielding a baseline resolution of the two species, the method may remain acceptable. The selection of the correct length of the column should be based on the goal of the separation. The 15-cm column operated at the typical flow rate of 0.35 mL/min yielded a backpressure of 11 Mpa, which was well within its maximum operable pressure and thus could be used in both HPLC and UHPLC systems.

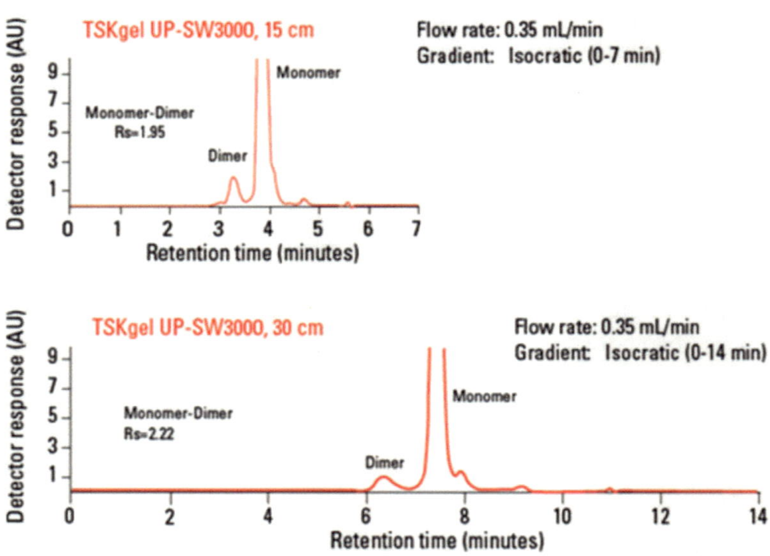

Figure 8. Effect of protein separation on the column length of SEC columns.

Factors considered when selecting an HPLC column supplier			
Factor	Respondents (Normalized %)		
	2007	2009	2011
Column-to-column reproducibility	21 } 37%	21 } 39%	19 } 34%
Column lifetime	16	17	15
Price	12	14	13
Reputation of company	14	12	9.6
Column plate number	8.7	9.1	9.1
Technical assistance	5.7	5.8	6.7
Variety of phases available	4.5	4.0	6.4
Tailing factor	6.3	5.4	5.0

Ref: LCGC: Jan 1, 2012; Article: Current trends in HPLC column usage – By: Ron Majors

Table 1. Factors that play a role in selecting a suitable HPLC column.

Reproducibility is important in SEC analysis of mAbs. The survey clearly showed the importance of column lifetime and reproducibility for column selection [29, 30]. The survey also shows how the same topic developed over a number of years. Factors which should be considered to select an HPLC column supplier are shown in **Table 1**.

Two different sources of silica can be a factor in lot-to-lot reproducibility. Vendors always maintain a strict quality control passing criteria if the silica source is different.

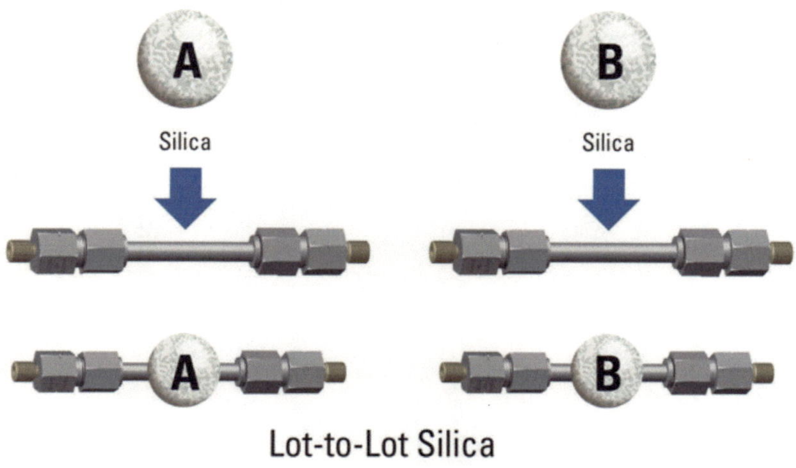

Bonding chemistry developed on the same silica at different times can also be a factor in lot-to-lot reproducibility.

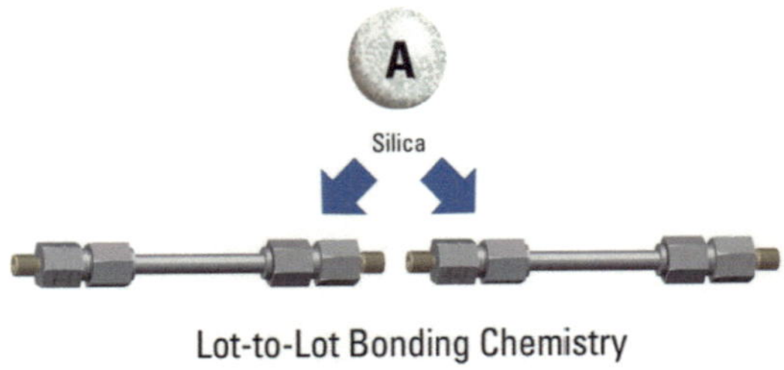

A robust method with a good SEC analytical column is critical for the analyst. A protein standard mixture can be used to confirm the lot-to-lot reproducibility of an SEC column. The protein standards are chosen to cover the whole range of calibration curve from total exclusion limit to total inclusion limit. A representative chromatogram of the analysis of a protein standard mixture using a TSKgel G3000SWXL, 5 μm, 7.8 mm ID ×30 cm column is shown in **Figure 9**. Thyroglobulin (700 kDa) is close to the total exclusion limit and para-amino-benzoic acid (PABA–137 Da) is near the total inclusion limit. Chromatographers use also vitamin B12 (1.4 kDa) in place of PABA. Vendors generally pass the packed SEC columns using a protein standard mixture and establish a QC pass criteria. For example, the specification for TSKgel G3000SWXL column passing QC is N (PABA) > 20,000 and As (PABA) = (0.7–1.6) where N represents the number of theoretical plates and As represents the peak asymmetry.

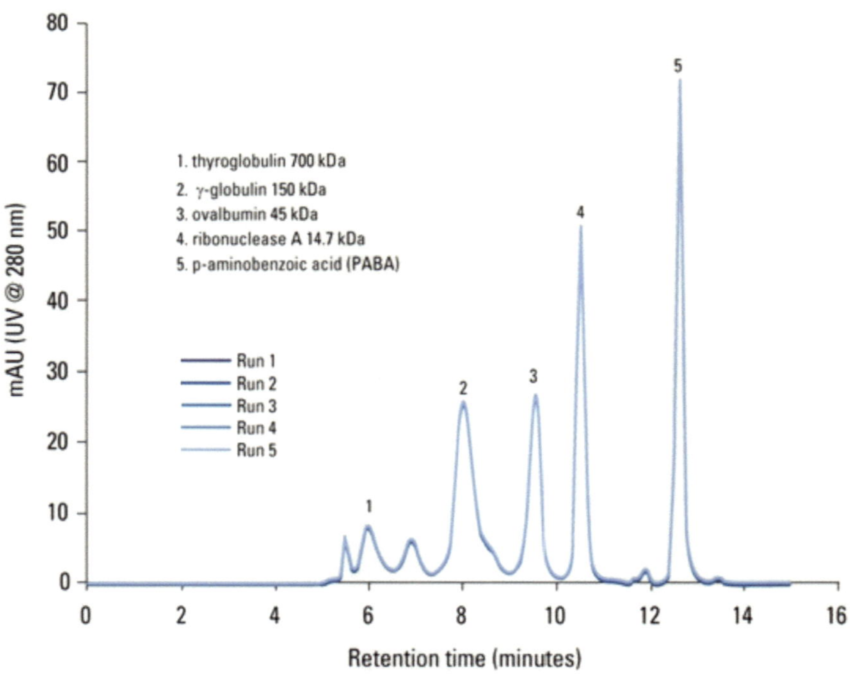

Figure 9. Retention time of five different proteins analyzed with a TSKgel G3000SWXL column was high reproducible. An overlay of five injections is shown.

Figure 9 [31] shows the reproducibility of five consecutive injections with low %RSD of all the peak parameters (data not shown here).

Reproducibility of the analysis of a protein standard mixture with low %RSD of the peak parameters such as retention time, peak area, peak asymmetry and number of theoretical plates and passing the vendor-defined QC criteria can be used for monitoring the column health. Routine users purifying a particular mAb with a particualr SEC column may use the same mAb as their internal standard to monitor the column quality and lifetime over a number of injections. Nowadays, mAb standards from USP and NIST are available for similar purpose.

Reproducibility of 15 consecutive injections during the analysis of a USP mAb using a 15-cm TSKgel UP-SW3000 column at 0.5 mL/min flow rate and phosphate buffer at pH 6.7 is shown in **Figure 10**.

The mAb monomer peak eluted at 2.717 min with good resolution between monomer and the dimer peaks as well as the fragments. Similar reproducibility is noticed in case of pH 6.2 (data not shown here).

Reproducibility in the analysis of the USP mAb in pH 6.2 conditions with 250 mM KCl at 0.3 mL/min using a 30 cm column is shown below—the overlay of the 15 consecutive injections demonstrated consistency (**Figure 11**) (all USP Reference Standards are provided as delivered and specified by the US Pharmacopeia). The monomer peak elution time was 8.367 min. Similar reproducibility was obtained using a 15-cm column at pH 6.7 (data not shown here).

Nonspecific absorption of antibodies onto the column gel matrix poses a challenge, and some newly engineered antibodies possess a high degree of hydrophobicity. The use of organic

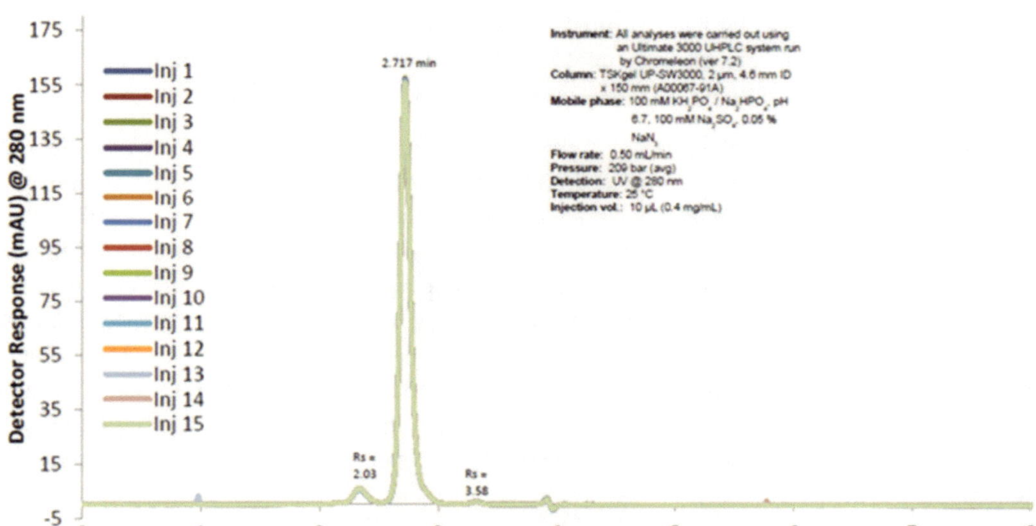

Figure 10. Reproducibility of 15 consecutive analytical injections of a USP mAb using a 15-cm TSKgel UP-SW3000 column at phosphate buffer pH 6.7. The overlay of 15 injections is shown.

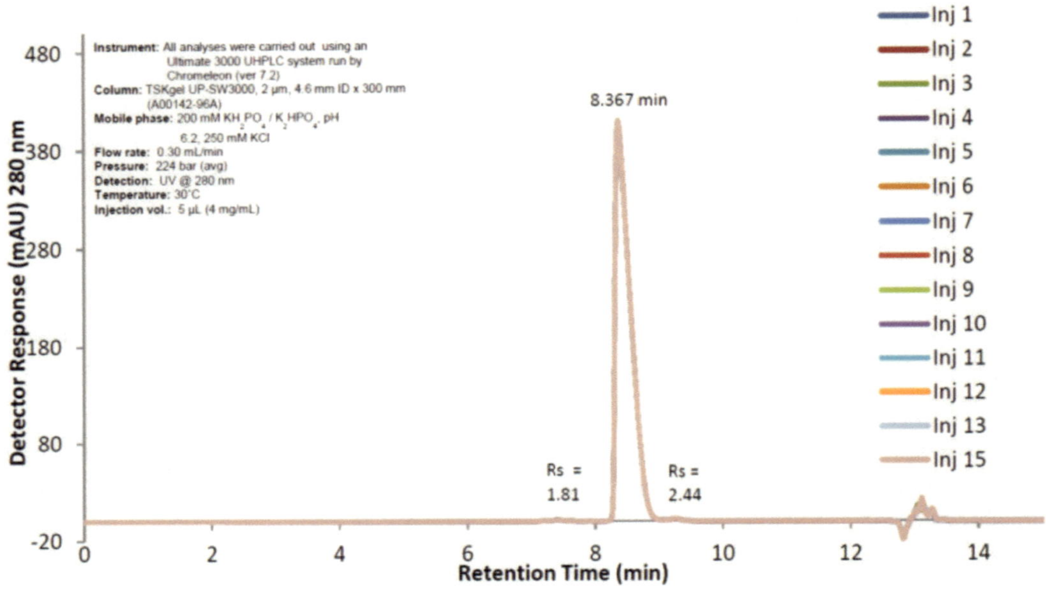

Figure 11. Reproducibility of 15 consecutive analytical injections of a USP mAb using a 30-cm TSKgel UP-SW3000 column at pH 6.2. The overlay of 15 injections is shown.

solvents such as isopropyl alcohol (IPA) or salts can decrease this interaction as reported by many scientists. However, the additives may alter the diffusion of these molecules, which results in retention time shift and poor peak resolution that did not occur in a typical aqueous buffer system, such as sodium phosphate buffer at neutral pH. The **Figure 12** and **Table 2** show that a TSKgel UP-SW3000, 2 μm SEC column was used for analyzing monoclonal antibodies (mAbs) with the addition of 15% IPA in sodium phosphate buffer, pH 6.7. As demonstrated, peak resolution and retention time shift were not impacted.

Similarly, **Figure 13** shows the overlay of the 15 consecutive injections of USP mAb at pH 6.7 with 15% IPA using a 30-cm column (**Figure 13** and **Table 3**). Improvement in the baseline was noticed after the first two injections. Overall, the analysis yielded excellent reproducibility. The monomer peak elution time was 8.338 min. As expected, there was no considerable difference here compared to the retention time obtained earlier at pH 6.2. The presence of IPA as additive obviously will yield a higher back pressure, and so long as the column is operated within its maximum operable pressure, this should not be an issue. The retention times of monomer, dimer, aggregates, and fragment peaks are nearly unchanged. Peak width and peak shape are very consistent from injection to injection. The baseline of the first injection (as shown in blue) indicate that the column takes only 1–2 injections to be stabilized. After that, all subsequent injections are overlaid perfectly.

The overlay indicates the similarities of peak retention times, peak width and peak height of dimer, monomer, aggregates and fragment peaks between the two different conditions. An appropriate percentage of organic solvent such as isopropyl alcohol (IPA) did not alter the diffusion of mAb molecules using a TSKgel UP-SW3000 column. As demonstrated, this column can be successfully operated with the addition of 15% IPA. Data indicate that the

http://dx.doi.org/10.5772/intechopen.73321

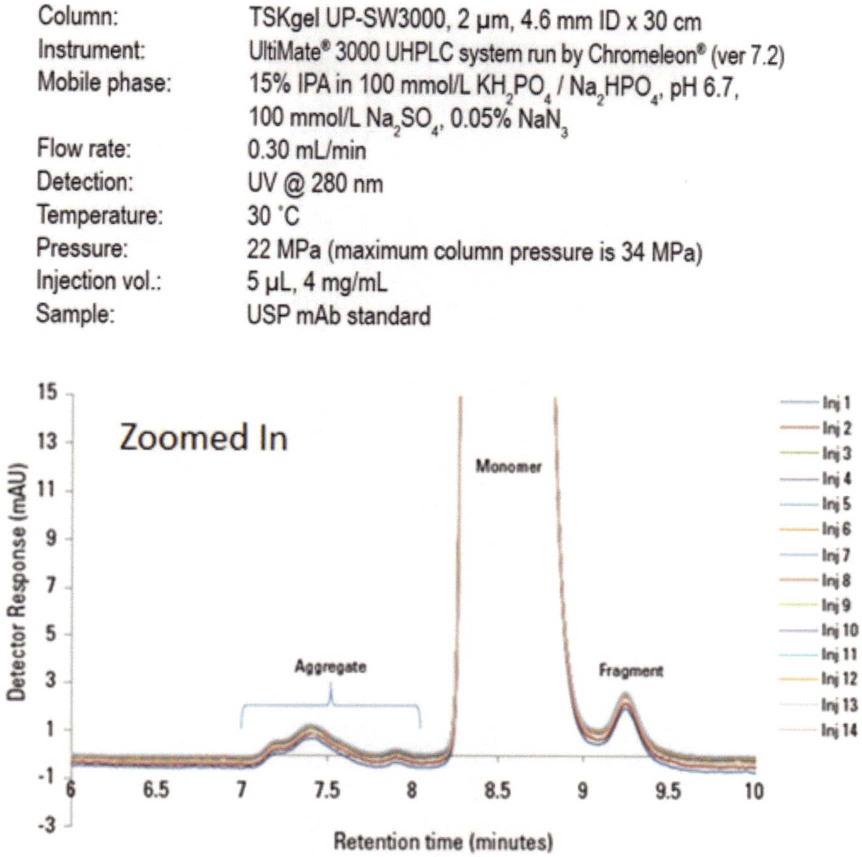

Figure 12. Reproducibility of 14 consecutive analytical injections of a USP mAb using a 30-cm TSKgel UP-SW3000, 2 μm SEC column at pH 6.7 with isopropyl alcohol. The overlay of 14 injections is shown.

column's particle chemistry and packing are optimized so that with the addition of an appropriate amount of selected organic solvents, there is no alteration of peak retention time or poor peak resolution [32].

2.5.1. Loading study

Sample load, in both volumetric load and absolute load, may affect SEC separation. Mass overload takes place when sample molecules no longer have free access to diffuse into and out of the pores, thus bypassing part of the column and thereby effectively reducing the length of the column that remains to fractionate the sample. If the height equivalent theoretical plates (HETP) are plotted against the load amount, the HETP values should remain constant as long as the column efficiency is not compromised. The loading capacity is the maximum load beyond which the HETP value starts increasing, as shown in **Figure 14** [33].

To obtain the capacity of an analytical SEC column as often the chromatographers like to do, a loading study plot HETP vs. load amount is shown above (**Figure 14**). The loading capacity of a SEC column with defined dimensions depends on the sample. The loading capacity can be

	Monomer peak		Dimer peak	
Injection	Ret. time (min)	Area (mAU*min)	Ret. time (min)	Area (mAU*min)
1	8.370	99.300	7.403	0.380
2	8.370	99.290	7.400	0.400
3	8.367	99.250	7.407	0.400
4	8.367	99.270	7.433	0.390
5	8.367	99.260	7.423	0.400
6	8.367	99.270	7.413	0.390
7	8.367	99.260	7.403	0.400
8	8.367	99.260	7.403	0.400
9	8.367	99.090	7.420	0.390
10	8.367	99.270	7.427	0.390
11	8.367	99.260	7.400	0.400
12	8.367	99.250	7.407	0.400
13	8.367	99.250	7.397	0.400
14	8.367	99.260	7.403	0.390
Average	**8.367**	**99.253**	**7.410**	**0.395**
Std Dev	**0.001**	**0.049**	**0.011**	**0.007**
%RSD	**0.013**	**0.049**	**0.153**	**1.647**

Table 2. Retention time and peak areas of the monomer and dimer peak (**Figure 12**).

increased by increasing the column length or diameter. Increasing column length also increases resolution and retention time, leading to an additional separation time and amount of mobile phase.

Below is the loading study of γ-globulin (150 kDa) using the TSKgel UP-SW3000 column. It is necessary to know the experimental range of loading where the retention time, peak shape, separation efficiency, etc., remain nearly unchanged over varying load concentrations. Please note that when a loading study is carried out, both volumetric loading and absolute loading amounts should be studied. In **Figure 15**, a volumetric loading study is shown. In any SEC analysis, by theory, the total volume injected should not be more than 3% of the column volume to avoid the effect of band broadening.

Figure 15 shows that even at larger volumetric load containing up to 160 μg proteins, the monomer peak remains well resolved from its dimer. Retention time is remaining constant over the experimental range. Excellent linearity of both monomer peak areas and dimer peak areas versus total load were obtained (data not shown here). So if the primary interest of the analyst is to separate the monomer from the dimer, 160 μg loading in 40 μL volume can be used. Now if the monoclonal antibody concentration can be increased so that 160 μg can be loaded in lower volume (e.g., 10 μL), then the peak shape can further be improved, if needed.

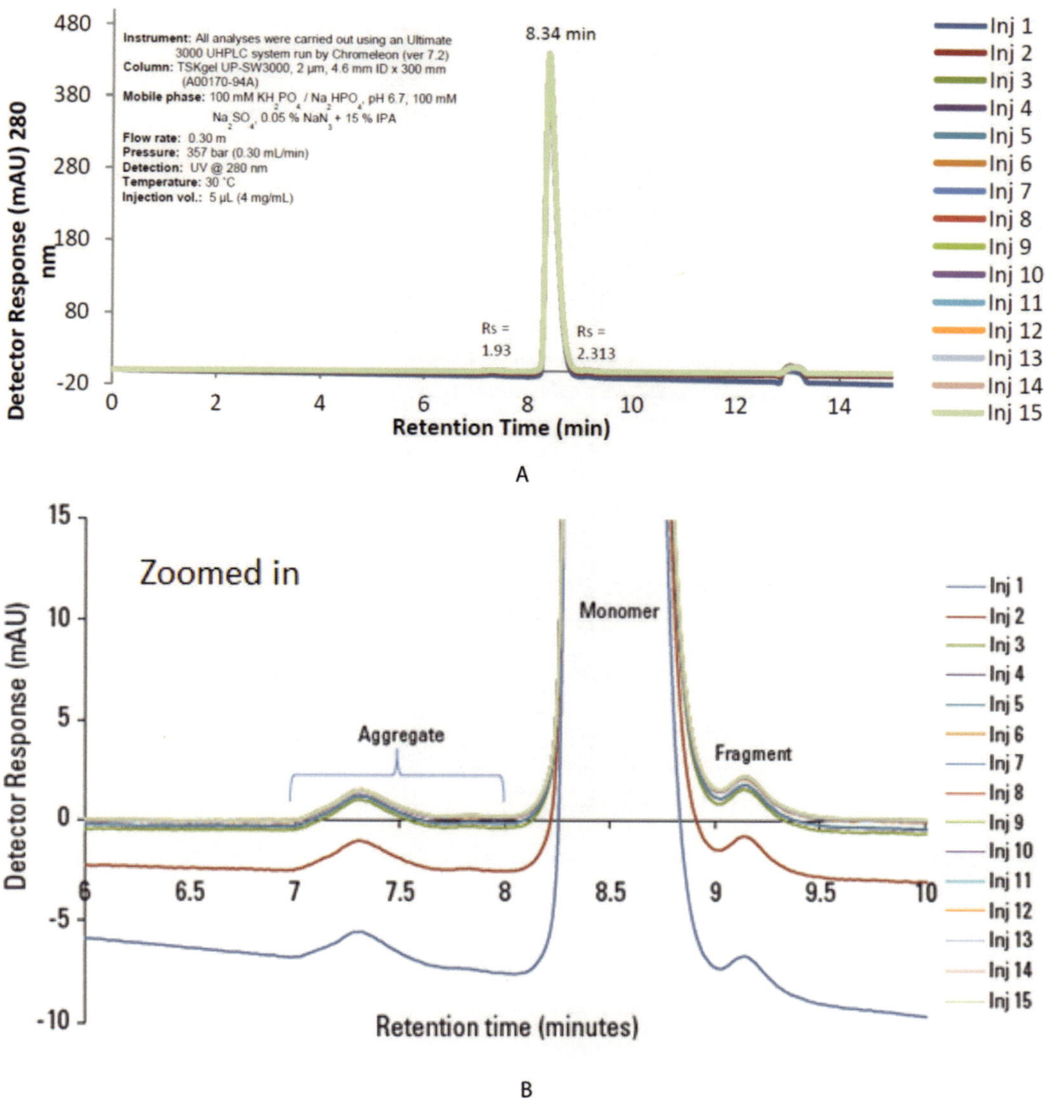

Figure 13. (A) Reproducibility of 15 consecutive analytical injections of a USP mAb using a 30-cm TSKgel UP-SW3000, 2 μm SEC column at pH 6.7 with 15% IPA. The overlay of 15 injections is shown. (B) Chromatogram of 13 a zoomed in.

Peak shape and efficiency were not affected when injecting 400 μg of a monoclonal antibody preparation during a loading study of a monoclonal antibody using a TSKgel G3000SWXL, 5 μm, 7.8 mm ID × 30 cm column (**Figure 16**). A 10-fold increase in total protein content did not affect the retention time, peak symmetry, or separation efficiency of the column [30]. Similar study using a TSKgel G2000SWXL, 5 μm, 7.8 mm ID × 30 cm analytical column even with a high load of Bovine Serum Albumin also yielded a well-resolved peak without any splitting [34].

As mentioned earlier, having an idea about the sample loading capacity will provide analyst the knowledge about the load range within which the desired sensitivity and resolution can be

	Monomer peak		Dimer peak	
Injection	Ret. time (min)	Area (mAU*min)	Ret. time (min)	Area (mAU*min)
1	8.340	97.110	7.417	0.470
2	8.340	98.280	7.410	0.460
3	8.340	98.420	7.410	0.470
4	8.340	98.400	7.407	0.490
5	8.340	98.440	7.417	0.470
6	8.340	97.940	7.413	0.500
7	8.337	98.010	7.420	0.470
8	8.337	98.030	7.437	0.470
9	8.337	98.110	7.407	0.470
10	8.337	98.110	7.423	0.470
11	8.337	98.120	7.413	0.460
12	8.337	98.220	7.417	0.470
13	8.337	98.130	7.420	0.480
14	8.337	98.220	7.413	0.460
15	8.367	98.260	7.413	0.390
Average	**8.338**	**98.120**	**7.416**	**0.471**
Std Dev	**0.002**	**0.317**	**0.008**	**0.012**
%RSD	**0.018**	**0.323**	**0.102**	**2.598**

Table 3. Retention time and peak areas of the monomer and dimer peak (**Figure 13**).

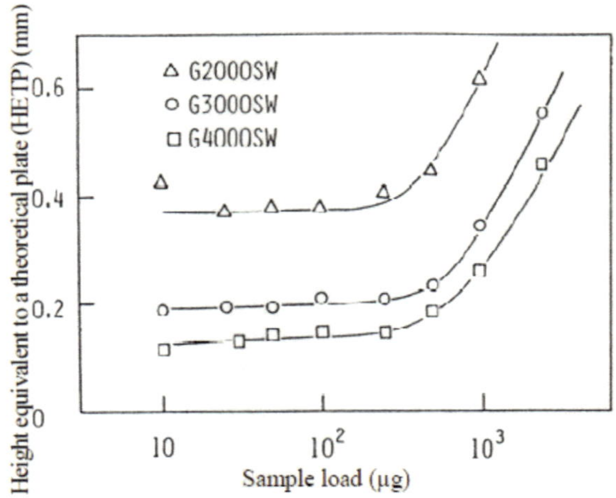

Figure 14. Influence of sample load on height equivalent theoretical plates (HEPT) using three different columns (G2000SW, G3000SW, G4000SW).

http://dx.doi.org/10.5772/intechopen.73321

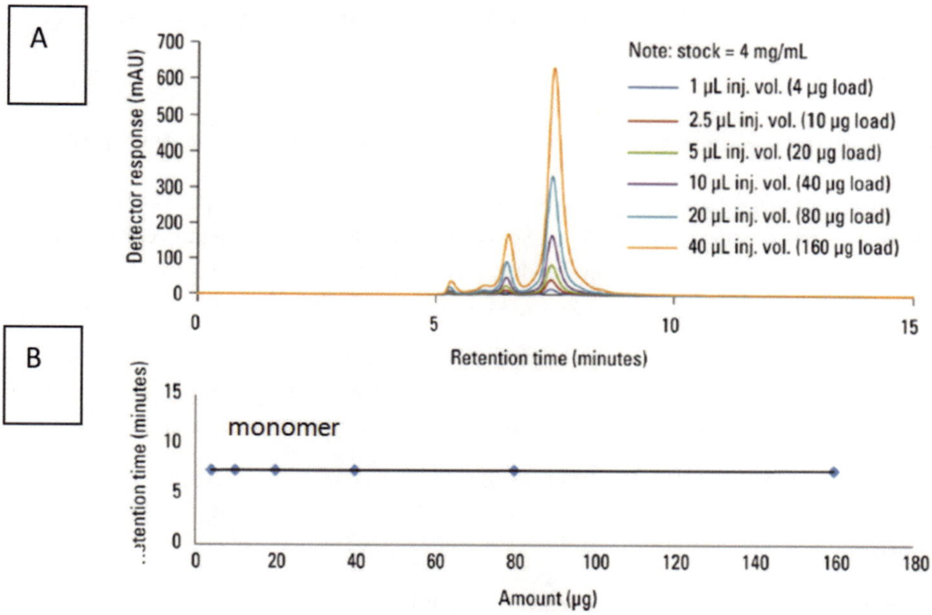

Figure 15. (A) Influence of peak resolution and retention time on the amount of γ-globulin loaded on a TSKgel UP-SW3000 column; (B) monomer retention time in dependence of the amount of sample.

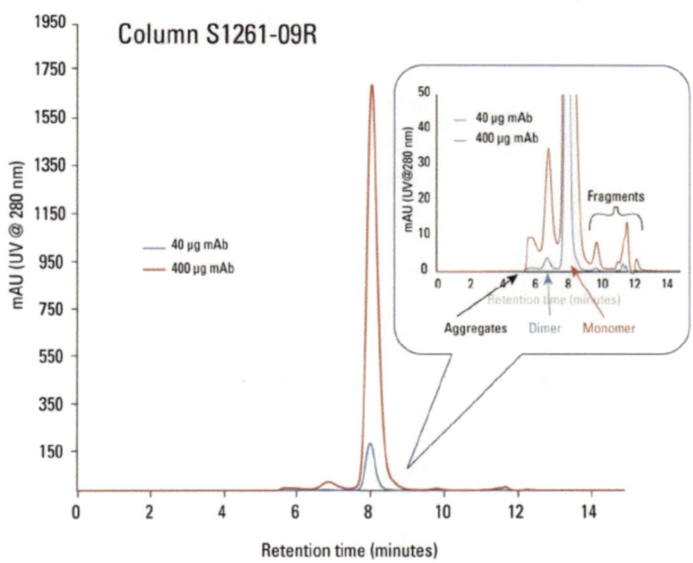

	Monoclonal antibody	
	40 µg Inj.	400 µg Inj.
t_R	8.023	8.061
N	4500	3508
AF	1.22	1.35

Figure 16. Influence of mAb loading on retention time, peak symmetry, or separation efficiency using a TSKgel G3000SWXL, 5 µm, 7.8 mm ID × 30 cm column.

achieved. The loading study can be extended to a lower range of detection to get the limit of detection (LOD) and limit of quantitation (LOQ) values for the column in the analysis of mAbs (data not shown here). Similarly, aggregation pattern of mAbs as a function of concentration can be monitored using SEC columns if a mAb is susceptible to aggregation at higher concentration.

2.6. Separation of digestion products of mAbs by size exclusion chromatography

IgG is a relatively large molecule (approx. 150 kDa), and in order to improve the penetration to the tissue, fragmentation is carried out. Digestion with papain or pepsin is commonly applied to obtain antibody fragments without the loss of activity. When papain is used for the antibody digestion, 2 Fab (50 kDa each) and 1 Fc (50 kDa) are obtained from one antibody (**Figure 17**).

When pepsin is used, a F(ab')2 is obtained. SEC can be used to analyze the separation of these fragments. The scope of this analysis by SEC is taken as an opportunity to explain how to select a column with right particle size, pore size, column dimensions, and so on.

In **Figures 18** and **19**, a set of four different SEC columns are compared during the separation of papain digestion products of a mAb to explain how to select the right SEC column for the right purpose [35].

For analyzing monoclonal antibody and other biopolymers 250 Å pore size, 5 μm, 7.8 mm ID × 30 cm SEC columns are widely considered. For example, TSKgel G3000SWxl columns

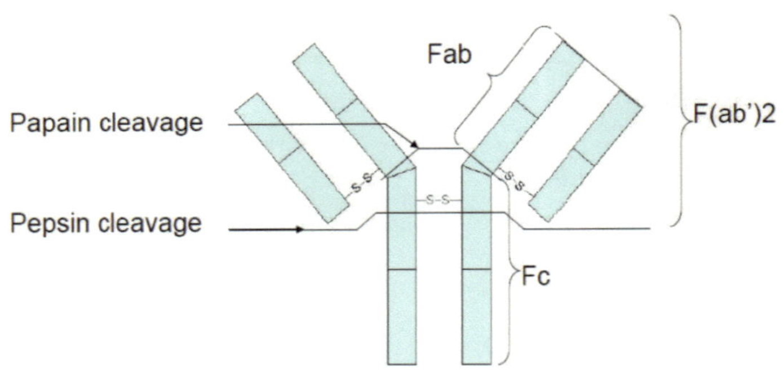

Figure 17. Cleavage of an IgG with papain or pepsin.

Columns	TSKgel SuperSW mAb HR	TSKgel SuperSW mAb HTP	TSKgel UltraSW Aggregate	TSKgel G3000SWXL
Column size	7.8 mm I.D.×30 cm	4.6 mm I.D.×15 cm	7.8 mm I.D.×30 cm	
Base material	Silica			
Ligand	Diol			
Particle size	4 μm		3 μm	5 μm
Pore size	25 nm		30 nm	25 nm
Exclusion limit (globular proteins)	800,000 Da		2,500,000 Da*)	800,000 Da
Separation range (globular proteins)	10,000−500,000 Da		10,000−1,500,000 Da	10,000−500,000 Da
Applications	High resolution of mAb dimer/monomer/fragments	High speed separation of mAb dimer/monomer	High resolution of mAb aggregates	Separation of proteins

*) Estimated value

Figure 18. Characteristics of the SEC columns used in the analysis of **Figure 19**.

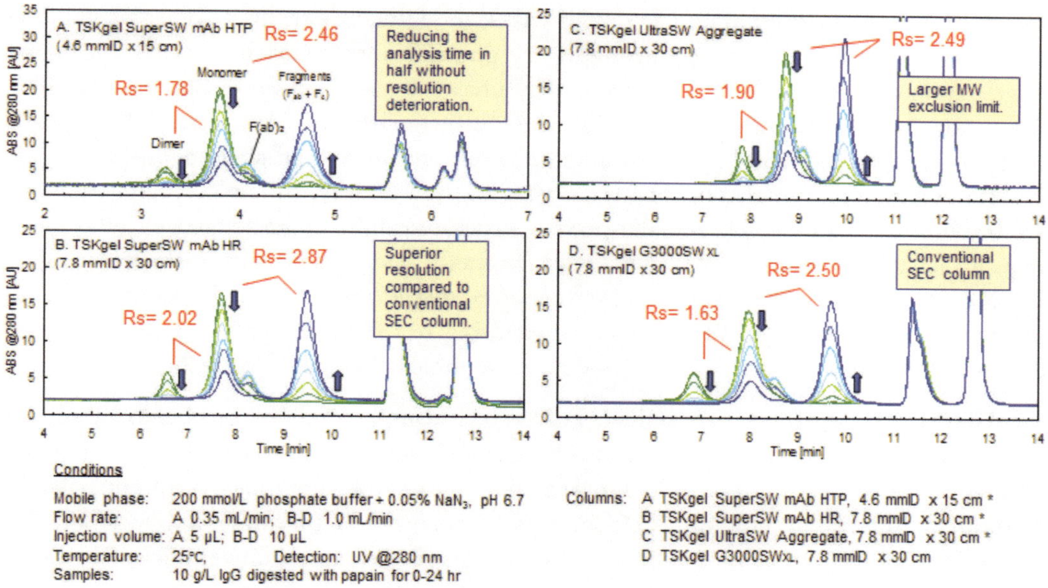

Figure 19. Separation of papain digestion products of a mAb using a set of four different SEC columns. Columns in panel A, B, and D are of 250 Å pore sizes, while column in panel D is of 300 Å pore size [35].

(Panel D) have a separation range for globular protein samples up to 500 kDa. The other SEC column is a 4-μm, 7.8 mm ID × 30 cm TSKgel SuperSW mAb HR SEC column (Panel B). It is smaller than the conventional 5 μm TSKgel G3000SWXL column. Smaller particle size and the optimized packing are expected to yield high-resolution analysis of mAb monomers, dimers, and fragments due to shallow calibration slope at the corresponding molar mass region of the mAb monomer (150 kDa). Monomer – dimer resolution increased from 1.63 to 2.02. Another SEC column (Panel A) is a 4-μm TSKgel SuperSW mAb HTP column which is smaller in dimensions, length, and ID (4.6 mm ID × 15 cm). This column offers high throughput analysis, separating the dimer and monomer in half the run time compared to all the other three columns in panels B, C, and D. Results are similar to the analysis of mAbs with a 5-μm conventional column (panel D). The fourth column (Panel C) discussed here is of even smaller particle size (3 μm) with higher molar mass exclusion limit (2500 kDa, globular proteins) than all other three columns (500 kDa, globular proteins). Due to the higher exclusion limit, this TSKgel UltraSW aggregate column (Panel C) is expected to yield higher resolution of mAb multimers and aggregates. Please see further discussion about this in Section 2.7.

2.7. Forced degradation study by SEC

Stability of the biotherapeutic proteins in formulation is very critical for candidate selection, characterization of the biotherapeutic, formulation and assay development, and so on. A forced degradation study, popularly known as stress testing, is considerably a faster way to monitor the stability of the therapeutic proteins. Stress is provided by increasing the temperature, changing the pH or a combination of both. Depending on the nature, individual mAbs can be susceptible to light, freeze–thaw conditions, mechanical stress, oxidation and so on. So, monitoring the stability from time to time is important. Literature reports: "Whereas stability-testing requirements are defined in regulatory guidelines, standard procedures for forced degradation of therapeutic proteins are largely unavailable, except for photo stability" [36]. Stress conditions induce unfolding of the native protein structure. As a result, the exposed hydrophobic patches may be able to interact with each other, leading to aggregation [37]. Protein degradation can also be measured using sodium dodecyl sulfate polyacrylamide gel electrophoresis (SDS PAGE), and the protein structure can be characterized by other techniques using Fourier transform infrared spectrometry and circular dichroism [38]. SEC is widely accepted as a great tool to monitor the forced degradation. Forced degradation by acid denaturation and heat denaturation analyzed using a TSKgel UltraSW Aggregate, 3 μm, 30 nm, 7.8 mm ID × 30 cm column is used as an example below [39] (**Figure 20**).

Acid denaturation: After reducing the pH of the IgG1 sample solution down to 4.7 by adding phosphoric acid, aliquots were analyzed at 5, 20, and 50 min, and the response was compared to that of the original sample solution. The blue trace shows the intact mAb and what is (presumably) its dimer eluting at 8.65 min when analyzed at flow rate of 1 mL/min. The degradation of the monoclonal antibody creates a larger MW entity (unidentified) that elutes directly after the dimer and before the monomer. Continued decay led to increase of both peaks. Clearly the dimer increases in size, while the peak height of the monomer decreases. Hints of higher order "multimers" are detected between 7 and 8 min [31].

Heat denaturation: Degradation of mAb at pH 5.5 and a temperature of 60°C were monitored. Fifty microliters of antibody in 0.1 M phosphate buffer (pH 6.0) was mixed with 50 μL of 0.1 mol/L phosphate buffer, pH 4.65; the final pH was 5.5; and 20 μL was injected [31]. Heating for 1 h at 60°C results in almost complete breakdown of the monoclonal antibody and the formation of very large aggregates (multimers) that extend to the exclusion volume of the column. The intensity of the multimer peaks increased as a function of the incubation period at 60°C. The larger the total exclusion volume of the column, the better the resolution of higher order aggregates. An SEC column with a 500-kDa exclusion limit may not be able to resolve the individual multimers such as trimers and tetramers. An SEC column with larger exclusion limit, for example, 2500 kDa, may be useful in such a case [31].

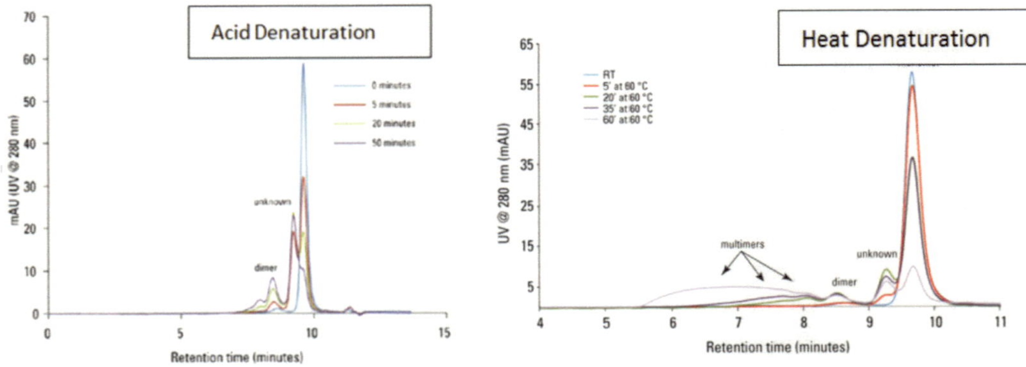

Figure 20. Analysis of forced degradation of IgG after acid and heat denaturation using a SEC TSKgel UltraSW aggregate, 3 μm, 30 nm, 7.8 mm ID × 30 cm column.

http://dx.doi.org/10.5772/intechopen.73321

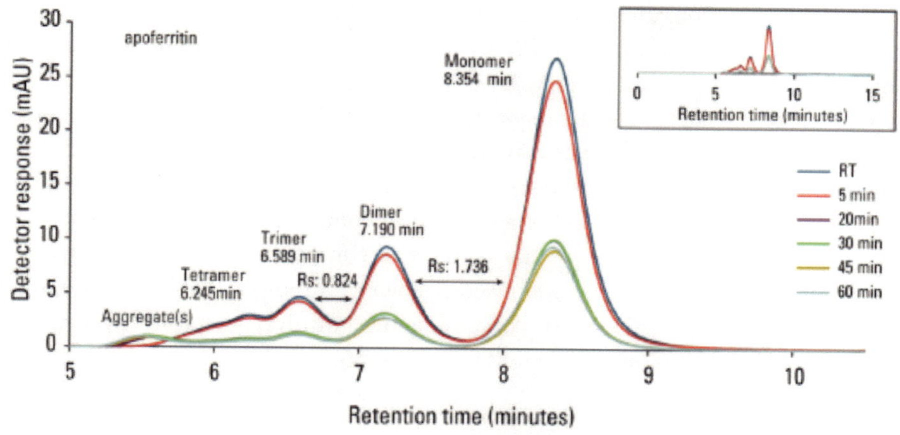

Figure 21. Analysis of Apo ferritin after heat denaturation using a TSKgel UltraSW aggregate column.

The analysis of a heat denatured, large hydrophobic metalloprotein, Apo ferritin, analyzed using a TSKgel UltraSW Aggregate column yielded high resolution between the monomer (450 kDa) and dimer (900 kDa) (**Figure 21**). The trimer (1350 kDa), tetramer (1800 kDa), and higher order aggregates of Apo ferritin were well separated. Tetramer of Apo ferritin is approximately equivalent to 13 mer of a mAb. Larger exclusion limit yielded better resolution of the higher order aggregates. [40].

3. Effect of mobile phase additives on the separation of monoclonal antibodies

The use of organic solvents such as isopropyl alcohol (IPA) or salts can decrease the secondary interaction as reported by many scientists and mentioned earlier briefly in this chapter in Section 2.5. Peak resolution and retention time shift were not impacted with the use of 15% IPA as demonstrated in the two examples (**Figure 12** and **Figure 13**). It is necessary to evaluate the individual SEC column regarding the impact of the additives since a stationary phase with minimum impact is always a favorable choice. After important mobile phase parameters have been set, such as pH, stationary phase, and ionic strength, significant improvements can, in fact, be made to separate mAb monomers from aggregates and fragments. There are no universal additives which can be applied for every mAb or protein purification. Other common additives are methanol and ethanol. Use of sodium perchlorate may also improve the separation and resolution. By switching from 0.2 mol/L sodium chloride to 0.2 mol/L of the more chaotropic sodium perchlorate salt, together with a twofold reduction in the buffer concentration, less peak tailing and distinct peaks for the dimer and trimer could be noticed [41]. Sodium dodecyl sulfate (SDS), urea, guanidine hydrochloride, etc., are sometimes used when the proteins need to be solubilized, leading to denaturation of the protein and breakage of the noncovalent bonds. The use of additives should be considered only when needed. In many cases, the performance of the column is irreversibly changed when a column is subjected to particular additives. Retention time may shift when the additive is added and the resolution may change, expectedly to a better resolution but these values should remain constant and the analysis should be reproducible. It is always better to dedicate the SEC column if the column is subjected to additives, since we still have no clear idea how the pore characteristic of the stationary phase may behave with and without additives. Analysts should check the operational and conditions (OCS) sheet for the column as provided by the vendor to make sure that additives are compatible with the stationary phase. If compatible the analyst should be aware of the percentage of organic solvent the column is compatible with. Generally, when the organic solvent is used, the column may need a slower ramping rate for proper equilibration of the column with the mobile phase containing the additive, generally by using gradual solvent changes using a shallow gradient at low flow rate.

4. Analysis of monoclonal antibody IgG1 by SEC using MS-friendly mobile phases

The use of mass spectrometry is becoming increasingly popular for scientists dealing with biomolecule separation to identify the individual peaks by molecular weight. The liquid chromatography-MS (LC–MS) system available nowadays is very robust and useful for routine mass determination. Reversed phase LC–MS or SEC-MS using organic solvents such as acetonitrile can be used for the mass spectrometric characterization of mAbs. But mAbs get denatured under these conditions.

There is a growing interest in the analysis of mAbs by online-SEC-MS under native conditions. Conventional SEC analysis of mAbs use phosphate buffers at pH 6.7—for example, the most common one is composed of 100 mmol/L phosphates (monobasic + dibasic) as buffering salts +100 mM Na_2SO_4 as neutral salt to adjust the ionic strength +0.05% NaN3 (as antibacterial agent). Both the buffering salts (phosphates) and neutral salt (sodium sulfate) are helpful in preventing secondary interaction of the proteins with the stationary phase. The concentration of these salts may need further optimization depending on the individual properties of the mAbs. But phosphate buffer is not suitable for the mass spectrometer and yields substantial noise and damage the MS system. So online SEC-MS is not possible in the presence of phosphate and other non-volatile salts. Use of volatile salts at lower concentration, which do not interfere with the MS system, can be applied and the method needs to be optimized as well. SEC columns should not exhibit particle shedding which will interfere with the MS signal.

The data below illustrate the effective use of MS-friendly mobile phase compositions in the online SEC-MS analysis of a monoclonal IgG1, IgG2 antibody, ADC and Bi-specific mAb using volatile salt environments (**Figure 22**).

The online LC–MS compatible chromatographic conditions used for the analysis of IgG1, IgG2, ADC, and a Bi-specific mAb is shown below.

Following the development of an optimized separation, liquid chromatography mass spectrometry (LC–MS) analysis was performed using a Q Exactive Plus mass spectrometer

- Column: TSKgel UP-SW3000 4.6mm ID x 30cm, 2µm
- Instrument: UHPLC Ultimate 3000
- Mobile Phase: 20mM Ammonium Acetate, 10mM Ammonium Bicarbonate; pH 7.2
- Gradient: 15 Minute Isocratic
- Flow rate: 0.350 mL/min
- Detection: UV@280nm
- Temperature - 30°C
- Sample: IgG1, IgG2, ADC, BI-Specific mAb

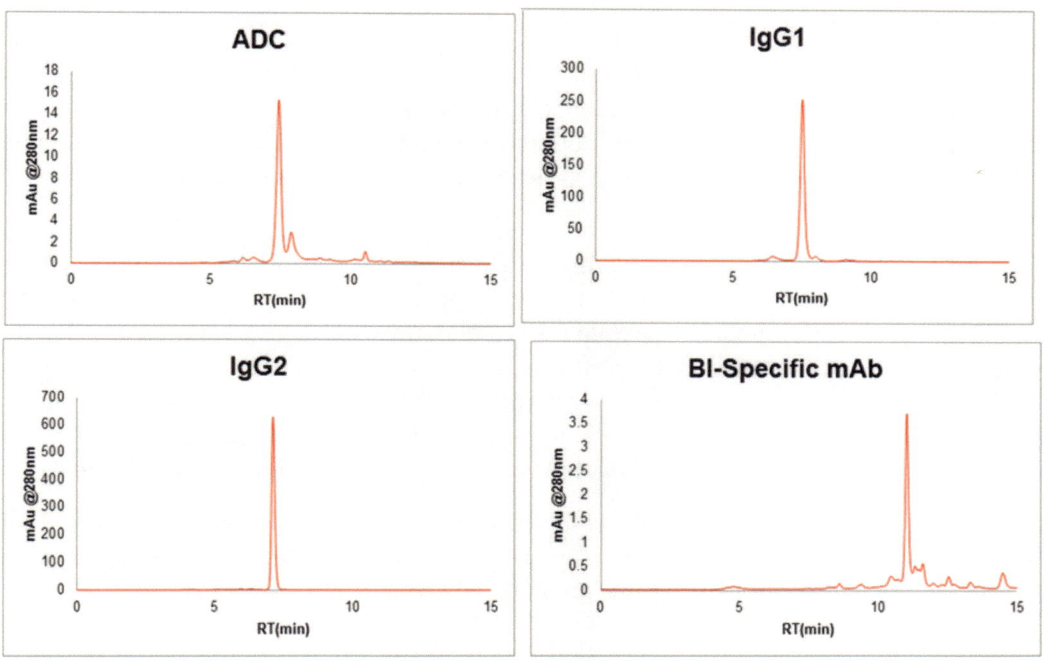

Figure 22. Separation of an ADC, two IgG1 and IgG2 mAbs, and the corresponding bi-specific mAb using a TSKgel UP-SW3000 column (2 µm, 4.6 mm ID x 30 cm).

(ThermoFisher Scientific) coupled to a Shimadzu Nexera XR UHPLC system. Samples were injected onto a TSKgel UP-SW3000 column (2 µm, 4.6 mm ID x 30 cm) and isocratically separated at 0.350 ml/min for 15 min with a mobile phase comprising 20 mM ammonium acetate and 10 mM ammonium bicarbonate, pH 7.2. A 15-min blank isocratic gradient was run between sample injections. No carryover was observed in the blank runs. Eluted proteins were analyzed by the mass spectrometer set to repetitively scan m/z from 800 to 6000 in a positive ion mode. The full MS scan was collected at 17,500 resolution, with spray voltage 4 kV, S-Lens RF 75, and in-source CID 80 eV. Protein mass deconvolution was performed using ProMass (Novatia). The (1) total ion chromatogram, (2) mass spectrum, and (3) deconvoluted mass spectrum of one mAb was evaluated. A main peak can be seen at m/z 149,264; adjacent peaks at m/z 149,426 and 149,592 correspond to different glycoforms.

Here we report the use of a TSKgel® UP-SW3000, 2 μm column for the separation of a bispecific antibody and the two parent mAbs (IgG1) followed by MS analysis. The Bispecific T cell Engager (BiTE®) technology was used in this study. BiTE is a fusion protein consisting of two single-chain variable fragments (scFvs)–CD19, a biomarker for normal and neoplastic B cells and CD3 (on T cells) – recombinantly linked by a nonimmunogenic five-amino-acid chain (**Figure 23**). BiTE is approximately 55 kDa in size. SEC/MS analysis was performed by the Wistar Proteomics and Metabolomics Facility (Philadelphia, PA) using a Nexera® XR UHPLC system (Shimadzu) coupled to a Q Exactive™ Plus mass spectrometer (Thermo Fisher Scientific) (**Figures 24–26**).

Prior to analysis, a blank injection was run in order to assess column particle shedding. The total ion chromatogram of a blank injection was run on a new TSKgel UP-SW3000 column. MS data indicate that there is no shedding from the TSKgel UP-SW3000 column prior to sample injection. Additionally a blank injection was run between each of the sample injections in order to monitor sample carryover.

Each mAb is different, and a method with the use of volatile salts needs to be optimized for reproducibility. There was a difference between the retention time of mAb1 under the isocratic mobile phase 20 mM ammonium acetate and 10 mM ammonium bicarbonate, pH 7.2 compared to 100 mM phosphate buffer containing 100 mM Na_2SO_4 and 0.05% NaN_3 pH 6.8. In an attempt to look for the condition where a MS compatible buffer yields a retention time similar to phosphate buffer, a comparison of elution profiles under 100 mM phosphate buffer and 100 mM ammonium acetate buffer both at pH 6.8 is shown below (**Figure 27** and **Table 4**).

Monomer peak areas remain constant under both conditions with high reproducibility of all the peak parameters. % RSD deviations of all the peak parameters were low. Mass spectrometric analysis under this chromatographic condition will be reported elsewhere.

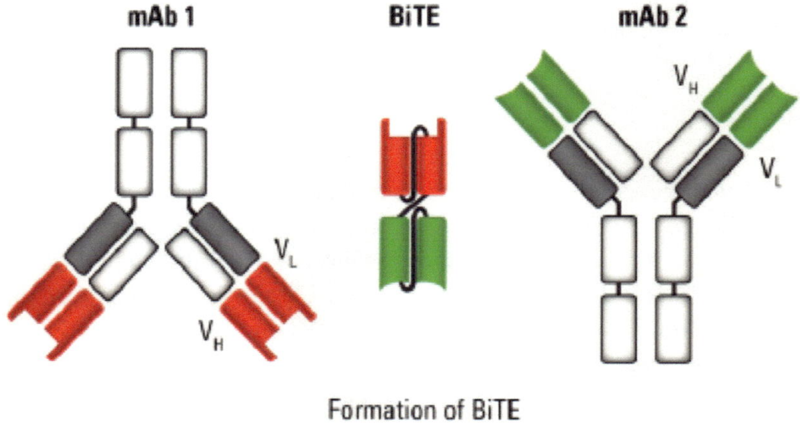

Figure 23. Scheme of a BiTE and corresponding original mAb 1 and mAb 2.

http://dx.doi.org/10.5772/intechopen.73321

Column: TSKgel UP-SW3000, 2 µm, 4.6 mm ID × 30 cm

Instrument: Dionex UltiMate® 3000 UHPLC system run by Chromeleon® (ver 7.2)

Mobile phase: 20 mmol/L ammonium acetate, 10 mmol/L ammonium bicarbonate; pH 7.2

Gradient: isocratic

Flow rate: 0.35 mL/min

Detection: UV @ 280 nm

Temperature: 30 °C

Injection vol.: 5.0 µL

Samples: BiTE, 0.3 mg/mL (*Creative Biolabs*)
parent mAb shown, 0.5 mg/mL (*Creative Biolabs*)

Mass Spectrometric Conditions

- **Eluted proteins were analyzed by the mass spectrometer set to repetitively scan m/z from 800 to 6000 in positive ion mode.**
- **The full MS scan was collected at 17,500 resolution, with spray voltage 4 kV, S-Lens RF 75, and in-source CID 80 eV. Protein mass deconvolution was performed using ProMass® (*Novatia*).**
- **Total ion chromatograms were collected; mass spectrum and peak deconvolution for the accurate mass are shown.**

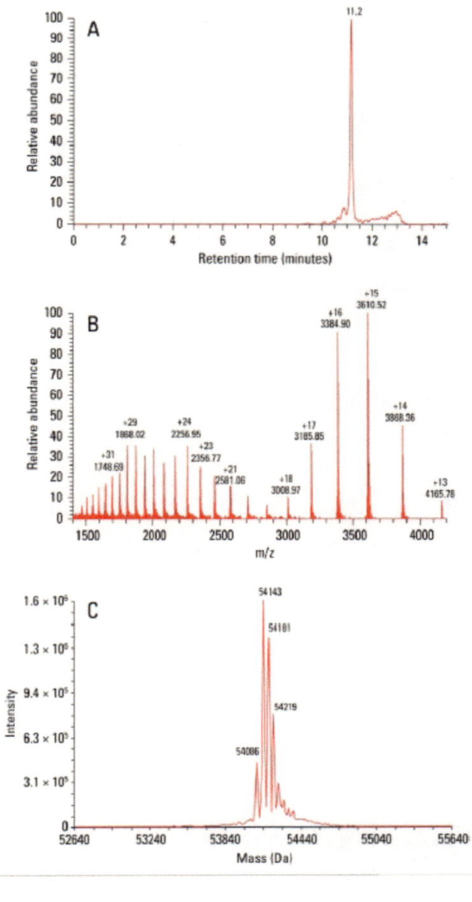

A: total ion chromatogram
B: mass spectrum
C: deconvoluted spectrum of BiTE

A main peak can be seen at m/z 54,143; adjacent peaks at m/z 54,181, 54,219 and 54,086 correspond to different salt adducts.

Figure 24. SEC/MS analysis of the CD19 X CD3 BiTE antibody.

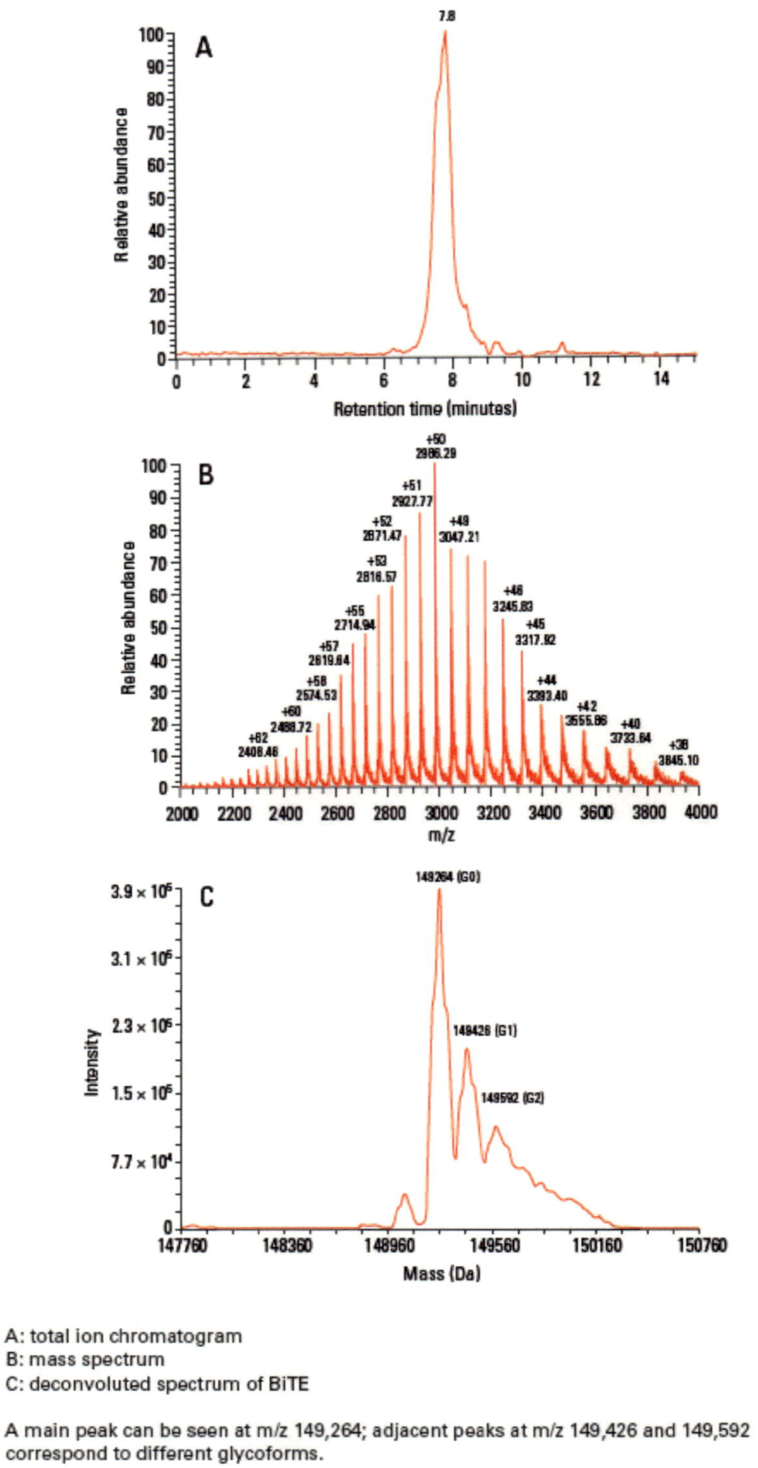

Figure 25. SEC/MS analysis of the original IgG1 mAb1.

http://dx.doi.org/10.5772/intechopen.73321

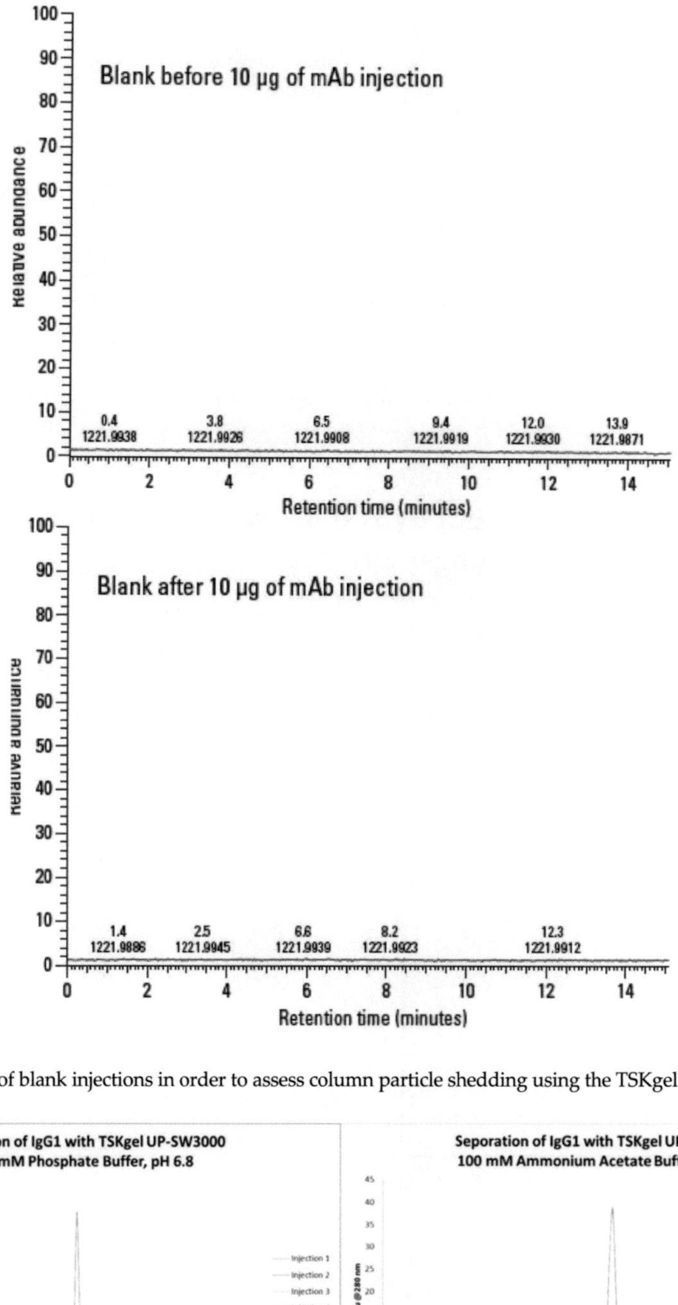

Figure 26. Analysis of blank injections in order to assess column particle shedding using the TSKgel UP-SW3000 column.

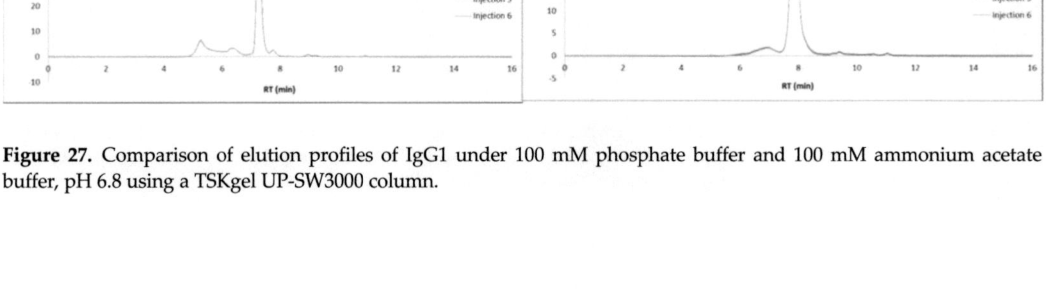

Figure 27. Comparison of elution profiles of IgG1 under 100 mM phosphate buffer and 100 mM ammonium acetate buffer, pH 6.8 using a TSKgel UP-SW3000 column.

Monomer						Monomer					
Phosphate Buffer IgG1: 2 g/L						100 mM Amm Ace pH 6.8 LC/MS Buffer IgG1: 2 g/L					
Injection	**RT**	**Area**	**Height**	**As**	**N**	**Injection**	**RT**	**Area**	**Height**	**As**	**N**
1	7.258	11.6	66.7	1.3	12104	**1**	7.872	11.9	37.3	1.2	4623
2	7.258	11.6	66.5	1.3	12083	**2**	7.877	11.9	37.4	1.2	4628
3	7.258	11.6	66.6	1.3	12058	**3**	7.875	11.9	37.7	1.2	4637
4	7.260	11.6	66.6	1.2	12074	**4**	7.875	12.0	37.9	1.2	4656
5	7.258	11.6	66.4	1.3	12042	**5**	7.878	12.0	38.2	1.2	4657
6	7.260	11.7	66.9	1.3	11974	**6**	7.878	12.1	38.5	1.2	4651
Avg	7.259	11.6	66.6	1.3	12056	**Avg**	7.876	12.0	37.8	1.2	4642
Std	0.0	0.0	0.2	0.0	45.3	**Std**	0.0	0.1	0.5	0.0	14.7
%RSD	0.0	0.4	0.3	0.5	0.4	**%RSD**	0.0	0.8	1.2	1.2	0.3

Table 4. Analysis of retention time, peak area, peak height, as (peak asymmetry) and N (theoretical plates) of the monomers. The average (Avg), standard deviation (Std) and relative standard deviation (RSD) are also shown.

5. Size exclusion chromatography and its orthogonal and complimentary modes for detection of heterogeneity

Two chromatographic modes are considered orthogonal techniques if the selectivity of the two modes are significantly different. Under ideal conditions without any secondary interaction, SEC should yield a characteristic Gaussian-shaped peak without the presence of any heterogeneity.

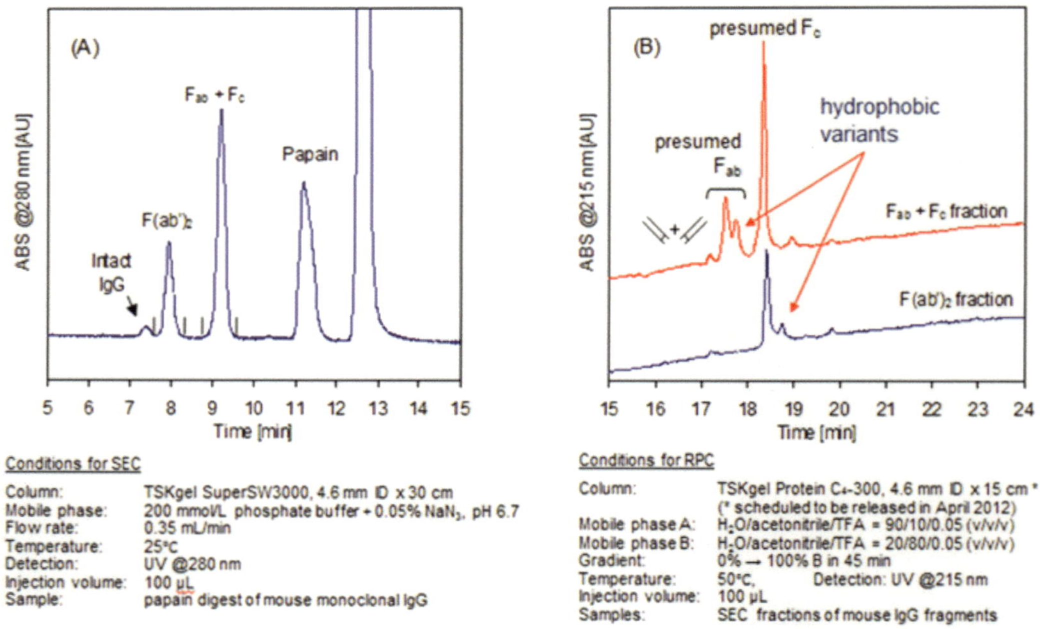

Figure 28. Analysis of papain digested IgG1 fragments. (A) Chromatogram of papain digested IgG1 fragments separated on a TSKgel SuperSW3000 column. (B) Individual peaks F (ab) 2 and Fab + Fc from the SEC separation (panel A) were applied to a reversed-phase chromatographic (RPC) TSKgel protein C4–300 column.

As shown in the figure below when individual peaks F (ab) 2 and Fab + Fc from SEC separation (panel A) were applied to the reversed-phase chromatographic (RPC) column, a number of hydrophobic variants eluted (panel B) in the increasing order of their hydrophobicity (**Figure 28**). Mechanism of papain digestion is discussed in Section 2.6. Though papain digestion yields primarily the Fab fragments, F(ab')2 fragment can be generated if the papain is first activated with 10 mM cysteine. Following the completion of the reaction, the excess needs to be removed by gel filtration. Size exclusion chromatography cannot differentiate these heterogenic impurities or hydrophobic variants, which are not sufficiently different in the size or hydrodynamic radii from each other. Similarly, a number of other chromatographic modes, other than RPC, can also be used as an orthogonal technique. The extent of the heterogeneity present in the SEC peak can only be confirmed by an orthogonal analysis.

Similarly, a reversed-phase chromatography column can also be used as a complimentary chromatography column along with SEC as shown below (**Figure 29**). The elution order of elution of the peaks is simply reversed as expected.

The PEG-conjugated species were more strongly retained by RPC, than the different forms of intact lysozyme. The order of elution in RPC is opposite to the order of size-based separation in SEC [35].

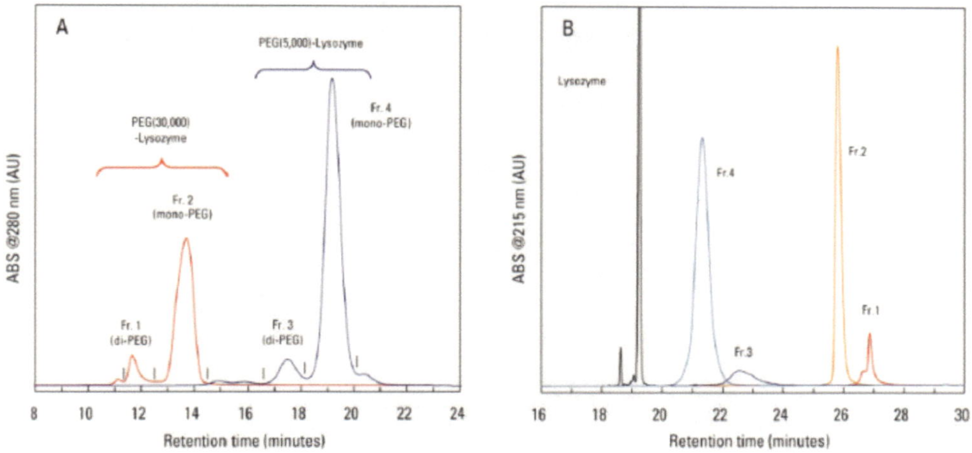

Conditions for SEC

Column:	TSKgel SuperSW3000, 4.6 mm ID × 30 cm × 2
Mobile phase:	200 mmol/L phosphate buffer, pH 6.7 + 0.05% NaN_3
Flow rate:	0.35 mL/min
Temperature:	25 °C
Detection:	UV @ 280 nm
Injection vol.:	50 μL
Samples:	5 g/L PEG(MW 5,000)-Lysozyme, 5 g/L PEG(MW 30,000)-Lysozyme

Conditions for RPC

Column:	TSKgel Protein C_4-300, 4.6 mm ID × 15 cm
Mobile phase A:	H_2O/acetonitrile/TFA = 90/10/0.05 (v/v/v)
Mobile phase B:	H_2O/acetonitrile/TFA = 20/80/0.05 (v/v/v)
Gradient:	0%→ 100% B in 45 min
Temperature:	40 °C
Detection:	UV @ 215 nm
Injection vol.	100 μL
Samples:	0.1 g/L lysozyme, SEC fractions 1~4 shown in the left figure.

Figure 29. Separation of PEG (MW 5000)-lysozyme and PEG (MW 30,000)-lysozyme on a SEC TSKgel SuperSW3000 column (A) followed by chromatography of the SEC fractions 1–4 using a reverse phase TSKgel protein C_4–300 column (B).

6. Method transfer

With the advancement of the liquid chromatographic instruments from HPLC to UHPLC and with the advancement in column packing technology with smaller particle sizes, an easy method transfer from HPLC to UHPLC is becoming necessary. UHPLC has much lower extra column volume and can withstand more than 1000 bar besides other optimized instrumental features while conventional HPLC has maximum operable pressure of 400 bars. Differences between HPLC and UHPLC instruments give rise to many challenges when a method needs to be transferred from one system to another and if equivalent separation profiles are obtained. On the other hand, there are analysts who do not possess the UHPLC but still want to get advantage of smaller particle size SEC columns while using a traditional HPLC instrument. The effect of extra column volume in band broadening in conventional HPLC needs to be reduced and optimized by reducing the diffusion in the tubing between the injection valve and the column and between the column and the UV cell by using smaller ID tubing and micro flow cell. A column compatible with both UHPLC and conventional HPLC instruments may be helpful for easy method transfer in both cases.

As an example, an SEC HPLC method for the separation of a mAb using 5 μm, 7.8 mm ID × 30 cm SEC column (TSKgel G3000SWXL) was transferred to a 2 μm, 4.6 mm ID × 30 cm SEC column (TSKgel UP-SW3000 SEC) on a UHPLC instrument (**Figure 30**). The mobile phase and other chromatographic parameters were not changed except the flow rate reduced for the 2-μm column.

A

B

- **Instrument:** All analyses were carried out using an Ultimate 3 system run by Chromeleon (ver 7.2) and Agilent un by Chemstation (ver B.04.02)
- **Column:** TSKgel UP-SW3000, 2 μm, 4.6 mm ID x 300 mm (A00115-89A) TSKgel G3000SWXL, 5 μm, 7.8 mm ID x 300 mm (A01905-07W)
- **Mobile phase:** 100 mM KH_2PO_4 / Na_2HPO_4, pH 6.7, 100 mM Na_2SO_4, 0.05 % NaN_3
- **Flow rate:** 0.35 mL/min (UHPLC), 1.0 mL/min (HPLC)
- **Pressure:** TSKgel UP-SW3000: 27.2 MPa [UHPLC], 26.7 MPa [HPLC] TSKgel G3000SWXL: 4.0 MPa [HPLC]
- **Detection:** UV @ 280 nm
- **Temperature:** 25 °C

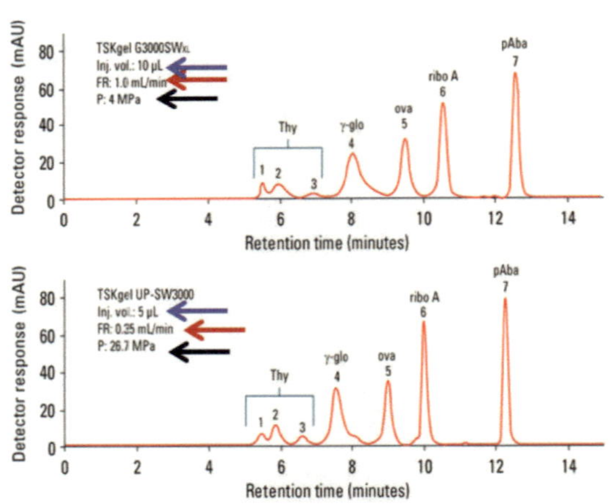

Peak resolutions	Rs 1-2	Rs 2-3	Rs 3-4	Rs 4-5	Rs 5-6	Rs 6-7
TSKgel UP-SW3000	0.89	1.68	1.94	3.32	3.35	8.75
TSKgel G3000SWXL	0.98	1.46	1.56	2.52	2.71	6.41

Figure 30. Comparison of the SEC HPLC method with the SEC UHPLC system. Separation efficiency of column TSKgel G3000SWXL (A) and column TSKgel UP-SW3000 SEC (B) was compared by loading a mixture of standard proteins (Thy = thyroglobulin bovine, γ-glo = γ-globulins from bovine blood, ova = albumin chicken egg grade VI, riboA = ribonuclease A type I-A from bovine pancreas, pAba = p-aminobenzoid acid) on both columns.

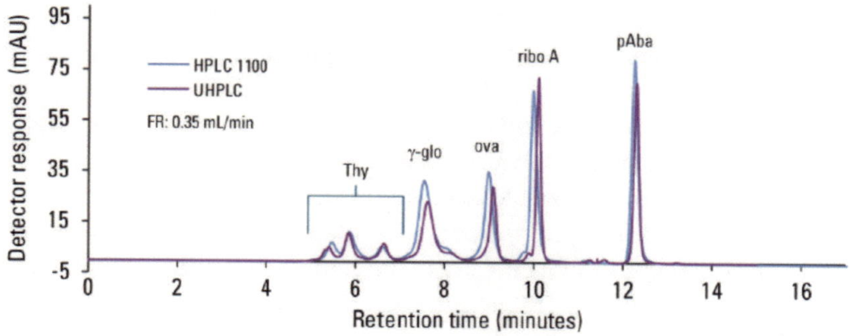

	Rs (Thy-γ-Glo)	Rs (γ-Glo-Ova)	Rs (Ribo A-pAba)
Agilent 1100 HPLC	3.52	3.22	10.23
Dionex UltiMate 3000RS UHPLC	4.46	3.85	11.61

Figure 31. Comparison of the separation efficiency of a 2-μm TSKgel UP-SW3000 column applied in HPLC and UHPLC mode. Conditions were the same as in **Figure 30**. The same standard protein mixture as in **Figure 30** was used.

TSKgel UP-SW3000 columns feature the same pore size as the well-established TSKgel G3000SWxl columns. With the use of the 2-μm column, the resolution between peaks 2–3, 3–4, 4–5, 5–6, and 6–7 increased respectively by 15, 25, 33, 24, and 37% compared to the 5-μm column. Retention time consistency was maintained, and similar separation profile was obtained at lower flow rate. A smaller 2-μm particle size column yielded a twofold higher sensitivity. The 2-μm columns yielded a back pressure acceptable for use in both HPLC and UHPLC.

Similarly, a method can be transferred directly from HPLC to UHPLC, without any change in conditions using 2 μm TSKgel UP-SW3000 columns as shown in **Figure 31** [42].

7. SEC for desalting

Desalting is a process to remove or reduce salt from the liquid, such as protein sample solution. Desalting by gel filtration chromatography (GFC) is the preferred method in biochemical laboratories to reduce the salt concentration or to exchange the buffer of a biopolymer solution. The main advantage of desalting by GFC over dialysis is the faster analysis time. Desalting may be needed for various reasons. Proteins eluting at high or elevated salt concentrations may need to be desalted to lower salt concentration prior to its use for the next step. Protein samples may also contain denaturants such as sodium dodecyl sulfate (SDS), guanidine hydrochloride, and urea which need to be removed. Desalting and buffer exchange of proteins or polynucleotides can also be performed by dialysis, ultra-filtration, or by using spin columns. Desalting columns are characterized by a low exclusion limit and a large pore volume. Salts can fully access all pores, while proteins and other high MW species are excluded. Analytical columns packed with conventional packing materials such as dextran, cellulose, and polyacrylamide have limited physical stability and are not suitable when fast desalting is desired. Requirements for a fast desalting SEC column are [1] an inert matrix, [2] a large pore volume that is fully accessible to common salts and buffer components, [3] a pore size distribution that excludes the component(s) of interest from accessing the pores, and [4] sufficient mechanical strength to allow the use of the column in standard HPLC equipment. As an example, a 15-μm particle size TSKgel BioAssist DS column is composed of a stationary phase where the mechanical strength of the polyacrylamide gel is fourfold higher as compared to conventional gel by urea cross-linking. Conventionally, polyacrylamide beads have been prepared by reversed-phase suspension polymerization or by using a spray dry method. The uniform and more pressure-stable polyacrylamide beads packed in TSKgel BioAssist DS columns were prepared using a normal phase suspension method as shown in **Figure 32** [43].

Fast desalting with excellent reproducibility could be carried out within 5 min using conventional HPLC system and TSKgel BioAssist DS Columns (4.6 mm ID and 10 mm ID) (**Figure 33**). All the proteins (see table below) eluted with the same retention time closer to void volume irrespective of their size (see the figures below), while salt and other small impurities eluted at longer retention time as a function of their size. Refractive index was used as a detector in this study since salts do not have any chromophore.

SEC columns designed for desalting using a HPLC instrument can be useful for the desalting of proteins and polynucleotides at analytical and semi-preparative scale.

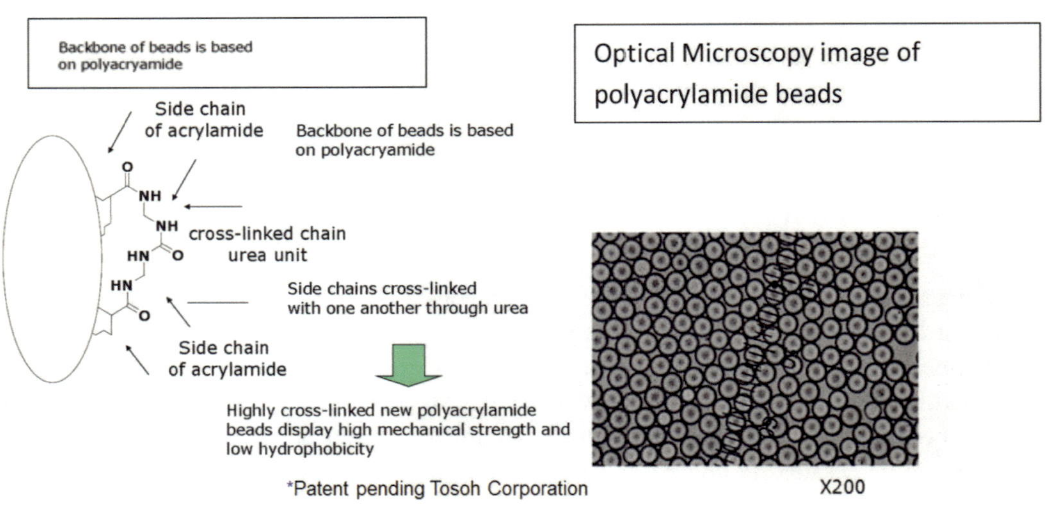

Figure 32. Principle of the generation of pressure-stable polyacrylamide beads which can be packed in TSKgel BioAssist DS columns.

Protein	MW (kDa)	Concentration* (g/L approx.)
ribonuclease A	14.7	19.5
thyroglobulin	670	11.3
γ-globulin	150	14.5
ovalbumin	45	13.1
α-chymotrypsinogen	25.6	13.1
β-lactoglobulin	18.4	10.8
lysozyme	14.7	11.6
myoglobin	16.7	14.5
cytochrome C	12.3	11.0
hemoglobin	68	11.9

*in 100 mmol/L Phosphate buffer, pH 6.7

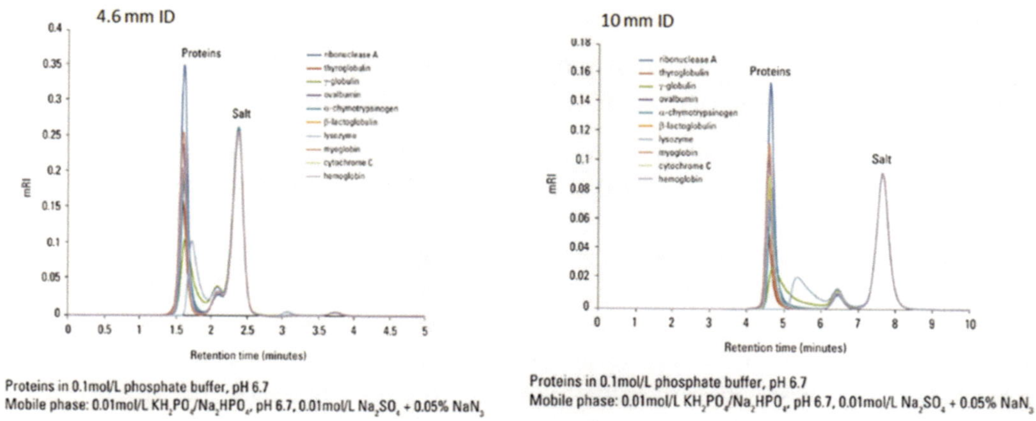

Figure 33. Desalting of proteins using a TSKgel BioAssist DS column with 4.6 mm ID or 10 mm ID packed with pressure-stable polyacrylamide beads. The retention times of standard proteins and salt are shown.

8. Size exclusion chromatography column in the HILIC mode

For many years, SEC columns have been used to separate various nucleic acid species such as DNA, RNA, and tRNA as well as their constituent bases, adenine, guanine, thymine, cytosine, and uracil. In medicine, several primary nucleobases are the basis for the nucleoside analogues and other synthetic analogs which are used as anticancer and antiviral agents. Nucleobase modifications are the basis of oligonucleotide-based therapeutics, making their purification very important.

Hydrophilic interaction chromatography (HILIC) is a variant of normal phase liquid chromatography which uses hydrophilic stationary phases with reversed-phase type eluents. It is applied for the separation of polar hydrophilic compounds.

Chemically bonded diol-coated phases in size exclusion chromatography (SEC) columns demonstrate high polarity and hydrogen bonding properties. They do not contain ionizable groups compared to the unreacted free residual silanols, making them appropriate for the HILIC mode.

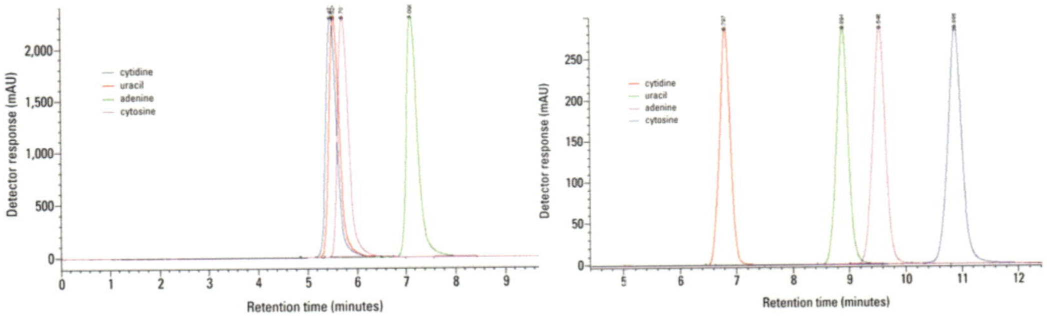

Figure 34. Separation of four nucleobases using a TSKgel SuperSW mAb HTP column under SEC condition (left panel) and in HILIC mode (right panel) at pH 7.4.

Figure 34 [44] shows the separation of four nucleobases using a TSKgel SuperSW mAb HTP Column under SEC condition and in HILIC mode at pH 7.4 (**Figure 34**).

As expected, due to the similarities in molecular masses between the four compounds, significant interference is observed among the peaks of interest, particularly the three pyrimidine derivatives, when separated on the TSKgel SuperSW mAb HTP column under SEC conditions. The late elution of adenine (relative to the other three compounds) may be attributed to possible interactions between the stationary phase and the derivatized purine compound, leading to a shift toward a longer retention time. When the same SEC column is used in the HILIC mode, the order of elution of the analytes does not correlate with their molecular mass (as in SEC separations), but instead is based on their relative hydrophilicity. This note demonstrates the benefits of using a SEC column in HILIC mode for the superior resolution of four nucleobases, as opposed to using the column in the SEC mode or using another type of a HILIC column.

9. Tips and tricks for size exclusion chromatography

It is a recommended practice to protect the column from potential sources of contamination during the SEC separation of mAbs and other proteins. Standards and mobile phases should be filtered through a 0.45-μm syringe filter. A frit filter used between injector and column will also be an additional help. The use of guard columns is highly recommended. Guard columns being short, of similar ID and with the same stationary phase do not possess any separation power. The slight change in the retention time due to small increase in length remains constant in consecutive injections. Using guard columns can prolong the lifetime of the analytical column. The guard column needs to be changed before the dirty material spills over to the analytical column. Frits at different parts of the HPLC instruments need to be changed intermittently. Please refer to the picture below which clearly shows how much dirty materials are trapped by these frits (**Figure 35**). Frequent changes of the frits are necessary to avoid spillage of the dirty materials to the columns. Phosphate buffer pH 6.8, very commonly used for the protein analysis by SEC is prone to bacterial growth. The column will get clogged and dirty, eventually leading to failure of the analysis and breakdown of the system. Previously I

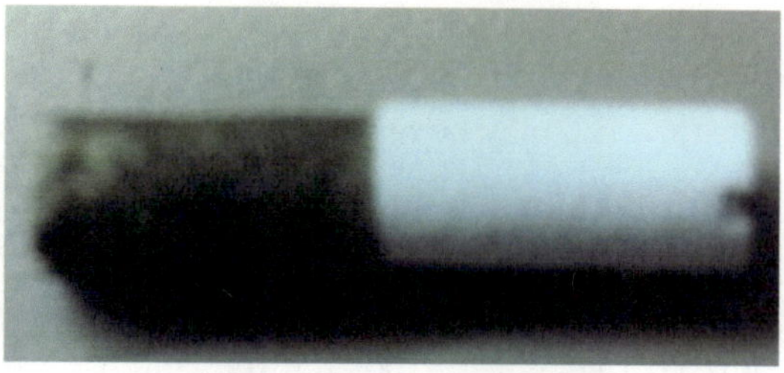

Figure 35. Comparison of a dirty frit with a new frit.

mentioned that sodium azide (NaN_3) was used as an antibacterial agent to prevent fouling of the phosphate buffer.

During the SEC of mAbs and proteins, mobile phases containing salts are constantly used and can deposit on the different parts of the HPLC system (**Figure 36**). The pump head assembly may get affected from the deposition of salts, resulting into a rise of back pressure as well as causing damage to the sapphire piston. The pump head assembly can be cleaned with distilled water and the back pressure issue is resolved. Mobile phase containing high salt or a combination of high salt and organic solvent can create this problem more than any other low salt aqueous mobile phases. The system should not remain idle with these types of mobile phases. The deposition may happen anywhere within the HPLC system and also inside the column, or in the pump, the injector, the in-line filter or the tubing.

The use of a surfactant is necessary for certain SEC applications as discussed earlier, but surfactants may change the bonding phase, so it may be necessary to dedicate the column for that particular application.

Occasionally protein samples are adsorbed onto the packing material. When this occurs, it is time to clean the SEC column. At the beginning of the separation, when the SEC column is new and operating correctly and the mAb monomer is yielding a well-resolved peak, it is better to establish baseline data and acceptable running conditions criteria. Then, if one of the performance

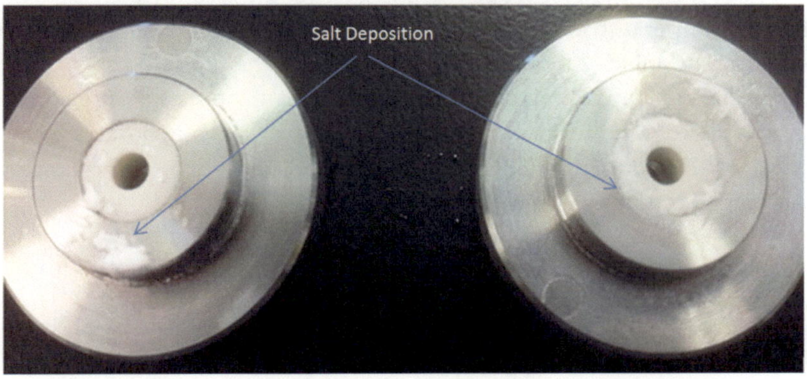

Figure 36. Salt depositions at screws of the column.

characteristics of the SEC column changes by 10% or more, it is prudent that cleaning is necessary. The acceptance criteria can be more stringent as needed. Similar cleaning of the whole system including the flow cell may be necessary.

If cleaning is necessary, it is better to try cleaning the column in reversed direction at half the flow rate while the column is detached from the detector to prevent detector damage since the proteins have a tendency to adhere to the quartz material of the detector. Since the dirty materials may remain trapped over the frit outside the column, cleaning in reversed flow direction may be the easiest way to clean the column. Once the column is cleaned using the vendor suggested protocol, the analyst must qualify the column using the QC method and QC pass criteria under normal flow direction.

It is always recommended to read the operational conditions and specification sheet (OCS) before the column is used. Occasionally, we may intend to use the column outside the specification for a short period of time, but it is the responsibility of the analyst to monitor if the column is functioning properly. For example, in Section 2.5, it has been shown that an analysis could be repeated to monitor the stability of the antibody over time using a TSKgel SuperSW mAb-HTP column at 0.75 mL/min. The used flow rate (0.75 mL/min) was higher than the recommended maximum flow rate of 0.5 mL/min, as mentioned in the operational conditions and specification (OCS) sheet for this column. Though the column could successfully be used at this higher flow rate without compromising the column health, the effect of the higher flow rate on the column lifetime for prolonged use was not investigated. It is always wise to operate within recommended maximum flow rate to remain in safe side in order to prolong the lifetime of the column. It is always necessary to keep an eye on the back pressure, peak parameters, and so on to monitor the column health.

HPLC system and analytical chromatography columns are costly. Method development is time-consuming and costly too. It is important to employ an HPLC system that is optimized with regard to extra-column band broadening to take full advantage of the high column efficiency that can be obtained on analytical columns. For any troubleshooting situation, the problem is one of the following: [1] the column, [2] the sample, [3] the mobile phases, [4] the instrumentation, and [5] personal errors. The same is true for size exclusion chromatography related troubleshooting issues too. Proper maintenance of the column and instrument is much more needed and important to avoid the troubleshooting in the beginning. Many troubleshooting issues can be avoided by taking proper handling the top three major components of any HPLC analysis. The importance of the use of a protein standard mixture and the standard mAb to monitor the column health from time to time is always a good idea as mentioned in brief in Section 2.5. Maintaining a SEC column is an art and good performance, which will result in a prolonged column lifetime.

10. Conclusions

Size-exclusion chromatography is a great tool for the purification of monoclonal antibodies. The secondary interaction of the stationary phase needs to be taken care of by controlling the stationary phase as well as by optimizing the mobile phase. The effect of particle size and pore size of the stationary phase on SEC separation needs to be clearly understood. A right column selection for the purification will depend on the separation range and the slope of the calibration curve. Separation of HMW and LMW species to purify the monomer is critical to get the pure mAb without heterogenic impurities, which might be immunogenic to human. Enzymatic digestion and forced degradations are necessary to characterize the monoclonal antibodies, and SEC columns need to be rightfully selected based on the separation goal. Mobile phase additives may be necessary to improve the separation, and few examples are discussed. Since online LC/MS is becoming popular, a mobile phase compatibility is needed as discussed in this chapter. Since size exclusion chromatography cannot separate the heterogenic species without much difference in hydrodynamic radii, an orthogonal technique is necessary. A similarly complimentary technique is also helpful for complete characterization of the monoclonal antibodies. SEC column developed, and optimization of surface and pore characteristics is critical for the separation of monoclonal antibodies and other proteins by HPLC and UHPLC instrument. With the advancement of UHPLC, an easy method transfer between HPLC and UHPLC is becoming necessary. Ease of method transfer using a column with dual functionality for its use in both HPLC and UHPLC is helpful. Desalting using a conventional SEC HPLC column can be very useful in removing the unwanted salts and additives. A robust separation with excellent reproducibility needs a size exclusion chromatography column with optimized packing as well as the knowledge about the tips and tricks to maintain the column lifetime.

Acknowledgements

Yoshimi Hashimoto, Toshiaki Nishi, Kazuaki Muranaka, Kosuke Araki, Yasutami Mitoma, Shigeru Nakatani, Hasegawa, Sachiyuki, Oscar Yamasaki, Toru Satoh – Tosoh Corporation, Separation Centre, Japan for their contributions in a number of references and overall support. Tosoh Bioscience LLC and Tosoh Corporation, Tosoh Bioscience LLC, Tosoh Bioscience Gmbh.

Author details

Atis Chakrabarti

Address all correspondence to: atis.chakrabarti@tosoh.com

Tosoh Bioscience LLC, USA

References

[1] Janeway CA Jr, Travers P, Walport M, et al. Immunobiology: The Immune System in Health and Disease. 5th ed. New York: Garland Science; 2001

[2] Elgert KD. Immunology: Understanding the Immune System, Chapter 04 Copyright ©. John Wiley & Sons, Inc; 1998

[3] Vidarsson G, Dekkers G, Rispens T. IgG subclasses and allotypes: From structure to effector functions. Frontiers in Immunology. 2014 Oct 20;**5**:520

[4] Starkie DO, Compson JE, Rapecki S, Lightwood DJ. Generation of recombinant monoclonal antibodies from immunised mice and rabbits via flow Cytometry and sorting of antigen-specific IgG+ memory B cells. PLoS One. March 29, 2016

[5] Morrow PR, Rennick DM, Leung CY, Benjamini E. The antibody response to a single antigenic determinant of the tobacco mosaic virus protein: Analysis using monoclonal antibodies, mutant proteins and synthetic peptides. Molecular Immunology. Apr 1984;**21**(4):301-309

[6] Beerli RR, Bauer M, Buser RB, Gwerder M, Muntwiler S, Maurer P, Saudan P, Bachmann MF. Isolation of human monoclonal antibodies by mammalian cell display. PNAS. September 23, 2008;**105**(38):14336-14341

[7] Reichert JM. Antibodies to watch in 2013: Mid-year update. MAbs. 2013;**5**:513-517

[8] Yang X, Wang F, Zhang Y, Wang L, Antonenko S, Zhang S, Zhang YW, Tabrizifard M, Ermakov G, Wiswell D, Beaumont M, Liu L, Richardson D, Shameem M, Ambrogelly A. Comprehensive analysis of the therapeutic IgG4 antibody Pembrolizumab: Hinge modification blocks half molecule exchange in vitro and in vivo. Journal of Pharmaceutical Sciences. Dec 2015;**104**(12):4002-4014

[9] Hong P, Koza S, ESP B. Size-exclusion chromatography for the analysis of protein biotherapeutics and their aggregates. Journal of Liquid Chromatography and Related Technologies. Nov 2012;**35**(20):2923-2950

[10] Coppola G, Underwood J, Cartwright G, Hearn MT. High-performance liquid chromatography of amino acids, peptides and proteins. XCIII. Comparison of methods for the purification of mouse monoclonal immunoglobulin M autoantibodies. Journal of Chromatography. 1989 Aug 4;**476**:269-290

[11] https://www.ncbi.nlm.nih.gov/pubmed

[12] Haberger M, Leiss M, Heidenreich A-K, Pester O, Hafenmair G, Hook M, Bonnington L, Wegele H, Haindl M, Reusch D, Bulau P. Rapid characterization of biotherapeutic proteins by size-exclusion chromatography coupled to native mass spectrometry. MAbs. 2016;**8**(2):331-339

[13] Ackers GK. Molecular exclusion and restricted diffusion processes in molecular-sieve chromatography. Biochemistry. 1964;**3**(5):723-730

[14] Eksteen R, Pardue KJ. Modified silica-based packing materials for size exclusion chromatography. In: Wu C-s, editor. Handbook of Size Exclusion Chromatography. Vol. 69. NY: Marcel Dekker; 1995. p. 453

[15] Arakawa T, Philo JS, Ejima D, Tsumoto K and Arisaka F. Bioprocess International, 2006 v4. (10) 42–43 (November 2006)

[16] Benner C, Chakrabarti A. Size exclusion chromatography column with larger exclusion limit useful for the separation of biomolecules using UHPLC and HPLC. Abstract #120–1, Session: Bioanalytical: LC Techniques; PITTCON 2016 Oral Presentation

[17] Separation Report SR 074, Tosoh Bioscience; visit: https://www.separations.us.tosohbioscience.com/literature

[18] Fesinmeyer RM, Hogan S, Saluja A, Brych SR, Kras E, Narhi LO, Brems DN, Gokarn YR. Effect of ions on agitation- and temperature-induced aggregation reactions of antibodies. Pharmaceutical Research. April 2009;**26**(4):903-913

[19] Wakankar A, Chen Y, Gokarn Y, Jacobson FS. Analytical methods for physicochemical characterization of antibody drug conjugates. MAbs. March/April 2011;**3**(2):161-172

[20] Amano M, Hasegawa J, Kobayashi N, Kishi N, Nakazawa T, Uchiyama S, Fukui K. Specific racemization of heavy-chain Cysteine-220 in the hinge region of immunoglobulin gamma 1 as a possible cause of degradation during storage. Analytical Chemistry. 2011; **83**:3857-3864

[21] Stathopulos PB, Scholz GA, Hwang Y-M, JAO R, Lepock JR, Meiering EM. Sonication of proteins causes formation of aggregates that resemble amyloid. Protein Science. Nov 2004;**13**(11):3017-3027

[22] https://www.fda.gov/downloads/drugs/guidancecomplianceregulatoryinformation/guidances/ucm073373.pdf

[23] Fischer N, Elson G, Magistrelli G, et al. Exploiting light chains for the scalable generation and platform purification of native human bispecific IgG. Nature Communications. 2015;**6**:7113

[24] Blatt NB, Bill RM, Glick GD. Characterization of a unique anti-DNA hybridoma. Hybridoma. Feb 1998;**17**(1):33-39

[25] Kungulovski G, Jeltsch A. Quality of histone modification antibodies undermines chromatin biology research. Protein Engineering, Design & Selection. 2015;**28**(10):303-305

[26] Zack DJ, Wong AL, Stempniak M, Weisbart RH. Two kappa immunoglobulin light chains are secreted by an anti-DNA hybridoma: Implications for isotypic exclusion. Molecular Immunology. Dec 1995;**32**(17–18):1345-1353

[27] Steve J, Chakrabarti A. High throughput and highly reproducible sub-separation of proteins and antibodies using size exclusion chromatography. Tosoh Bioscience LLC; Poster #212, Session – HPLC of Peptides, Proteins and Other Biomolecules Eastern Analytical Symposium 2014

[28] Application Note AN95 Tosoh Bioscience; https://www.separations.us.tosohbioscience.com/HPLC_Columns/id-8306/TSKgel_UP-SW3000

[29] Majors R. Current trends in column usage. LCGC. Jan 1, 2012

[30] Chakrabarti A. Troubleshooting tricks and tips about column maintenance and Improving column lifetime of aqueous size exclusion chromatography columns m Poster. HPLC 2012. Anaheim, CA

[31] Chakrabarti A. Three novel prototype SEC columns for the separation of an antibody monomer from its dimer, higher aggregates, and antibody fragments Poster – Fall ACS. 2012

[32] Application note: AN 97; visit: https://www.separations.us.tosohbioscience.com/HPLC_Columns/id-8306/TSKgel_UP-SW3000 Tosoh Bioscience

[33] Separation Report SR 046. visit: https://www.separations.us.tosohbioscience.com/literature

[34] Gayen-Betal S, Chakrabarti A. Separation of BSA monomer from its dimer and aggregates using a 125 Å pore size diol coated 7.8 mm ID × 30 cm, 5 μm gel filtration column. Poster, HPLC 2012 Anaheim, CA

[35] Kawai Y, Yamasaki H and Moriyama H. Separation Center, TOSOH Corporation, Kaisei-cho 4560 Shunan, Yamaguchi 746–8501, Japan; New silica-based SEC columns designed for the separation of mAb monomers and their impurities; Poster – PITTCON 2012

[36] Hawe A, Wiggenhorn M, van de Weert M, Garbe JH, Mahler HC, Jiskoot W.; Forced degradation of therapeutic proteins, Journal of Pharmaceutical Sciences Mar 2012;**101**(3): 895-913

[37] Hughes H, Morgan C, Brunyak E, Barranco K, Cohen E, Edmunds T, Lee KA. Multi-tiered analytical approach for the analysis and quantitation of high-molecular-weight aggregates in a recombinant therapeutic glycoprotein. The AAPS Journal. June 2009;**11**(2):335-341

[38] Greenfield NJ. Using circular dichroism spectra to estimate protein secondary structure. Nature Protocols. 2006;**1**(6):2876-2890

[39] Chakrabarti A et al. Separation of Monoclonal Antibody and Protein Aggregates Induced by Thermal Denaturation, using a Novel Size Exclusion Chromatography Column, Poster Fall ACS. 2013

[40] Chakrabarti A et al Characterization of Two Novel Analytical Chromatographic Columns for Orthogonal Analysis of Monoclonal Antibodies and Protein Aggregates and Their Isoforms, Poster ISPPP 2013

[41] Chakrabarti A. A brief overview of the analysis of biomolecules using gel filtration chromatography (GFC): common issues in method development and troubleshooting Oral Presentation, PITTCON 2012

[42] Benner C, Chakrabarti A, et al. Characterization Of New 2 μm Particle Size, 25 nm Pore Size Analytical Size Exclusion Chromatography Column With Larger Exclusion Limit Useful For The Separation Of Biomolecules Using UHPLC And HPLC–Poster, ESF New York Biotechnology Symposium 2016

[43] Hashimoto Y, Nishi T, Muranaka K, Araki K, Mitoma Y, Higley TJ, Nakatani S. The Characteristic of New Desalting Column for Biomolecule. PITTCON: Poster; 2005

[44] Application Note AN064, Separation of Nucleobases using TSKgel® SuperSW mAb HTP column in HILIC mode, visit https://www.separations.us.tosohbioscience.com/literature

Chapter 8

The Development of Single Domain Antibodies for Diagnostic and Therapeutic Applications

Chiuan Herng Leow, Qin Cheng, Katja Fischer and James McCarthy

Additional information is available at the end of the chapter

http://dx.doi.org/10.5772/intechopen.73324

Abstract

Monoclonal antibodies have become increasingly accepted as diagnostics and therapeutics for various human diseases due to their high affinity and specificity. However, several practical drawbacks are apparent for the reagents based on conventional IgG antibodies. With the emergence of antibody engineering, many problems were overcome when the recombinant antibody fragments such as Fabs, scFvs, diabodies and single domain antibodies (sdAbs), are developed. These fragments not only retain the specificity of the whole monoclonal antibodies, but are also easy to express and produce in prokaryotic expression systems. Rather unexpectedly, the natural sdAbs namely V_{HH}s, V_{NAR}s and variable lymphocyte receptors (VLRs) that comprise excellent biological activities were recently discovered in camelids, cartilaginous fish and lampreys, respectively. Due to their unique characteristics, including small size, high thermostability, stable folding in the nucleus and cytosol and long CDR3 regions which have access to cavities or clefts on the surface of proteins, these new binders are now investigated extensively as a substitute for conventional antibodies. This review describes the potential of sdAbs selected using *in vitro* display systems and their use in multiple applications.

Keywords: recombinant antibody, single domain antibody, diagnostic and therapeutic single domain antibody, scFv, IgNAR, V_{HH}, VLR, V_{NAR}s

1. Introduction

In research applications, antibodies are widely used as binders due to their high specificity and high affinity. Antibodies can be classified into three different categories such as polyclonal antibodies, monoclonal antibodies and recombinant antibodies [1]. Polyclonal antibodies

INTECH
open science | open minds

© 2018 The Author(s). Licensee InTech. This chapter is distributed under the terms of the Creative Commons Attribution License (http://creativecommons.org/licenses/by/3.0), which permits unrestricted use, distribution, and reproduction in any medium, provided the original work is properly cited. (cc) BY

(polyclonal Abs) are heterogeneous antibody mixtures that are derived from multiple plasma cell lines. Because polyclonal antibodies comprise a mixture of different antibodies carrying numerous paratopes, they have excellent properties for recognizing antigens [2]. A monoclonal antibody (mAb) is a homogeneous antibody generated from a single B lymphocyte clone. Antibodies produced in mAb format have an extremely high specificity against a single epitope on antigens [3]. Recombinant antibodies (rAbs) are antibodies generated using molecular biology techniques. They are aimed to improve the sensitivity, selectivity, stability and immobilization properties in diagnostic applications, for example, in biosensors [4]. In making decision to use or generate polyclonal, monoclonal or recombinant antibodies, several factors should be considered, including commercial availability, possibility to raise animals, types of applications, time length of a project and costs [1]. Although a vast number of rAbs has been proposed [5–8], the natural sdAb fragments that were recently discovered from camelids (V_{HH}s), sharks (V_{NAR}s) and lampreys (VLRs) have shown to possess extraordinary features that are not found in conventional antibodies, such as a small dimension, an elevated stability and the capability of recognizing cavities and clefts on the surface of proteins that cannot be reached by conventional recombinant antibodies [9–11]. This chapter will discuss the availability of new binders derived from vertebrates and give an overview of their applications in a biomedical platform by recognizing specified targets from various diseases.

2. Monoclonal antibodies and their limitations

The first description of monoclonal antibody (mAbs) production was published by Nobel prize winners, Kohler and Milstein in 1984 [12]. The fusion technique developed between splenic B cells and myeloma cells is termed the hybridoma technique has revolutionized immunology and medicine. The production of mAbs is not influenced by sources of animal used, making mAbs having better homogeneity in scale-up production [13]. The mAb technology has been widely applied in biomedical research and pharmaceutical industries.

Unlike polyclonal Abs, the monospecificity of a mAb enables targeting of a single epitope. This enables a range of applications, including targeting specific members of a protein family and evaluating changes in molecular conformation and targeting protein-protein interactions. However, the specificity and sensitivity of mAbs can be reduced by small changes in the structure of the antigen determining regions, or even by minor changes in pH or salt concentration. An advantage is that, mAbs can be produced at a greater concentration and much higher purity than polyclonal Abs [13].

The conventional mAb predominantly produced as IgG after an immune response, is represented in **Figure 1**. As determined by their structural and biological properties, IgG molecules have specific features, namely their large size compared to recombinant antibody fragments, higher synthesis rate and longer half-life. IgGs are the most widely used immunoglobulins for antibody-based diagnostic and therapeutic development. Generally, conventional IgGs are characterized by having a high affinity (K_a) ranging from 10^{-2} to 10^{1} nM, and excellent specificity for its cognate target epitope [14]. The high degree in variations of antibody specificities is

http://dx.doi.org/10.5772/intechopen.73324

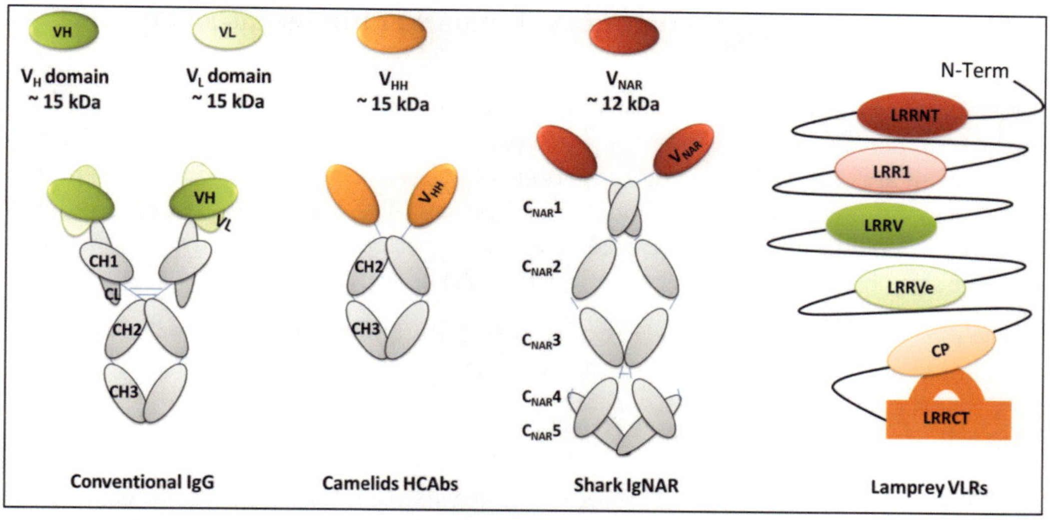

Figure 1. Schematic representation of conventional antibodies and natural single domain antibodies. The conventional IgGs derive from mammals while the natural single domain antibodies derive from camelids, sharks and lampreys, respectively. Single V domains are presented as colored ovals; C domains are shown gray colored. The domains in lamprey variable lymphocyte receptor (VLR) are demonstrated on the right. VLRs consist of an N-terminal cap (LRRNT), the first LRR (LRR1), multiple (usually up to seven) 24-residue variable LRRs (LRRVs), a terminal or end LRRV (LRRVe), a connecting peptide (CP) and a C-terminal cap (LRRCT), followed by an invariant 3′-terminal region.

conferred by the variable amino acid sequences in the variable regions of the heavy and light chain (VH and VL). Each variable domain is comprised of three hypervariable (HV) regions, separated by four framework regions (FR). The HV regions are known as complementarity-determining regions (CDRs), and are responsible for the identification of the specific epitope of the cognate antigen. The FR regions are major components of the backbone structure for VH and VL regions in antibodies and can potentially influence the conformation of the antigenic binding loops [15].

However, several practical drawbacks are apparent for diagnostic reagents based on conventional IgG antibodies. The complex architecture and large molecular size (~150 kDa) may result in weak binding when small size protein antigens are not easily recognized by the concave surfaces of CDR loops [16]. Initial attempts to generate single domain antibody fragments by separating expression of individual human VH or VL units was reported to result in solubility problems in aqueous solvents, higher cost and more time consuming process and the requirements for sophisticated protein engineering approaches [17]. Moreover, the failure of recognition of selected mAbs on conserved epitopes of specific antigens due to unbound reactivities mediated by the Fc region may hinder their utility for diagnostic applications [18, 19].

With the emergence of DNA engineering, surface display has been widely used to discover new antibody fragments as a means for diagnostic and therapeutic applications. An overview of principles in phage display technology, including antibody library construction, biopanning, types of bacteriophages used and antibody fragments applications are further discussed in the following sessions.

3. Phage display technology for new biomarker binder discovery

Screening phage display libraries are a powerful tool for identifying specific binders from libraries containing a large diversity of phage surface expressed molecules [20, 21]. Libraries construction are achieved by fusing a repertoire of genes (genotype) encoding the peptides/proteins to a gene encoding a capsid structural protein. The "displayed" peptides/proteins (phenotypes) are included in the capsid layer on the phage surface. Ideally, these proteins should not be interfered with the phage structure [22].

The display technologies have enabled exploration of new antibodies from humans or animals, including shark, camel, llama and lamprey [23–26] that may not otherwise be discovered.

3.1. Antibody phage display library

Antibody phage display libraries have been extensively used for isolation of specific high affinity binders against unique antigens from different targets [27–31]. Three types of antibody library are typically constructed: naïve, synthetic and immunized libraries [32]. A naïve antibody library refers to the repertoire of antibody genes derived from non-immunized donors. Synthetic antibody libraries are constructed using synthesized mutated CDRs and synthetic frameworks whereas immunized libraries are based on a host immunized with a target antigen of disease [33].

The function of the phagemid vector is akin to that of a plasmid whereby the genes of interest can be cloned directly into the multiple cloning sites upstream of the capsid structural phage protein after digestion by appropriate restriction enzymes. Phage display technology has facilitated the selection of different antibody fragments using genetic engineering approaches [34]. Many antibody fragments created (Fab, scFv and diabody) were used to overcome the limitations of conventional IgG antibodies derived from higher organism [19]. Furthermore, the presentation of single domain antibodies (sdAb) of heavy chains derived from different animals are being widely investigated, including camelids V_{HH} or Nanobodies®, sharks V_{NAR} region of IgNAR [35] and the antibody of variable-like lymphocytes (VLRs) from lamprey fish [36].

3.2. Biopanning of phage display

The selection of high binding clones from antibody libraries using phage display can be undertaken *in vitro* via a process called biopanning. In this process, the antibody fragments displayed on the surface of phages are incubated with an antigen of interest that is immobilized on a surface [37, 38]. Generally, immunoabsorbent ELISA microplates, uncoated cell culture dishes and immunotubes are commonly used for ligand immobilization [39]. Non-specific or unbound phages are removed by washing, whereas phage that binds specifically to the target is eluted by changing the binding conditions, depending on types of bacteriophages used in the experiment. For instance, acidic solutions of HCl or glycine buffer are used for M13 bacteriophage [40]. Other methods include use of basic solutions of triethylamine [41], enzymatic cleavage of protease site incorporated in the recombinant coat protein [42], competition with excess antigen [38] and direct bacterial elution [43] have been reported for the elution of M13 bacteriophage. For T7 phage display system, the elution buffer is 1% SDS [44].

The amplification of eluted phage is carried out by infecting the exponential growth phase of *Escherichia coli*. To assembly and produce the recombinant phage a helper phage is added [45], whereas T7 phages can be directly released from the host by cell lysis [46]. Successive rounds of biopanning varied by types of library and target antigen used. In practice, the enrichment of phages of interest can be obtained within three to six rounds of biopanning. Further rounds of selection may potentially lead to bias by the enrichment of non-specific background phages [47, 48].

Phage display is a powerful technology for the generation of antibodies for medical applications. Nowadays, approximately 30 monoclonal antibodies have been approved by FDA for use in clinical practice with many more currently being tested in clinical trials. [49, 50]. The principle of the phage display is represented in **Figure 2**, indicating the workflows of library construction, biopanning and clone screening prior to purification for functional assays.

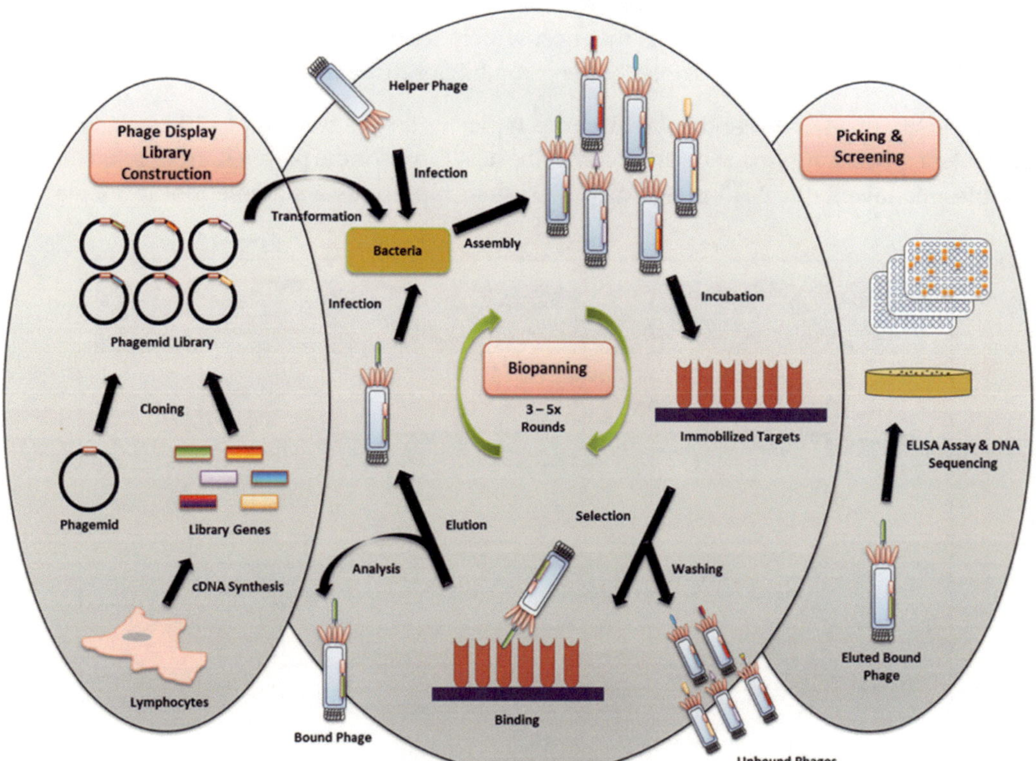

Figure 2. Principle of filamentous bacteriophage M13 phage display using a phagemid vector. Antibody genes encoding for millions of variants of libraries are cloned into a phagemid vector carrying the gene encoding for one of five phage coat proteins (pIII). Large phage libraries can be obtained by transforming *E. coli* with phagemids and rescue of phages with helperphage. Hence, phages displaying the specific antibodies against immobilized targets can be selected and isolated by several rounds of biopanning. These steps involve binding, washing, elution, infection and amplification. The eluted bound phages are subsequently screened by ELISA assay and followed by DNA sequencing prior to their protein expression and purification.

3.3. Types of bacteriophage utilized in phage display system

In phage display systems, different bacteriophages have been used to display a range of proteins on surface. M13 filamentous bacteriophage [51, 52] and T7 lytic phage are the most commonly used for displaying and production of antibody fragments [53, 54]. A comparison between M13 bacteriophage and T7 lytic phage are discussed in the following section and summarized in **Table 1**.

3.3.1. Filamentous bacteriophage M13 system

The filamentous phage M13 is the most extensively used phage for antibody phage display [55]. Other classes of filamentous phages that have been studied include F1 and Ff phages [56, 57]. In the mature virus particle, filamentous phage M13 have a cylindrical-shaped structure, about 930 nm in length and phage proteins are encoded by a circular single-stranded DNA genome. Foreign peptides are typically displayed on the N-terminal of the minor p3 coat protein or on the major p8 coat protein with the copy numbers from 5 to more than 2000 depending on type of vectors used. However, type 3 is the most widely used display format [56, 58]. Generally, this leads to expression of 1–3 copies of the recombinant fusion protein on the phage surface.

The diversity of M13 phage display libraries typically ranges from 10^5 to 10^{12}, and is greatly dependent on the transformation efficiency of the host *E. coli*. As the proteins are secreted through periplasmic layers, the M13 phage display system represents a suitable tool to display the

Parameters	M13 filamentous phage	T7 phage
Structure diagram	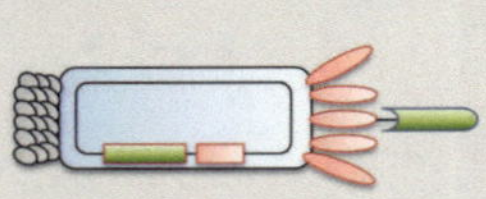	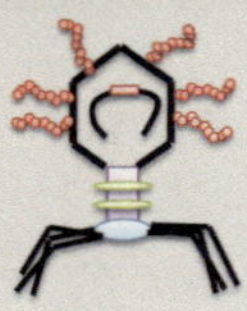
Virus behavior	Temperate phage • Colonies • Host cell = male (F-pilus)	Virulent phage • Plagues • Host cell = female
Rate of growing	Slow (~ 16 hours)	Fast (1.5 – 3 hours)
Stability range of pH	pH 1.5 – 10	pH 4 – 10
Bias of displayed peptide / protein	Physical limitation (periplasmic transport required)	Less bias than M13 phage (secreted by cell lysis)
Displaying platform	pIII or pIV protein	Capsid protein

Table 1. Comparison of M13 filamentous phage with T7 phage.

appropriately folded proteins containing disulfide bonds. Hence, many functional antibody fragments, enzymes and inhibitors have been displayed and selected using this system [28, 59, 60]. However, it also has the minor limitation of poor display of cytoplasmic proteins on the membrane [61]. Moreover, the removal of stop codons in the DNA library can facilitate correct display of the foreign proteins on the coat protein at the N-terminus of M13 bacteriophage [56].

3.3.2. *T7 bacteriophage system*

The bacteriophage display and cloning system using T7, T4 and λ phage was introduced in 1990s, and has several advantageous features over other phage display systems [62–64]. As a lytic phage, the T7 phage contains a linear double-stranded DNA genome. It has a diameter of 55 nm, with the capsid shaped in an icosahedron structure. The Novagen's T7Select® is the commercially available phage display system that takes advantage of the properties of bacteriophage T7. There are three types of vectors available in this system: for peptide display with up to 50 amino acids in high-copy number (415 per phage); 1200 amino acids display in mid-copy number (5–15 phage) and 1200 amino acids display in low-copy number (0.1–1 per phage) [64].

Fusion proteins are displayed at the C-terminal end of the T7 capsid protein (gene 10); the removal of the stop codon from foreign genes is not necessary, resulting in ease construction of a library. The diversity of T7 phage display is often dependent on the packaging efficiency into the capsid. Nevertheless, a successfully constructed library could encode a library of the size 10^7–10^8 clones [64]. In contrast to bacteriophage M13, the secretion of library proteins through the periplasmic layer of the host cell does not occur in the T7 phage display system. This may lead to the reduction of physiochemical restriction and less bias in the library peptide diversity [65]. In addition, the T7 phage system has the advantages of being able to display a cytoplasmic protein, a major limitation of the M13 filamentous phage [61, 66].

However, folding of cytoplasmic proteins with disulfide bonds in T7 bacterial phage system do not occur quite well. This problem can be resolved by using the complementing hosts such as BLT5615 or BLT 5403 *E. coli* strain included in the T7Select® kit [65, 67, 68]. In term of general features, T7 phage grows much faster than M13. After infection, clear plaques (lawns) of T7 phages can usually be observed within 2–3 h on an LB plate at 37°C. Furthermore, the purification process of T7 phage for ELISA and DNA sequencing is also simple to perform, with only PEG/NaCl precipitation required to recover the purified phage [47, 65].

4. Engineered sdAb fragments from vertebrates

With the advent of recombinant DNA technology, antibody genes can be selected and amplified using phage display, yeast display, bacterial display, ribosome display, mRNA display, DNA display or mammalian cell surface display [69–73] and see chapter in this book: "Display technologies for the selection of monoclonal antibodies for clinical use" by Tsuruta et al. A range of mammalian V-gene libraries have been used to undertake *in vitro* recombinant antibodies screening projects using phage display. These include mouse [74], rabbit [75], sheep [76] and human [77]. Unlike hybridoma technology, the direct link between the genotype and the phenotype of displayed antibodies during selection (biopanning) can facilitate the identification of binding antibodies and corresponding antibody genes. Further, the gene encoding the desired antibody can be manipulated to improve affinity, specificity and expression or fusion to a carrier protein can be performed [38, 48, 78].

An advantage of sdAb fragments is their ease of genetic manipulation due to their smaller size, in addition ease of expression in bacterial system, low lot-to-lot variation and easy scaled-up production [79, 80] . Moreover, sdAb production is not influenced by species-specific cell fusion partner incompabilities. Nowadays, the desired sdAb repertoire can be developed from shark, camels and humans with an appropriate set of specific primers [81] . However, an additional step of point mutations in framework regions and CDR randomization is required to construct human V_H and V_L sdAbs [81]. Regardless, the generation of sdAbs by bacterial fermentation is significantly cheaper, simpler and quicker than conventional polyclonal Abs or mAbs production [80, 82–84]. The general features of some natural sdAb fragments are described in the following section.

4.1. V_{HH} heavy-chain domain in camelids

Conventional immunoglobulins comprise two major parts such as the antigen-binding fragment (Fab region) and fragment crystallisable region (Fc region), with a typical molecular weight of 150 kDa. The Fab domain is responsible for antigen binding and therefore its specificity. This domain is divided into heavy (H) and light (L) chains with the molecular weights of 25 kDa each [85]. The stability of the molecular complex of an immunoglobulin is conferred by four inter-domain disulfide bonds in the hinge regions. The heavy chain can be subdivided into one variable (VH) region and three constant (C) regions (CH1, CH2 and CH3) while the light chain contains one variable region (VL) and only one constant region (CL). Lacking direct antigen-binding functions, the main role of the Fc domain is to provide effector functions such as binding to cellular receptors on macrophages and complement activation, and determination of the half-life of an antibody [86].

In addition to conventional heterotetrameric antibodies, the sera of Camelidae were discovered to possess special IgG antibodies known as heavy-chain antibodies (HCAbs). Although HCAbs contain both a constant (Fc) and variable domain, these antibodies are slightly different from conventional IgG by devoid of the L chain polypeptide and the first constant domain (CH1) (**Figure 1**). Therefore, the isolated variable domain region of camelids HCAbs is known as V_{HH} (variable domain of the heavy chain of HCAbs) or Nanobody® (Nb; Ablynx) [87]. V_{HH} constitutes a binding surface to interact with the target antigen. The molecular weight of V_{HH} is 15 kDa, 10 times lower than that of a conventional antibody. It was thereby considered the smallest possible antibody fragment and has attracted the interests of many scientists [88, 89]. Moreover, the capability of camelid antibodies to retain the reversibility and binding activity after heat denaturation has enabled new applications where transient heating may occur [90].

The major advantage of a V_{HH} antibody is their greater solubility compared to classical VH [17]. This is due to the hydrophilic amino acid substitution present in the framework 2 region. Meanwhile, the single coding exon of less than 450 base pairs facilitates genetic engineering of V_{HH} fragments [91]. In addition, on account of its smaller antigen binding surface area, the unique CDR3 region enables the heavy domain of camelids to penetrate into antigen cleft regions that are not easily recognized by conventional antibodies [92, 93]. From a phylogenetic prospect, since camelids are related to the primate lineage [94] it is possible to produce humanized V_{HH}, a process that may be easier to perform than the complicated manipulation required to "humanize" murine or other more distant species to reduce an alloresponse, such as the human anti-mouse antibody (HAMA) response [95].

Furthermore, due to their high intrinsic domain stability, camelids V_{HH} are now under investigation as probes for diagnostics [18, 96]. The diagnostic potential of camelids V_{HH} as probes in immunodetection systems offers the possibilities of improving the diagnosis of infection [97], cancers [98] and food contaminants [99]. Although V_{HH}s do not originate from humans, the humanizations strategies of V_{HH}s have successfully been undertaken by designing a humanized scaffold region onto the antigen-binding loops (CDRs) of specific V_{HH}s can be grafted [100]. In addition, non-humanized and humanized V_{HH}s with therapeutic potential have been applied in multiple areas, including hematology [101], inflammatory diseases [102], infectious diseases [103], *in vivo* imaging [104], neurological disorders [105] and oncology [106, 107].

4.2. V_{NAR} heavy-chain domain in sharks

A class of naturally occurring antibodies comprising a variable domain of a heavy chain (V_{NAR}) without a variable light chain domain was discovered in the serum of elasmobranch cartilaginous fish during early of 1990s [108–110]. These natural functional antibody repertoires were termed as immunoglobulin new antigen receptors (IgNARs). IgNARs are an unconventional and unique class of proteins found in sharks, including nurse sharks (*Ginglymostoma cirratum*) [111], wobbegong sharks (*Orectolobus maculatus*) [112], smooth dogfish (*Mustelus canis*) [113], banded hound sharks (*Triakis scyllium*) [68] and horn shark (*Heterodontus francisci*) [114]. Investigations have revealed that IgNARs function as antibody and immune response mediators in sharks. However, until now it is not clear if the IgNARs as single domain antibodies arise from TCR domains/L chains or primitive cell surface molecules [109, 115].

Several desirable biological properties of IgNAR V domains have been identified, and their potential as alternative antigen binders explored [112, 113, 116]. The natural habitat of sharks has resulted in evolving extraordinary stable antibodies such that the functionality of antibodies can be retained in a harsh environment [117]. Electron microscopic studies have indicated that the intact IgNAR exists as a disulfide-bonded homodimer that consists of a polyprotein with one variable domain (V_{NAR}) and five constant domains (C_{NAR}) (**Figure 1**) [118].

Similar to the camelid V_{HH}, the V_{NAR} has only a heavy-chain domain. However, the cross-species conservation of the amino acid sequence with a human VH is extremely low in a V_{NAR} domain (~25%), whereas it is more than 80% homologous to V_{HH} scaffolds in camelids V_{HH} [110, 119]. It is hypothesized that IgNARs lack many residues that exist in conventional antibodies. These are replaced by other hydrophilic residues. The greatly truncated CDR2 region, herein defined as HV2 region, has created a signature hallmark for shark V_{NAR}. Due to this unusual structure, the single variable heavy domain proteins of shark IgNARs are currently the smallest antibody fragments observed in animal kingdoms, having a size of only 12 kDa.

Yet, in combination with the peculiar feature of a long CDR3 region, these V_{NAR} domains tend to more readily penetrate cleft regions of antigens, thereby increasing the opportunity to target small target epitopes that may not be accessible to conventional IgG [120].

In terms of heat stability, V_{NAR} also possess refolding properties as found in camelids V_{HH}. The ability of retaining fully functional antigen-binding activity after exposure up to 95°C may make V_{NAR} ideally suited to protein array and diagnostic applications where transient heating may occur as part of the protein immobilization process [9, 113]. It is partly due to the presence of cysteine residues in these single domain antibodies, resulting in an extraordinary conformation [35].

V_{NAR} domains are more easily produced as recombinant proteins compared to conventional antibodies. Additionally, due to hydrophilic residues present within V_{NAR} surfaces, high yields of expressed proteins associated with high solubility, are achievable and thus they can be easy produced in prokaryotic systems [112]. Therefore, the potential utility of V_{NARs} as alternative binders for clinical applications is now being investigated in a variety of areas.

4.3. VLRs immunoglobulin-like domains in lamprey

Lamprey and hagfish are the only surviving groups of jawless fish, having appeared since the Cambrian period. The adaptive immune system of jawless vertebrates was recognized as unique due to the rearrangement of antigen receptors which is completely different from that used by jawed vertebrates [121]. The somatic rearrangement of the variable (V) gene segments, diversity (D) segments, joining (J) segments and constant (C) segments is commonly observed in conventional Ig-based Ag receptors. However, the immune system in jawless vertebrates is predominantly regulated by recombination activating gene (RAG)-independent combinatorial assembly to generate leucine-rich repeats (LRR) cassettes for Ag recognition. Owing to these differences, antibodies in jawless fish were termed as variable lymphocyte receptors (VLRs) rather than Ig superfamily (**Figure 1**) [122].

In comparison to CDR loops used by Ig-based antibodies and T-cell receptors in many animals, the antigen-binding regions of VLRs have evolved into variable β-strands and C-terminal loop structural motifs, resulting in a crescent-shaped protein conformation [123, 124]. Due to the prevalence of this unusual pattern, VLRs tend to be more useful for microbial recognition [36]. Thus far, two VLR genes have been identified in lamprey and hagfish, namely VLRA and VLRB. However, the VLRB gene in lamprey shows more complexity in terms of coding sequence analysis [125].

Sequences analysis has revealed that each VLR consists of a signal peptide (SP), hypervariable LRR regions, consisting of a 27–34 residue N-terminal LRR (LRRNT), the first 24-residue LRR (LRR1), up to nine 24-residue variable LRRs (LRRV), one 24-residue end LRRV (LRRVe), one 16-residue connecting peptide LRR (LRRCP) and a 48–63 residue C-terminal LRR (LRRCT) [126]. The assembly of VLRs entails greater recombination events in LRR modules and can efficiently generate more than 10^{14} unique repertoires at a level comparable to mammalian Ig. Thus, VLRs may be a source of single-chain domains alternative to conventional Ig-based antibodies [123]. Nevertheless no single domain antibody comprising only one engineered VLR domain has been so far reported.

Having undergone evolution over millions of years, VLRs appear to have been optimized as suitable antigen receptors for humoral protection. Further analysis indicates that VLRs are extremely stable in harsh environments. Their antigen binding capability remained unchanged even after it was eluted from a column at a very basic pH (>11) [11]. In addition, the heat stability of VLRs is similar to shark IgNARs and camelids V_{HH}. For example, eluted VLRs can be stored over 1 year at 4°C, 1 month at room temperature and 36 h at 56°C. However, the degradation of Ag-binding activity occurred when the incubation period was prolonged more than 1 h at 70°C [126].

Although VLRs were discovered less than a decade ago [122], they have provided new insights into the potential of ancestral antibodies in biotechnogical applications. Owing to a greater VLR library diversity as well as associated self-tolerance ability, VLRs can be efficiently used to detect antigens that may not be recognized by mammalian Ig, for example, the sensitivity of VLRB mAb targeting against *Bacillus anthracis* (BclA) was superior to that of a high affinity conventional murine IgG [11]. Furthermore, the simple modular single polypeptide structures facilitate the production of VLRs antibodies through DNA engineering. VLRs combinatorial libraries of high affinity binders can be constructed through *in vitro* random mutagenesis and loop shuffling using a surface display technology approach, for instance, yeast display system [36]. Thus, VLRs may become alternatives for the developments of new reagents in diagnostic applications to overcome the lack of Ag recognition ability of conventional monoclonal antibodies made from mammals.

5. Use of different recombinant antibodies for specific applications

To date, humans and mice remain the main source of complete antibodies for targeting diseases. However, with the aid of DNA technology, a number of new antibody fragments have been engineered as smaller single domain fragments to improve immunoassays, immunosensors and imaging probes in various applications. As described recently, the discovery of natural single heavy domain antibodies from camelids V_{HH} and shark V_{NAR}, and in addition lamprey VLRs offers some advantages over conventional antibodies. This range of natural antibodies is expected to open various applications: to trace molecule trafficking and to inhibit protein function inside the cell as intrabody, to apply them as therapeuticum and they can be used as detection units in biosensors or immunodiagnostics. In this section, we will review the deployment of different binders in specific diagnostic applications and to what extent these binders are used.

5.1. Applications of camelids V_{HH} domains or nanobodies®

To monitor infections, single domain antibodies naturally derived from camelids (nanobodies) may enable superior species-specific antigen detection than classical monoclonal antibodies in immunodiagnostic tests. Trypanosome infection causes African sleeping sickness and Chagas disease. Both are severe parasitic diseases caused by protozoa of the genus *Trypanosoma*. Sleeping sickness disease is mainly found in rural Africa. The antigenic variation strategy adopted by this parasite represents a major barrier to the immune system to eliminate it. Consequently, it is difficult for specific mAbs to detect genus-specific antigens [127]. By adoption of an *in vitro* selection method, novel nanobody clones were isolated that showed specificity to *T. evansi* at species level, and genus-specific reactivity against various *Trypanosoma* species [128].

Cysticercosis is a serious tissue infection caused by larval cysts of the pork tapeworm, which is prevalent in many low-income countries [129]. Monoclonal antibodies that are currently deployed in sandwich ELISAs are mainly genus-specific against *Taenia* sp., but poorly specific at a species level to identify *Taenia solium*, the major *Taenia* species threatening human health [130, 131]. To circumvent such limitations, an *in vitro* selection of nanobodies from immunized dromedaries was developed to recognize a specific marker on *T. solium*. After *in vitro* selection, the nanobodies showed no cross-reactivity against other livestock *Taenia* species, while having a very specific response to a specific 14 kDa glycoprotein (Ts14) in *T. solium*. Therefore, nanobodies showed potential as an alternative to genus-species mAb for developing unambiguous ELISA tests for human cysticercosis [97].

Apart from diagnostic reagents for infectious diseases, nanobodies have been identified as alternative binders to analyze the compositions of substances in food and beverages industries. Due to their excellent thermal stability, nanobodies showed superior behavior to classical mouse mAbs in ELISA to measure caffeine concentration in hot and cold beverages [132].

Camelid sdAbs have recently been applied in ELISA methods to detect a wide range of small molecules, including explosive materials (trinitroluene or TNT) [133], agents of bioterrorism (Botulinum A neurotoxin) [90], toxins (ricin, cholera and staphylococcal enterotoxin B) [134], scorpion toxin [135] and viruses (HIV, rotavirus, Vaccinia and Marburg) [136–138]. Owing to the combination of several favorable properties, camelid nanobodies have also been employed as molecules to diagnose diseases. In small molecule development, the advanced features of highly stable and unique conformational structure of nanobodies have permitted overcoming many problems faced by traditional whole antibodies and scFv fragments such as cross-reactivity and nanoparticle agglutination. The development of biosensors coupled with nanobodies (nanoconjugates system) has enabled significant improvement in the performance of a device to identify harmful bacteria (*Staphylococcus aureus*) to a nanometer scale within 10 min [139].

Nevertheless, mAbs remain the common binding agents to identify and trace tumor-associated proteins for noninvasive *in vivo* imaging. However, limitations, particularly large size (150 kDa) and Fc regions, result in mAbs poorly penetrating into solid tumors [140]. The emergence of nanobodies offers the possibility of resolving such problems, and thereby enables nanobodies to diagnose tumor markers such as EGF receptor [141]. This will enable cancer staging predictions in blood circulation such as prostate-specific antigen [142]. More applications using camelids V_{HH} targeting antigens from various diseases are summarized in **Table 2**.

5.2. Applications of shark V_{NAR} domains

Evidence that IgNAR is part of the shark adaptive immune response was demonstrated in a work where increasing levels of hen egg lysozyme (HEL) led to the development of specific IgNARs developed in the shark sera after 4–5 months of immunization [25]. The peculiar structure of the shark IgNAR variable domain renders it amenable to create synthetic peptide mimetics to target specific epitopes that are inaccessible to conventional antibodies [118]. Therefore, V_{NAR} may be suitable as new molecular reagents for research, diagnostic and immunotherapeutic applications.

Target antigens	Diseases	Applications	Reference
VEGF-A_{165}	Neoangiogenesis	Diagnostic and therapeutic	[143]
HER2	Breast cancer	Diagnostic	[144, 145]
HPV-16 L1 protein	Cervical cancer	Diagnostic and therapeutic	[146, 147]
HSP-60	Brucellosis (livestock)	Diagnostic and vaccine	[23, 148]
VCAM1	Atherosclerotic lesions	Molecular imaging	[149–151]
VEGFR2	Angiogenesis	Therapeutic	[152]
TNT	Explosive	Diagnostic	[133, 153]
SEB	Toxin	Sensor and diagnostic	[134]
Ricin	Toxin	Sensor and diagnostic	[134]
BoNT/A	Toxin	Sensor and diagnostic	[90, 154, 155]
Scorpion AahII	Toxin	Neutralizing and therapeutic	[135]
EGFR	Tumors	Detection and imaging	
DARC	Malaria (by *P. vivax*)	Diagnostic or therapeutic	
LMM, ES, CSE, TSB, LLGPs, VF of *T. solium*	Neurocysticercosis	Immunodiagnosis	[97]
Heat-killed *B. melitensis* Riv1 lysates	Brucellosis	Vaccination, diagnostic, therapeutic	[141, 156–158]
Poliovirus type 1 Sabin strain particles	Poliomyelitis	Diagnostic and therapeutic	[159, 160]
CEA	Colon cancer	*In vivo* imaging	[161–163]
RSV protein F	Acute lower respiratory tract	Therapeutic	[164]
CD105	Angiogenesis related tumors	Diagnostic and therapeutic	[165, 166]
Ts14 glycoprotein	*T. solium* cysticercosis	Diagnostic	[97]
vWF	Thrombosis	Therapeutic	www.ablynx.com
TNFα, IL-6R, IgE	Rheumatoid arthritis	Therapeutic	www.ablynx.com
RANKL	Bone metastasis	Therapeutic	www.ablynx.com
RSV	Bronchiolitis and pneumonia	Therapeutic	www.ablynx.com
DR5	Solid tumors	Therapeutic	www.ablynx.com
Not stated	Alzheimer's disease	Therapeutic	www.ablynx.com

Table 2. The applications of camelids V_{HH} against specified antigens from various diseases.

Apical membrane antigen-1 (AMA1) is a highly polymorphic 83 kDa merozoite surface protein that is essential for erythrocyte invasion in malaria parasites [143]. A V_{NAR} isolated from a wobbegong shark showed high-binding affinity to *Plasmodium falciparum* AMA1 through its unique CDR3 region after undergoing affinity maturation [144]. The binding specificity of a monovalent V_{NAR} clone to *P. falciparum* AMA1 was comparable with commercially available binding reagents, derived from conventional polyclonal sera, monoclonal antibodies, small fragments (Fab and scFv) and peptides [145]. Foley and co-workers demonstrated the heat stability of purified recombinant V_{NAR} was superior to that of conventional mAbs by targeting immobilized *P. falciparum* AMA1 in various formats at 45°C, and the refolding property of V_{NAR} was retained when the temperature increased to 80°C. The excellent stability property at extreme pH and resistance to proteolytic cleavage was further evidenced by incubating V_{NAR} with homogenized murine stomach tissues under *in vivo* conditions [9]. From this point of view, it was purposed that V_{NAR} domains have potential for development as alternate binders for malaria diagnostic platforms.

Human periodontal disease is an advanced gingivitis caused by the bacterial pathogen *Porphyromonas gingivalis* [146]. Late treatments often lead to dental loss due to the accumulation of lysine gingipain (KgP). KgP is a high molecular weight polyprotease produced by *P. gingivalis* [147]. This bacterial toxin is responsible for destruction of dental tissue of host by suppressing the secretion of specific lytic enzymes from the immune system [148]. Nuttall and co-workers [149] identified two distinct clones specific to KgP from a naïve wobbegong shark V_{NAR} phage display library with synthetic CDR3 loops. The high stability and binding affinity toward *P. gingivalis* KgP indicated the potential for V_{NAR} sdAbs as a valuable source of single domain binding reagents [149].

In recent studies, shark V_{NAR} domains have been reported to detect markers from viral diseases at greater sensitivity compared to mAbs and scFvs. Ebola virus hemorrhagic fever (EVHF) is a highly lethal disease caused by Bundibugyo virus (BDBV), Sudan virus (SUDV), Tai Forest virus (TAFV) and Zaire Ebolavirus (ZEBOV) [150–152]. Shark V_{NAR} and murine scFv phage display libraries have been generated against specified markers on Zaire Ebolavirus. The results indicated that the sensitivity and thermal stability of shark V_{NAR} sdAbs against viral nucleoprotein (NP) of ZEBOV was superior in comparison to murine mAbs and scFvs. [116].

As in the case with camelids nanobodies, highly diversified shark V_{NAR} libraries have also been used to detect different kind of toxins, including staphylococcal enterotoxin B (SEB), ricin and botulinum toxin A (BoNT/A) complex toxoid [153] and cholera toxin (CT) [113]. In addition, V_{NAR} sdAbs have been reported to recognize immunosilent targets in human, for example, the 70 kDa translocase of outer membrane (Tom70) [154]. Owing to the findings of negligible cross-reactivity with other antigens and superior heat stability, shark V_{NAR} domains may be a potent source of sdAbs with thermal stability over conventional antibodies in diagnostic and biotherapeutic applications [155, 156]. The applications of recombinant shark V_{NAR} sdAbs against specified antigens from various diseases are summarized in **Table 3**.

5.3. Applications of lamprey VLRs

The variable lymphocyte receptors (VLRs) discovered from jawless fish had recently attracted interests and is leading to the development of new monoclonal antibodies for biomedical applications [11, 36, 157]. Despite possessing an unusual structure, VLRs have been shown to have excellent binding ability to specified targets (**Table 4**).

Cooper and co-workers demonstrated high specificity of recombinant VLRs for BclA, a major anthrax spore coat which could be produced from an immunized sea lamprey (*Petromyzon*

Target antigens	Diseases	Applications	Reference
Kgp protease (*P. gingivalis*)	Periodontal disease	Neutralization	[173]
rhTNFα	Pro-inflammatory cytokine	Therapeutic	[114, 181]
AMA1 (*P. falciparum*)	Malaria	Diagnostic	[168, 169]
Nonfibrillar oligomer formation	Alzheimer's disease	Modeling	[182]
Zaire ebolavirus viral nucleoprotein	Ebolavirus Haemorrhagic Fever	Diagnostic	[116]
HBeAg	Hepatitis B virus	Immunolocalization and diagnostic	[183]
Cholera toxin	Toxin	Diagnostic	[113]
SEB	Toxin	Sensor and diagnostic	[177]
Ricin	Toxin	Sensor and diagnostic	[177]
BoNT/A	Toxin	Sensor and diagnostic	[177]
Tom70	Human immunosilent target processes	Detection	[178]
GPCR's ion channels		Therapeutic	www.adalta.com.au
Anti-thrombotic drug targets	Cardiovacular disease	Diagnostic and therapeutic	www.adalta.com.au
			www.adalta.com.au
	Blood brain barrier	Therapeutic	www.ossianix.com
	Gastrointestinal tract	Therapeutic	www.ossianix.com
Myostatin	Neurological disease	Therapeutic	www.ossianix.com
	Uveitis	Therapeutic	www.elasmogen.com

Table 3. The applications of shark V_{NAR} against specified antigens from various diseases.

marinus) using hybridoma technology [11]. *Bacillus anthracis* is the causative agent for anthrax and the only pathogenic species in the genus *Bacillus* [158]. Due to their extreme dormancy and durability, anthrax spores have long been considered ideal biological weapons [159–161]. In this work, the recombinant monoclonal VLRs were shown to be capable of identifying bacteria at a genus level, by differentiating the C-terminal domain of BclA *Bacillus anthracis* from non-coated bacteria of *Bacillus cereus* [11].

Target antigens	Diseases	Applications	Reference
BclA glycoprotein	*B. anthracis* spores (anthrax)	Diagnostic	[11]
HEL, β-gal, cholera toxin subunit B, R-phycoerythrin, and B-trisaccharide	Complex protein antigens	Affinity determination	[39, 189]
C1q and C3 proteins	Cytotoxicity for bacteria and tumor cells	Binding interaction	[190]

Table 4. The applications of lamprey VLRs against specified antigens from various diseases.

In another study, a large library of recombinant VLRs was constructed to target lysozyme, β-gal, cholera toxin subunit B, R-phycoerythrin and B-trisaccharide antigens using yeast surface display technologies [36]. This high-throughput technology platform offers the potential of rapid identification and isolation of monoclonal VLRs that specifically bind to target antigens with affinities in the micromolar to nanomolar range [36]. Using such display methods, the specificity of selected VLR antibodies can recognize the target antigen with high binding affinity up to 100-fold compared to conventional mouse mAb [36]. These data indicate that the function of VLRs is comparable or perhaps better than that of mammalian IgG antibodies. Therefore, it is speculated that VLRs may be an alternative reagent for the future development of therapeutic and diagnostic applications.

6. Conclusion

The fields of antibody engineering have undergone major advancements in the past few decades. New surface display technologies, in particular phage display and yeast display, are powerful tools that could facilitate the isolation of new antibodies with high specificities for a broad range of targets. Due to their affinity, which often is similar to conventional antibodies and reliable production, recombinant antibodies are becoming increasingly important in the field of diagnosis and therapy for targeting a wide range of diseases such as cancer, inflammatory, autoimmune and viral diseases. In view of natural scaffold design, previous studies showed that the sdAbs repertoires derived from animals such as camelid V_{HH}s, shark V_{NAR}s and lamprey VLRs contain several advantages over conventional antibodies. One of the unusual characteristics shared among the sdAbs is that they possess better penetration ability. This feature allows the sdAbs to effectively penetrate into antigen clefts (enzyme active sites, viral capsids and cell surface receptors) which are not easily recognized by the concave surfaces of CDR loops of complex conventional antibodies. To date, due to their ability to target both refractory antigens and immunosilent epitopes, the engineered antibody fragments coupled with latest screening technologies have extensively been used in positron emission tomography and high-sensitivity (nonradioactive, noninvasive) laser technologies for medical imaging. To sum up, it is believed that with rapid progress in antibody engineering technologies, sdAbs will become indispensable as clinical and research reagents in the next decades.

Acknowledgements

The authors would like to acknowledge support from University of Queensland, QIMR Berghofer Medical Research Institute in Australia and Malaysian Government, including Malaysian Ministry of Higher Education the Higher Institutions Centre of Excellence Program (Grant no.: 311/CIPPM/4401005), RUI Grant no.: RU(1001/CIPPM/811296) and USM Short Term (Grant no.: 304/CIPPM/6313191).

Author details

Chiuan Herng Leow[1]*, Qin Cheng[2,3], Katja Fischer[2,4] and James McCarthy[2,4]

*Address all correspondence to: herng.leow@usm.my

1 Institute for Research in Molecular Medicine (INFORMM), Universiti Sains Malaysia, Penang, Malaysia

2 QIMR Berghofer Medical Research Institute, Brisbane, Australia

3 Australian Army Malaria Institute, Brisbane, Australia

4 University of Queensland, Brisbane, Australia

References

[1] Conroy PJ, Hearty S, Leonard P, O'Kennedy RJ. Antibody production, design and use for biosensor-based applications. Semin Cell Dev Biol 2009;**20**:10-26

[2] Newcombe C, Newcombe AR. Antibody production: polyclonal-derived biotherapeutics. J Chromatogr B Analyt Technol Biomed Life Sci 2007;**848**:2-7

[3] Milstein C. 12th Sir Hans Krebs Lecture. From antibody diversity to monoclonal antibodies. Eur J Biochem 1981;**118**:429-436

[4] Torrance L, Ziegler A, Pittman H, Paterson M, Toth R, Eggleston I. Oriented immobilisation of engineered single-chain antibodies to develop biosensors for virus detection. J Virol Methods 2006;**134**:164-170

[5] Moon SA, Ki MK, Lee S, Hong ML, Kim M, Kim S, Chung J, Rhee SG, Shim H. Antibodies against non-immunizing antigens derived from a large immune scFv library. Mol Cells 2011;**31**:509-513

[6] Proba K, Wörn A, Honegger A, Plückthun A. Antibody scFv fragments without disulfide bonds made by molecular evolution. J Mol Biol 1998;**275**:245-253

[7] Dong J, Ihara M, Ueda H. Antibody Fab display system that can perform open-sandwich ELISA. Anal Biochem 2009;**386**:36-44

[8] Zhang MY, Shu Y, Phogat S, Xiao X, Cham F, Bouma P, Choudhary A, Feng YR, Sanz I, Rybak S, et al. Broadly cross-reactive HIV neutralizing human monoclonal antibody Fab selected by sequential antigen panning of a phage display library. J Immunol Methods 2003;**283**:17-25

[9] Griffiths K, Dolezal O, Parisi K, Angerosa J, Dogovski, C, Barraclough M, Sanalla A, Casey J, González I, Perugini M, Nuttall S, Foley M. Shark Variable New Antigen Receptor (VNAR) Single Domain Antibody Fragments: Stability and Diagnostic Applications. Antibodies 2013;**2**:66-81

[10] Muyldermans S, Baral TN, Retamozzo VC, De Baetselier P, De Genst E, Kinne J, Leonhardt H, Magez S, Nguyen VK, Revets H, et al. Camelid immunoglobulins and nanobody technology. Vet Immunol Immunopathol 2009;**128**:178-183

[11] Herrin BR, Alder MN, Roux KH, Sina C, Ehrhardt GR, Boydston JA, Turnbough CL, Jr., Cooper MD. Structure and specificity of lamprey monoclonal antibodies. Proc Natl Acad Sci U S A 2008;**105**:2040-2045

[12] Kohler G, Milstein C. Continuous cultures of fused cells secreting antibody of predefined specificity. Nature 1975;**256**:495-497

[13] Lipman NS, Jackson LR, Trudel LJ, Weis-Garcia F. Monoclonal versus polyclonal antibodies: distinguishing characteristics, applications, and information resources. ILAR J 2005;**46**:258-268

[14] Correia IR. Stability of IgG isotypes in serum. MAbs 2010;**2**:221-232

[15] Janeway CA, Travers JP, WAlport M, Schlomchik M. Immunology. New York: Garland Science; 2001

[16] Wesolowski J, Alzogaray V, Reyelt J, Unger M, Juarez K, Urrutia M, Cauerhff A, Danquah W, Rissiek B, Scheuplein F, et al. Single domain antibodies: promising experimental and therapeutic tools in infection and immunity. Med Microbiol Immunol 2009;**198**:157-174

[17] Barthelemy PA, Raab H, Appleton BA, Bond CJ, Wu P, Wiesmann C, Sidhu SS. Comprehensive analysis of the factors contributing to the stability and solubility of autonomous human VH domains. J Biol Chem 2008;**283**:3639-3654

[18] Huang L, Reekmans G, Saerens D, Friedt JM, Frederix F, Francis L, Muyldermans S, Campitelli A, Van Hoof C. Prostate-specific antigen immunosensing based on mixed self-assembled monolayers, camel antibodies and colloidal gold enhanced sandwich assays. Biosens Bioelectron 2005;**21**:483-490

[19] Hudson PJ, Souriau C. Engineered antibodies. Nat Med 2003;**9**:129-134

[20] Hoogenboom HR. Selecting and screening recombinant antibody libraries. Nat Biotechnol 2005;**23**:1105-1116

[21] Jostock T, Vanhove M, Brepoels E, Van Gool R, Daukandt M, Wehnert A, Van Hegelsom R, Dransfield D, Sexton D, Devlin M, et al. Rapid generation of functional human IgG antibodies derived from Fab-on-phage display libraries. J Immunol Methods 2004;**289**:65-80

[22] McCafferty J, Griffiths AD, Winter G, Chiswell DJ. Phage antibodies: filamentous phage displaying antibody variable domains. Nature 1990;**348**:552-554

[23] Abbady AQ, Al-Mariri A, Zarkawi M, Al-Assad A, Muyldermans S. Evaluation of a nanobody phage display library constructed from a *Brucella*-immunised camel. Vet Immunol Immunopathol 2011;**142**:49-56

[24] Dolk E, van der Vaart M, Lutje Hulsik D, Vriend G, de Haard H, Spinelli S, Cambillau C, Frenken L, Verrips T. Isolation of llama antibody fragments for prevention of dandruff by phage display in shampoo. Appl Environ Microbiol 2005;**71**:442-450

[25] Dooley H, Flajnik MF, Porter AJ. Selection and characterization of naturally occurring single-domain (IgNAR) antibody fragments from immunized sharks by phage display. Mol Immunol 2003;**40**:25-33

[26] Xu G, Tasumi S, Pancer Z. Yeast surface display of lamprey variable lymphocyte receptors. Methods Mol Biol 2011;**748**:21-33

[27] Hussack G, Arbabi-Ghahroudi M, Mackenzie CR, Tanha J. Isolation and characterization of *Clostridium difficile* toxin-specific single-domain antibodies. Methods Mol Biol 2012;**911**:211-239

[28] Liu Y, Regula LK, Stewart A, Lai JR. Synthetic Fab fragments that bind the HIV-1 gp41 heptad repeat regions. Biochem Biophys Res Commun 2011;**413**:611-615

[29] Shui X, Huang J, Li YH, Xie PL, Li GC. Construction and selection of human Fab antibody phage display library of liver cancer. Hybridoma (Larchmt) 2009;**28**:341-347

[30] Sowa KM, Cavanagh DR, Creasey AM, Raats J, McBride J, Sauerwein R, Roeffen WF, Arnot DE. Isolation of a monoclonal antibody from a malaria patient-derived phage display library recognising the Block 2 region of *Plasmodium falciparum* merozoite surface protein-1. Mol Biochem Parasitol 2001;**112**:143-147

[31] Yang GH, Yoon SO, Jang MH, Hong HJ. Affinity maturation of an anti-hepatitis B virus PreS1 humanized antibody by phage display. J Microbiol 2007;**45**:528-533

[32] Carmen S, Jermutus L. Concepts in antibody phage display. Brief Funct Genomic Proteomic 2002;**1**:189-203

[33] Brichta J, Hnilova M, Viskovic T. Generation of hapten-specific recombinant antibodies: antibody phage display technology: a review. Veterinarni Medicina 2005;**50**:231-252

[34] Hoogenboom HR, de Bruine AP, Hufton SE, Hoet RM, Arends JW, Roovers RC. Antibody phage display technology and its applications. Immunotechnology 1998;**4**:1-20

[35] Flajnik MF, Deschacht N, Muyldermans S. A case of convergence: why did a simple alternative to canonical antibodies arise in sharks and camels? PLoS Biol 2011;**9**:e1001120

[36] Tasumi S, Velikovsky CA, Xu G, Gai SA, Wittrup KD, Flajnik MF, Mariuzza RA, Pancer Z. High-affinity lamprey VLRA and VLRB monoclonal antibodies. Proc Natl Acad Sci USA 2009;**106**:12891-12896

[37] Ehrlich GK, Berthold W, Bailon P. Phage display technology. Affinity selection by biopanning. Methods Mol Biol 2000;**147**:195-208

[38] Clackson T, Hoogenboom HR, Griffiths AD, Winter G. Making antibody fragments using phage display libraries. Nature 1991;**352**:624-628

[39] Takakusagi Y, Takakusagi K, Sugawara F, Sakaguchi K. Use of phage display technology for the determination of the targets for small-molecule therapeutics. Expert Opin Drug Discov 2010;**5**:361-389

[40] Goletz S, Christensen PA, Kristensen P, Blohm D, Tomlinson I, Winter G, Karsten U. Selection of large diversities of antiidiotypic antibody fragments by phage display. J Mol Biol 2002;**315**:1087-1097

[41] Wang X, Zhong P, Luo PP, Wang KC. Antibody engineering using phage display with a coiled-coil heterodimeric Fv antibody fragment. PLoS One 2011;**6**:e19023

[42] Ward RL, Clark MA, Lees J, Hawkins NJ. Retrieval of human antibodies from phage-display libraries using enzymatic cleavage. J Immunol Methods 1996;**189**:73-82

[43] Wind T, Stausbol-Gron B, Kjaer S, Kahns L, Jensen KH, Clark BF. Retrieval of phage displayed scFv fragments using direct bacterial elution. J Immunol Methods 1997;**209**:75-83

[44] Nowak JE, Chatterjee M, Mohapatra S, Dryden SC, Tainsky MA. Direct production and purification of T7 phage display cloned proteins selected and analyzed on microarrays. Biotechniques 2006;**40**:220-227

[45] Soltes G, Barker H, Marmai K, Pun E, Yuen A, Wiersma EJ. A new helper phage and phagemid vector system improves viral display of antibody Fab fragments and avoids propagation of insert-less virions. J Immunol Methods 2003;**274**:233-244

[46] Sharma SC, Memic A, Rupasinghe CN, Duc AC, Spaller MR. T7 phage display as a method of peptide ligand discovery for PDZ domain proteins. Biopolymers 2009;**92**:183-193

[47] Fukunaga K, Taki M. Practical tips for construction of custom Peptide libraries and affinity selection by using commercially available phage display cloning systems. J Nucleic Acids 2012;**2012**:295719

[48] Hoogenboom HR. Overview of antibody phage-display technology and its applications. Methods Mol Biol 2002;**178**:1-37

[49] Nelson AL, Dhimolea E, Reichert JM. Development trends for human monoclonal antibody therapeutics. Nat Rev Drug Discov 2010;**9**:767-774

[50] Reichert JM. New biopharmaceuticals in the USA: trends in development and marketing approvals 1995-1999. Trends Biotechnol 2000;**18**:364-369

[51] Tikunova NV, Morozova VV. Phage display on the base of filamentous bacteriophages: application for recombinant antibodies selection. Acta Naturae 2009;**1**:20-28

[52] Tuckey CD, Noren CJ. Selection for mutants improving expression of an anti-MAP kinase monoclonal antibody by filamentous phage display. J Immunol Methods 2002;**270**: 247-257

[53] Ohtani M, Hikima J, Jung TS, Kondo H, Hirono I, Takeyama H, Aoki T. Variable domain antibodies specific for viral hemorrhagic septicemia virus (VHSV) selected from a randomized IgNAR phage display library. Fish Shellfish Immunol 2013;**34**:724-728

[54] Sun D, Shi H, Chen J, Shi D, Zhu Q, Zhang H, Liu S, Wang Y, Qiu H, Feng L. Generation of a mouse scFv library specific for porcine aminopeptidase N using the T7 phage display system. J Virol Methods 2012;**182**:99-103

[55] Smith GP. Filamentous fusion phage: novel expression vectors that display cloned antigens on the virion surface. Science 1985;**228**:1315-1317

[56] Smith GP, Petrenko VA. Phage Display. Chem Rev 1997;**97**:391-410

[57] Rader C, Barbas CF, 3rd: Phage display of combinatorial antibody libraries. Curr Opin Biotechnol 1997;**8**:503-508

[58] Sidhu SS. Engineering M13 for phage display. Biomol Eng 2001;**18**:57-63

[59] Love KR, Swoboda JG, Noren CJ, Walker S. Enabling glycosyltransferase evolution: a facile substrate-attachment strategy for phage-display enzyme evolution. Chembiochem 2006;**7**:753-756

[60] Zani ML, Moreau T. Phage display as a powerful tool to engineer protease inhibitors. Biochimie 2010;**92**:1689-1704

[61] Takakusagi Y, Ohta K, Kuramochi K, Morohashi K, Kobayashi S, Sakaguchi K, Sugawara F. Synthesis of a biotinylated camptothecin derivative and determination of the binding sequence by T7 phage display technology. Bioorg Med Chem Lett 2005;**15**:4846-4849

[62] Castagnoli L, Zucconi A, Quondam M, Rossi M, Vaccaro P, Panni S, Paoluzi S, Santonico E, Dente L, Cesareni G. Alternative bacteriophage display systems. Comb Chem High Throughput Screen 2001;**4**:121-133

[63] Jespers LS, De Keyser A, Stanssens PE. LambdaZLG6: a phage lambda vector for high-efficiency cloning and surface expression of cDNA libraries on filamentous phage. Gene 1996;**173**:179-181

[64] Rosenberg A, Griffin K, Stiduer FW, et al. T7 Phage Display System: a powerful new protein display system based on bacteriophage T7. *inNovations* 1998;**6**:1-6

[65] Krumpe LR, Atkinson AJ, Smythers GW, Kandel A, Schumacher KM, McMahon JB, Makowski L, Mori T. T7 lytic phage-displayed peptide libraries exhibit less sequence bias than M13 filamentous phage-displayed peptide libraries. Proteomics 2006;**6**:4210-4222

[66] McKenzie KM, Videlock EJ, Splittgerber U, Austin DJ. Simultaneous identification of multiple protein targets by using complementary-DNA phage display and a natural-product-mimetic probe. Angew Chem Int Ed Engl 2004;**43**:4052-4055

[67] Du XJ, Wu YN, Zhang WW, Dong F, Wang S. Construction and quality examination of murine naive T7 phage display antibody library. Food and Agricultural Immunology 2010;**21**:81-90

[68] Ohtani M, Hikima J, Jung TS, Kondo H, Hirono I, Aoki T. Construction of an artificially randomized IgNAR phage display library: screening of variable regions that bind to hen egg white lysozyme. Mar Biotechnol (NY) 2013;**15**:56-62

[69] Colby DW, Kellogg BA, Graff CP, Yeung YA, Swers JS, Wittrup KD. Engineering antibody affinity by yeast surface display. Methods Enzymol 2004;**388**:348-358

[70] Dantas-Barbosa C, de Macedo Brigido M, Maranhao AQ. Antibody phage display libraries: contributions to oncology. Int J Mol Sci 2012;**13**:5420-5440

[71] Zhou C, Jacobsen FW, Cai L, Chen Q, Shen WD. Development of a novel mammalian cell surface antibody display platform. MAbs 2010;**2**:508-518

[72] Bessette PH, Rice JJ, Daugherty PS. Rapid isolation of high-affinity protein binding peptides using bacterial display. Protein Eng Des Sel 2004;**17**:731-739

[73] Zhou C, Shen WD. Mammalian cell surface display of full length IgG. Methods Mol Biol 2012;**907**:293-302

[74] Sommavilla R, Lovato V, Villa A, Sgier D, Neri D. Design and construction of a naive mouse antibody phage display library. J Immunol Methods 2010;**353**:31-43

[75] Rader C. Generation and selection of rabbit antibody libraries by phage display. Methods Mol Biol 2009;**525**:101-128, xiv

[76] Li Y, Kilpatrick J, Whitelam GC. Sheep monoclonal antibody fragments generated using a phage display system. J Immunol Methods 2000;**236**:133-146

[77] Solforosi L, Mancini N, Canducci F, Clementi N, Sautto GA, Diotti RA, Clementi M, Burioni R. A phage display vector optimized for the generation of human antibody combinatorial libraries and the molecular cloning of monoclonal antibody fragments. New Microbiol 2012;**35**:289-294

[78] Johns M. Phage display technology. Methods Mol Med 2000;**40**:53-62

[79] Harmsen MM, De Haard HJ. Properties, production, and applications of camelid single-domain antibody fragments. Appl Microbiol Biotechnol 2007;**77**:13-22

[80] Leow CH, Fischer K, Leow CY, Cheng Q, Chuah C, McCarthy J. Single Domain Antibodies as New Biomarker Detectors. Diagnostics (Basel) 2017;**7**

[81] Boldicke T. Single domain antibodies for the knockdown of cytosolic and nuclear proteins. Protein Sci 2017;**26**:925-945

[82] Doyle PJ, Arbabi-Ghahroudi M, Gaudette N, Furzer G, Savard ME, Gleddie S, McLean MD, Mackenzie CR, Hall JC. Cloning, expression, and characterization of a single-domain antibody fragment with affinity for 15-acetyl-deoxynivalenol. Mol Immunol 2008;**45**:3703-3713

[83] Shriver-Lake LC, Goldman ER, Zabetakis D, Anderson GP. Improved production of single domain antibodies with two disulfide bonds by co-expression of chaperone proteins in the Escherichia coli periplasm. J Immunol Methods 2017;**443**:64-67

[84] Liu JL, Goldman ER, Zabetakis D, Walper SA, Turner KB, Shriver-Lake LC, Anderson GP. Enhanced production of a single domain antibody with an engineered stabilizing extra disulfide bond. Microb Cell Fact 2015;**14**:158

[85] Mian IS, Bradwell AR, Olson AJ. Structure, function and properties of antibody binding sites. J Mol Biol 1991;**217**:133-151

[86] O'Kennedy R, Roben P. Antibody engineering: an overview. Essays Biochem 1991;**26**: 59-75

[87] Huang L, Muyldermans S, Saerens D. Nanobodies(R): proficient tools in diagnostics. Expert Rev Mol Diagn 2010;**10**:777-785

[88] Muyldermans S, Atarhouch T, Saldanha J, Barbosa JA, Hamers R. Sequence and structure of VH domain from naturally occurring camel heavy chain immunoglobulins lacking light chains. Protein Eng 1994;**7**:1129-1135

[89] Muyldermans S. Single domain camel antibodies: current status. J Biotechnol 2001;**74**: 277-302

[90] Goldman ER, Anderson GP, Conway J, Sherwood LJ, Fech M, Vo B, Liu JL, Hayhurst A. Thermostable llama single domain antibodies for detection of botulinum A neurotoxin complex. Anal Chem 2008;**80**:8583-8591

[91] Saerens D, Ghassabeh GH, Muyldermans S. Single-domain antibodies as building blocks for novel therapeutics. Curr Opin Pharmacol 2008;**8**:600-608

[92] De Genst E, Silence K, Decanniere K, Conrath K, Loris R, Kinne J, Muyldermans S, Wyns L. Molecular basis for the preferential cleft recognition by dromedary heavy-chain antibodies. Proc Natl Acad Sci U S A 2006;**103**:4586-4591

[93] Desmyter A, Transue TR, Ghahroudi MA, Thi MH, Poortmans F, Hamers R, Muyldermans S, Wyns L. Crystal structure of a camel single-domain VH antibody fragment in complex with lysozyme. Nat Struct Biol 1996;**3**:803-811

[94] Vincke C, Loris R, Saerens D, Martinez-Rodriguez S, Muyldermans S, Conrath K. General strategy to humanize a camelid single-domain antibody and identification of a universal humanized nanobody scaffold. J Biol Chem 2009;**284**:3273-3284

[95] Line BR, Breyer RJ, McElvany KD, Earle DC, Khazaeli MB. Evaluation of human anti-mouse antibody response in normal volunteers following repeated injections of fanolesomab (NeutroSpec), a murine anti-CD15 IgM monoclonal antibody for imaging infection. Nucl Med Commun 2004;**25**:807-811

[96] Vo-Dinh T, Kasili P, Wabuyele M. Nanoprobes and nanobiosensors for monitoring and imaging individual living cells. Nanomedicine 2006;**2**:22-30

[97] Deckers N, Saerens D, Kanobana K, Conrath K, Victor B, Wernery U, Vercruysse J, Muyldermans S, Dorny P. Nanobodies, a promising tool for species-specific diagnosis of *Taenia solium* cysticercosis. Int J Parasitol 2009;**39**:625-633

[98] Roovers RC, Laeremans T, Huang L, De Taeye S, Verkleij AJ, Revets H, de Haard HJ, van Bergen en Henegouwen PM. Efficient inhibition of EGFR signaling and of tumour growth by antagonistic anti-EFGR Nanobodies. Cancer Immunol Immunother 2007;**56**:303-317

[99] Franco EJ, Sonneson GJ, DeLegge TJ, Hofstetter H, Horn JR, Hofstetter O. Production and characterization of a genetically engineered anti-caffeine camelid antibody and its use in immunoaffinity chromatography. J Chromatogr B Analyt Technol Biomed Life Sci 2010;**878**:177-186

[100] Moutel S, Bery N, Bernard V, Keller L, Lemesre E, de Marco A, Ligat L, Rain JC, Favre G, Olichon A, Perez F. NaLi-H1: A universal synthetic library of humanized nanobodies providing highly functional antibodies and intrabodies. Elife 2016;**5**

[101] Peyvandi F, Callewaert F. Caplacizumab for Acquired Thrombotic Thrombocytopenic Purpura. N Engl J Med 2016;**374**:2497-2498

[102] Behar G, Siberil S, Groulet A, Chames P, Pugniere M, Boix C, Sautes-Fridman C, Teillaud JL, Baty D. Isolation and characterization of anti-FcgammaRIII (CD16) llama single-domain antibodies that activate natural killer cells. Protein Eng Des Sel 2008;**21**:1-10

[103] McCoy LE, Rutten L, Frampton D, Anderson I, Granger L, Bashford-Rogers R, Dekkers G, Strokappe NM, Seaman MS, Koh W, et al: Molecular evolution of broadly neutralizing Llama antibodies to the CD4-binding site of HIV-1. PLoS Pathog 2014;**10**:e1004552

[104] Li T, Vandesquille M, Koukouli F, Dudeffant C, Youssef I, Lenormand P, Ganneau C, Maskos U, Czech C, Grueninger F, et al. Camelid single-domain antibodies: A versatile tool for in vivo imaging of extracellular and intracellular brain targets. J Control Release 2016;**243**:1-10

[105] Nabuurs RJ, Rutgers KS, Welling MM, Metaxas A, de Backer ME, Rotman M, Bacskai BJ, van Buchem MA, van der Maarel SM, van der Weerd L. In vivo detection of amyloid-beta deposits using heavy chain antibody fragments in a transgenic mouse model for Alzheimer's disease. PLoS One 2012;**7**:e38284

[106] Araste F, Ebrahimizadeh W, Rasooli I, Rajabibazl M, Mousavi Gargari SL. A novel VHH nanobody against the active site (the CA domain) of tumor-associated, carbonic anhydrase isoform IX and its usefulness for cancer diagnosis. Biotechnol Lett 2014;**36**:21-28

[107] Yu Y, Li J, Zhu X, Tang X, Bao Y, Sun X, Huang Y, Tian F, Liu X, Yang L. Humanized CD7 nanobody-based immunotoxins exhibit promising anti-T-cell acute lymphoblastic leukemia potential. Int J Nanomedicine 2017;**12**:1969-1983

[108] Diaz M, Greenberg AS, Flajnik MF. Somatic hypermutation of the new antigen receptor gene (NAR) in the nurse shark does not generate the repertoire: possible role in antigen-driven reactions in the absence of germinal centers. Proc Natl Acad Sci USA 1998;**95**:14343-14348

[109] Greenberg AS, Avila D, Hughes M, Hughes A, McKinney EC, Flajnik MF. A new antigen receptor gene family that undergoes rearrangement and extensive somatic diversification in sharks. Nature 1995;**374**:168-173

[110] Roux KH, Greenberg AS, Greene L, Strelets L, Avila D, McKinney EC, Flajnik MF. Structural analysis of the nurse shark (new) antigen receptor (NAR): molecular convergence of NAR and unusual mammalian immunoglobulins. Proc Natl Acad Sci USA 1998;**95**:11804-11809

[111] Dooley H, Stanfield RL, Brady RA, Flajnik MF. First molecular and biochemical analysis of *in vivo* affinity maturation in an ectothermic vertebrate. Proc Natl Acad Sci USA 2006;**103**:1846-1851

[112] Nuttall SD, Krishnan UV, Hattarki M, De Gori R, Irving RA, Hudson PJ. Isolation of the new antigen receptor from wobbegong sharks, and use as a scaffold for the display of protein loop libraries. Mol Immunol 2001;**38**:313-326

[113] Liu JL, Anderson GP, Delehanty JB, Baumann R, Hayhurst A, Goldman ER. Selection of cholera toxin specific IgNAR single-domain antibodies from a naive shark library. Mol Immunol 2007;**44**:1775-1783

[114] Camacho-Villegas T, Mata-Gonzalez T, Paniagua-Solis J, Sanchez E, Licea A. Human TNF cytokine neutralization with a vNAR from *Heterodontus francisci* shark: a potential therapeutic use. MAbs 2013;**5**:80-85

[115] Streltsov VA, Varghese JN, Carmichael JA, Irving RA, Hudson PJ, Nuttall SD. Structural evidence for evolution of shark Ig new antigen receptor variable domain antibodies from a cell-surface receptor. Proc Natl Acad Sci USA 2004;**101**:12444-12449

[116] Goodchild SA, Dooley H, Schoepp RJ, Flajnik M, Lonsdale SG. Isolation and characterisation of Ebolavirus-specific recombinant antibody fragments from murine and shark immune libraries. Mol Immunol 2011;**48**:2027-2037

[117] Barelle C, Gill DS, Charlton K. Shark novel antigen receptors--the next generation of biologic therapeutics? Adv Exp Med Biol 2009;**655**:49-62

[118] Stanfield RL, Dooley H, Flajnik MF, Wilson IA. Crystal structure of a shark single-domain antibody V region in complex with lysozyme. Science 2004;**305**:1770-1773

[119] Muyldermans S, Cambillau C, Wyns L. Recognition of antigens by single-domain antibody fragments: the superfluous luxury of paired domains. Trends Biochem Sci 2001;**26**:230-235

[120] Streltsov VA, Carmichael JA, Nuttall SD. Structure of a shark IgNAR antibody variable domain and modeling of an early-developmental isotype. Protein Sci 2005;**14**:2901-2909

[121] Cooper MD, Alder MN. The evolution of adaptive immune systems. Cell 2006;**124**:815-822

[122] Pancer Z, Amemiya CT, Ehrhardt GR, Ceitlin J, Gartland GL, Cooper MD. Somatic diversification of variable lymphocyte receptors in the agnathan sea lamprey. Nature 2004;**430**:174-180

[123] Alder MN, Rogozin IB, Iyer LM, Glazko GV, Cooper MD, Pancer Z. Diversity and function of adaptive immune receptors in a jawless vertebrate. Science 2005;**310**:1970-1973

[124] Kim HM, Oh SC, Lim KJ, Kasamatsu J, Heo JY, Park BS, Lee H, Yoo OJ, Kasahara M, Lee JO. Structural diversity of the hagfish variable lymphocyte receptors. J Biol Chem 2007;**282**:6726-6732

[125] Rogozin IB, Iyer LM, Liang L, Glazko GV, Liston VG, Pavlov YI, Aravind L, Pancer Z. Evolution and diversification of lamprey antigen receptors: evidence for involvement of an AID-APOBEC family cytosine deaminase. Nat Immunol 2007;**8**:647-656

[126] Herrin BR, Cooper MD. Alternative adaptive immunity in jawless vertebrates. J Immunol 2010;**185**:1367-1374

[127] Pays E, Vanhamme L, Perez-Morga D. Antigenic variation in *Trypanosoma brucei*: facts, challenges and mysteries. Curr Opin Microbiol 2004;**7**:369-374

[128] Saerens D, Stijlemans B, Baral TN, Nguyen Thi GT, Wernery U, Magez S, De Baetselier P, Muyldermans S, Conrath K. Parallel selection of multiple anti-infectome Nanobodies without access to purified antigens. J Immunol Methods 2008;**329**:138-150

[129] Hernandez M, Beltran C, Garcia E, Fragoso G, Gevorkian G, Fleury A, Parkhouse M, Harrison L, Sotelo J, Sciutto E. Cysticercosis: towards the design of a diagnostic kit based on synthetic peptides. Immunol Lett 2000;**71**:13-17

[130] Dorny P, Brandt J, Zoli A, Geerts S. Immunodiagnostic tools for human and porcine cysticercosis. Acta Trop 2003;**87**:79-86

[131] Garcia HH, Harrison LJ, Parkhouse RM, Montenegro T, Martinez SM, Tsang VC, Gilman RH. A specific antigen-detection ELISA for the diagnosis of human neurocysticercosis. The Cysticercosis Working Group in Peru. Trans R Soc Trop Med Hyg 1998;**92**:411-414

[132] Ladenson RC, Crimmins DL, Landt Y, Ladenson JH. Isolation and characterization of a thermally stable recombinant anti-caffeine heavy-chain antibody fragment. Anal Chem 2006;**78**:4501-4508

[133] Anderson GP, Goldman ER. TNT detection using llama antibodies and a two-step competitive fluid array immunoassay. J Immunol Methods 2008;**339**:47-54

[134] Goldman ER, Anderson GP, Liu JL, Delehanty JB, Sherwood LJ, Osborn LE, Cummins LB, Hayhurst A. Facile generation of heat-stable antiviral and antitoxin single domain antibodies from a semisynthetic llama library. Anal Chem 2006;**78**:8245-8255

[135] Hmila I, Abdallah RB, Saerens D, Benlasfar Z, Conrath K, Ayeb ME, Muyldermans S, Bouhaouala-Zahar B. VHH, bivalent domains and chimeric Heavy chain-only antibodies with high neutralizing efficacy for scorpion toxin AahI'. Mol Immunol 2008;**45**: 3847-3856

[136] Strokappe N, Szynol A, Aasa-Chapman M, Gorlani A, Forsman Quigley A, Hulsik DL, Chen L, Weiss R, de Haard H, Verrips T. Llama antibody fragments recognizing various epitopes of the CD4bs neutralize a broad range of HIV-1 subtypes A, B and C. PLoS One 2012;**7**:e33298

[137] Vanlandschoot P, Stortelers C, Beirnaert E, Ibanez LI, Schepens B, Depla E, Saelens X. Nanobodies(R): new ammunition to battle viruses. Antiviral Res 2011;**92**:389-407

[138] Pant N, Marcotte H, Hermans P, Bezemer S, Frenken L, Johansen K, Hammarstrom L. *Lactobacilli* producing bispecific llama-derived anti-rotavirus proteins *in vivo* for rotavirus-induced diarrhea. Future Microbiol 2011;**6**:583-593

[139] Ryan S, Kell AJ, van Faassen H, Tay LL, Simard B, MacKenzie R, Gilbert M, Tanha J. Single-domain antibody-nanoparticles: promising architectures for increased *Staphylococcus aureus* detection specificity and sensitivity. Bioconjug Chem 2009;**20**:1966-1974

[140] Kenanova V, Wu AM. Tailoring antibodies for radionuclide delivery. Expert Opin Drug Deliv 2006;**3**:53-70

[141] Huang L, Gainkam LO, Caveliers V, Vanhove C, Keyaerts M, De Baetselier P, Bossuyt A, Revets H, Lahoutte T. SPECT imaging with 99mTc-labeled EGFR-specific nanobody for in vivo monitoring of EGFR expression. Mol Imaging Biol 2008;**10**:167-175

[142] Pleschberger M, Saerens D, Weigert S, Sleytr UB, Muyldermans S, Sara M, Egelseer EM. An S-layer heavy chain camel antibody fusion protein for generation of a nanopatterned sensing layer to detect the prostate-specific antigen by surface plasmon resonance technology. Bioconjug Chem 2004;**15**:664-671

[143] Tillib SV, Ivanova TI, Lyssuk EY, Larin SS, Kibardin AV, Korobko EV, Vikhreva PN, Gnuchev NV, Georgiev GP, Korobko IV. Nanoantibodies for detection and blocking of bioactivity of human vascular endothelial growth factor A(165). Biochemistry (Mosc) 2012;**77**:659-665

[144] Pruszynski M, Koumarianou E, Vaidyanathan G, Revets H, Devoogdt N, Lahoutte T, Zalutsky MR. Targeting breast carcinoma with radioiodinated anti-HER2 Nanobody. Nucl Med Biol 2013;**40**:52-59

[145] Vaneycken I, Devoogdt N, Van Gassen N, Vincke C, Xavier C, Wernery U, Muyldermans S, Lahoutte T, Caveliers V. Preclinical screening of anti-HER2 nanobodies for molecular imaging of breast cancer. FASEB J 2011;**25**:2433-2446

[146] Minaeian S, Rahbarizadeh F, Zarkesh-Esfahani SH, Ahmadvand D, Broom OJ. Neutralization of human papillomavirus by specific nanobodies against major capsid protein L1. J Microbiol Biotechnol 2012;**22**:721-728

[147] Vosjan MJ, Vercammen J, Kolkman JA, Stigter-van Walsum M, Revets H, van Dongen GA. Nanobodies targeting the hepatocyte growth factor: potential new drugs for molecular cancer therapy. Mol Cancer Ther 2012;**11**:1017-1025

[148] Abbady AQ, Al-Daoude A, Al-Mariri A, Zarkawi M, Muyldermans S. Chaperonin GroEL a *Brucella* immunodominant antigen identified using Nanobody and MALDI-TOF-MS technologies. Vet Immunol Immunopathol 2012;**146**:254-263

[149] Leung K: 99mTc(CO)3-Anti-vascular cell adhesion molecule-1 nanobody cAbVCAM1-5. In Molecular Imaging and Contrast Agent Database (MICAD). Bethesda (MD)2004

[150] Leung K. Microbubbles conjugated with anti-vascular cell adhesion molecule-1 nanobody cAbVCAM1-5. In Molecular Imaging and Contrast Agent Database (MICAD). Bethesda (MD)2004

[151] Broisat A, Hernot S, Toczek J, De Vos J, Riou LM, Martin S, Ahmadi M, Thielens N, Wernery U, Caveliers V, et al. Nanobodies targeting mouse/human VCAM1 for the nuclear imaging of atherosclerotic lesions. Circ Res 2012;**110**:927-937

[152] Behdani M, Zeinali S, Khanahmad H, Karimipour M, Asadzadeh N, Azadmanesh K, Khabiri A, Schoonooghe S, Habibi Anbouhi M, Hassanzadeh-Ghassabeh G, Muyldermans S. Generation and characterization of a functional Nanobody against the vascular endothelial growth factor receptor-2; angiogenesis cell receptor. Mol Immunol 2012;**50**:35-41

[153] Anderson GP, Moreira SC, Charles PT, Medintz IL, Goldman ER, Zeinali M, Taitt CR. TNT detection using multiplexed liquid array displacement immunoassays. Anal Chem 2006;**78**:2279-2285

[154] Goldman ER, Anderson GP, Bernstein RD, Swain MD. Amplification of immunoassays using phage-displayed single domain antibodies. J Immunol Methods 2010;**352**:182-185

[155] Swain MD, Anderson GP, Zabetakis D, Bernstein RD, Liu JL, Sherwood LJ, Hayhurst A, Goldman ER. Llama-derived single-domain antibodies for the detection of botulinum A neurotoxin. Anal Bioanal Chem 2010;**398**:339-348

[156] Altintas I, Kok RJ, Schiffelers RM. Targeting epidermal growth factor receptor in tumors: from conventional monoclonal antibodies via heavy chain-only antibodies to nanobodies. Eur J Pharm Sci 2012;**45**:399-407

[157] Chopra A: [99mTc]Epidermal growth factor receptor-specific nanobody. In Molecular Imaging and Contrast Agent Database (MICAD). Bethesda (MD)2004

[158] Friedman M, Stahl S. Engineered affinity proteins for tumour-targeting applications. Biotechnol Appl Biochem 2009;**53**:1-29

[159] Thys B, Saerens D, Schotte L, De Bleeser G, Muyldermans S, Hassanzadeh-Ghassabeh G, Rombaut B. A simple quantitative affinity capturing assay of poliovirus antigens and subviral particles by single-domain antibodies using magnetic beads. J Virol Methods 2011;**173**:300-305

[160] Thys B, Schotte L, Muyldermans S, Wernery U, Hassanzadeh-Ghassabeh G, Rombaut B. *in vitro* antiviral activity of single domain antibody fragments against poliovirus. Antiviral Res 2010;**87**:257-264

[161] Leung K: 99mTc(CO)3-Anti-carcinoembryonic antigen (CEA) humanized CEA5 graft nanobody. In Molecular Imaging and Contrast Agent Database (MICAD). Bethesda (MD)2004

[162] Sukhanova A, Even-Desrumeaux K, Kisserli A, Tabary T, Reveil B, Millot JM, Chames P, Baty D, Artemyev M, Oleinikov V, et al: Oriented conjugates of single-domain antibodies and quantum dots: toward a new generation of ultrasmall diagnostic nanoprobes. Nanomedicine 2012;**8**:516-525

[163] Vaneycken I, Govaert J, Vincke C, Caveliers V, Lahoutte T, De Baetselier P, Raes G, Bossuyt A, Muyldermans S, Devoogdt N. *In vitro* analysis and *in vivo* tumor targeting of a humanized, grafted nanobody in mice using pinhole SPECT/micro-CT. J Nucl Med 2010;**51**:1099-1106

[164] Hultberg A, Temperton NJ, Rosseels V, Koenders M, Gonzalez-Pajuelo M, Schepens B, Ibanez LI, Vanlandschoot P, Schillemans J, Saunders M, et al. Llama-derived single domain antibodies to build multivalent, superpotent and broadened neutralizing anti-viral molecules. PLoS One 2011;**6**:e17665

[165] Ahmadvand D, Rasaee MJ, Rahbarizadeh F, Kontermann RE, Sheikholislami F. Cell selection and characterization of a novel human endothelial cell specific nanobody. Mol Immunol 2009;**46**:1814-1823

[166] Ahmadvand D, Rasaee MJ, Rahbarizadeh F, Mohammadi M. Production and characterization of a high-affinity nanobody against human endoglin. Hybridoma (Larchmt) 2008;**27**:353-360

[167] Narum DL, Thomas AW. Differential localization of full-length and processed forms of PF83/AMA-1 an apical membrane antigen of *Plasmodium falciparum* merozoites. Mol Biochem Parasitol 1994;**67**:59-68

[168] Nuttall SD, Humberstone KS, Krishnan UV, Carmichael JA, Doughty L, Hattarki M, Coley AM, Casey JL, Anders RF, Foley M, et al. Selection and affinity maturation of IgNAR variable domains targeting *Plasmodium falciparum* AMA1. Proteins 2004;**55**:187-197

[169] Henderson KA, Streltsov VA, Coley AM, Dolezal O, Hudson PJ, Batchelor AH, Gupta A, Bai T, Murphy VJ, Anders RF, et al. Structure of an IgNAR-AMA1 complex: targeting a conserved hydrophobic cleft broadens malarial strain recognition. Structure 2007;**15**:1452-1466

[170] Slots J, Ting M. *Actinobacillus actinomycetemcomitans* and *Porphyromonas gingivalis* in human periodontal disease: occurrence and treatment. Periodontol 2000 1999;**20**:82-121

[171] Kadowaki T, Nakayama K, Okamoto K, Abe N, Baba A, Shi Y, Ratnayake DB, Yamamoto K. *Porphyromonas gingivalis* proteinases as virulence determinants in progression of periodontal diseases. J Biochem 2000;**128**:153-159

[172] Aduse-Opoku J, Davies NN, Gallagher A, Hashim A, Evans HE, Rangarajan M, Slaney JM, Curtis MA. Generation of lys-gingipain protease activity in *Porphyromonas gingivalis* W50 is independent of Arg-gingipain protease activities. Microbiology 2000;**146**(PT 8):1933-1940

[173] Nuttall SD, Krishnan UV, Doughty L, Nathanielsz A, Ally N, Pike RN, Hudson PJ, Kortt AA, Irving RA. A naturally occurring NAR variable domain binds the Kgp protease from Porphyromonas gingivalis. FEBS Lett 2002;**516**:80-86

[174] Papaneri AB, Wirblich C, Cooper K, Jahrling PB, Schnell MJ, Blaney JE. Further characterization of the immune response in mice to inactivated and live rabies vaccines expressing Ebola virus glycoprotein. Vaccine 2012;**30**:6136-6141

[175] Kondratowicz AS, Maury WJ. Ebolavirus: a brief review of novel therapeutic targets. Future Microbiol 2012;**7**:1-4

[176] Fausther-Bovendo H, Mulangu S, Sullivan NJ. Ebolavirus vaccines for humans and apes. Curr Opin Virol 2012;**2**:324-329

[177] Liu JL, Anderson GP, Goldman ER. Isolation of anti-toxin single domain antibodies from a semi-synthetic spiny dogfish shark display library. BMC Biotechnol 2007;**7**:78

[178] Nuttall SD, Krishnan UV, Doughty L, Pearson K, Ryan MT, Hoogenraad NJ, Hattarki M, Carmichael JA, Irving RA, Hudson PJ. Isolation and characterization of an IgNAR variable domain specific for the human mitochondrial translocase receptor Tom70. Eur J Biochem 2003;**270**:3543-3554

[179] Kovaleva M, Ferguson L, Steven J, Porter A, Barelle C. Shark variable new antigen receptor biologics - a novel technology platform for therapeutic drug development. Expert Opin Biol Ther 2014;**14**:1527-1539

[180] Zielonka S, Empting M, Grzeschik J, Konning D, Barelle CJ, Kolmar H. Structural insights and biomedical potential of IgNAR scaffolds from sharks. MAbs 2015;**7**:15-25

[181] Bojalil R, Mata-Gonzalez MT, Sanchez-Munoz F, Yee Y, Argueta I, Bolanos L, Amezcua-Guerra LM, Camacho-Villegas TA, Sanchez-Castrejon E, Garcia-Ubbelohde WJ, et al: Anti-tumor necrosis factor VNAR single domains reduce lethality and regulate underlying inflammatory response in a murine model of endotoxic shock. BMC Immunol 2013;**14**:17

[182] Streltsov VA, Varghese JN, Masters CL, Nuttall SD. Crystal structure of the amyloid-beta p3 fragment provides a model for oligomer formation in Alzheimer's disease. J Neurosci 2011;**31**:1419-1426

[183] Walsh R, Nuttall S, Revill P, Colledge D, Cabuang L, Soppe S, Dolezal O, Griffiths K, Bartholomeusz A, Locarnini S. Targeting the hepatitis B virus precore antigen with a novel IgNAR single variable domain intrabody. Virology 2011;**411**:132-141

[184] Yu C, Ali S, St-Germain J, Liu Y, Yu X, Jaye DL, Moran MF, Cooper MD, Ehrhardt GR. Purification and identification of cell surface antigens using lamprey monoclonal antibodies. J Immunol Methods 2012;**386**:43-49

[185] Steichen C, Chen P, Kearney JF, Turnbough CL. Identification of the immunodominant protein and other proteins of the *Bacillus anthracis* exosporium. J Bacteriol 2003;**185**: 1903-1910

[186] Tasota FJ, Henker RA, Hoffman LA. Anthrax as a biological weapon: an old disease that poses a new threat. Crit Care Nurse 2002;**22**:21-32, 34; quiz 35-26

[187] Witkowski JA, Parish LC. The story of anthrax from antiquity to the present: a biological weapon of nature and humans. Clin Dermatol 2002;**20**:336-342

[188] Inglesby TV, O'Toole T, Henderson DA, Bartlett JG, Ascher MS, Eitzen E, Friedlander AM, Gerberding J, Hauer J, Hughes J, et al. Anthrax as a biological weapon, 2002: updated recommendations for management. JAMA 2002;**287**:2236-2252

[189] Velikovsky CA, Deng L, Tasumi S, Iyer LM, Kerzic MC, Aravind L, Pancer Z, Mariuzza RA. Structure of a lamprey variable lymphocyte receptor in complex with a protein antigen. Nat Struct Mol Biol 2009;**16**:725-730

[190] Wu F, Chen L, Liu X, Wang H, Su P, Han Y, Feng B, Qiao X, Zhao J, Ma N, et al. Lamprey variable lymphocyte receptors mediate complement-dependent cytotoxicity. J Immunol 2013;**190**:922-930

Chapter 9

Use, Applications and Mechanisms of Intracellular Actions of Camelid VHHs

Anneleen Steels, Laurence Bertier and
Jan Gettemans

Additional information is available at the end of the chapter

http://dx.doi.org/10.5772/intechopen.70495

Abstract

The discovery of heavy-chain-only antibodies (HCAbs) in *camelids* and *sharks* led to the rise of a new research field in which single-domain antibodies are used for various applications. Single-domain antibodies are the antigen-binding fragments derived from HCAbs showing several beneficial properties (e.g., small size, specificity, stability under extreme conditions, cost-effective production, and ease of engineering). Importantly, they are stable in reducing cytoplasmic environment, which allows their use as an intrabody to target a wide range of intracellular targets. In this chapter, we discuss both the therapeutic potential of camelid single-domain antibodies (nanobodies) and their use as a research tool with the main focus on its intracellular employment. Targeting intracellular proteins using nanobodies as a therapeutic per se is, up to now, limited due to its incapacity to traverse the cellular membrane. They can however serve as a stepping stone to small compound development, since they directly target a resident, endogenous protein, similar to how a conventional drug acts. In addition, nanobodies are highly adaptable tools and possess interesting properties for more fundamental research objectives like the elucidation of protein function, the tracking and visualization of endogenous proteins in an in vivo setting, and the assessment of protein-protein interactions.

Keywords: VHH, single-domain antibody, nanobody, intrabody, therapy, research tool

1. Nanobodies: a concise introduction

In 1993, Hamers-Casterman discovered the presence of heavy-chain-only antibodies in the sera of Camelidae and assessed that these antibodies are still capable of recognizing an extensive repertoire of antigens despite the absence of the light chain. Single-domain antibodies from camels are called nanobodies. They stated that this discovery could be of inestimable

INTECH
open science | open minds

© 2018 The Author(s). Licensee InTech. This chapter is distributed under the terms of the Creative Commons Attribution License (http://creativecommons.org/licenses/by/3.0), which permits unrestricted use, distribution, and reproduction in any medium, provided the original work is properly cited. (cc) BY

value to the development and engineering of soluble V_H domains or new immunological molecules for diagnostic, therapeutic, and biochemical purposes [1]. This discovery gave rise to a whole new research field in which single-domain antibodies are used for a wide range of applications. Some of these will be reviewed in the current chapter.

The structural properties of conventional IgG antibodies are well known. These consist of two heavy-chain polypeptides and two light-chain polypeptides, each of which is folded into four and two domains, respectively. A variable domain is situated at the N-terminus of both chains (VH and VL) and, as the name suggests, its sequence diverges between IgG antibodies. Paired VH-VL domains make up the variable fragment (Fab) and are responsible for the recognition and binding of the target antigen. The sequence of the other domains is well conserved between IgGs, which led to the designation of these domains as constant domains. Heavy-chain-only antibodies differ from conventional IgG antibodies by the lack of a light-chain polypeptide and the first constant domain of the heavy-chain polypeptide (CH1). Consequently, the antigen-binding fragment of heavy-chain antibodies from camels consists of one single domain, termed the VHH domain. This unit forms the functional and structural equivalent of the Fab in conventional IgG antibodies [2]. The smallest antibody fragment that can be produced from conventional IgG antibodies is a short-chain variable fragment (ScFv, ±27 kDa), which consists of a VH and VL domain linked via a polypeptide. In the continuous search for smaller antibody formats, HCAbs were a thrilling novelty, because their discovery allowed researchers to produce an even smaller antibody fragment of only ±15 kDa. This antibody format derived from camels consists of an isolated VHH domain also known as a single-domain antibody or a nanobody (Nb) (**Figure 1**). In addition, human single-domain antibodies VH and VL have been engineered from human conventional antibodies [3–5], and sharks develop heavy-chain-only antibodies (HCAbs) too [6].

The structural features of nanobodies are quite similar to those of the variable domain of conventional IgGs. The core structure of the immunoglobulin domain is formed by four framework regions (FR), whereas antigen binding occurs through three complementarity-determining regions (CDRs). The latter are located in loops in between β-strands that form the variable immunoglobulin domain. Importantly, FR2 of the VHH domain often contains amino acid substitutions of residues that are involved in hydrophobic interactions between the VH and the VL domains of conventional IgGs (V37 → F/Y, G44 → E/Q, L45 → R, and W47 → G/F/L; Kabat numbering). These substitutions lie at the heart of the single-domain nature of nanobodies because they reduce the hydrophobicity of the former VL interface and improve the nonstickiness of the domain. There are other examples of amino acid substitutions that frequently take place, but these appear to be of less importance [7, 8]. Since nanobodies only consist of one domain, one might wonder whether nanobodies have a diverse antibody repertoire. After all, they lack the VH-VL combinatorial diversity in the antigen-binding site. Nanobodies have counterbalanced the absence of the three hypervariable loops of the VL domain by an *extension* of the hypervariable loops in the VHH domain. These loops show substantial variation in both conformation and length compared with the corresponding loops of the VH domain. This implies that a larger structural repertoire and thus a sufficient diversification in antigen-binding sites can be obtained [9]. More specifically, the introduction of additional Cys residues in the CDRs creates extra disulfide bridges within the VHH domain,

http://dx.doi.org/10.5772/intechopen.70495

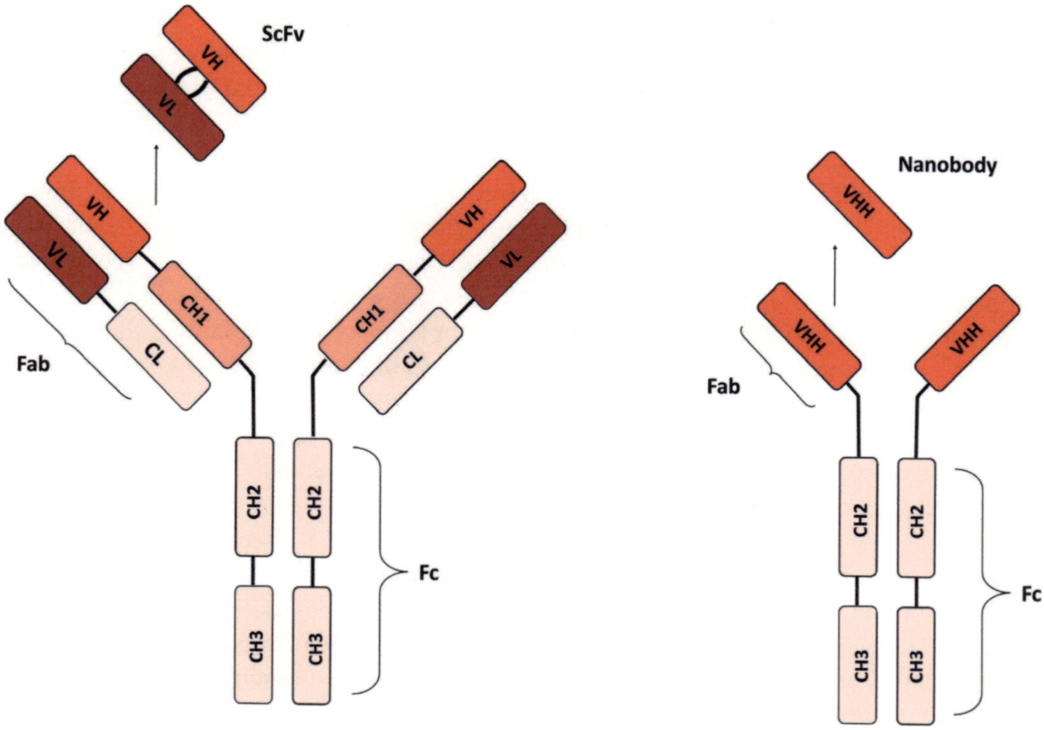

Figure 1. Schematic representation of a conventional IgG antibody and a camelid heavy-chain-only antibody (HCAb). For both antibody formats, the smallest producible antibody fragment is depicted: a short-chain variable fragment (ScFv, ±27 kDa) and a nanobody (Nb, ±15 kDa), respectively.

and these are in part responsible for the diversification of the structural repertoire. The disulfide bridges crosslink the antigen-binding loops, resulting not only in the stabilization of the domain but also in the induction of constraints in CDR1 or CDR3. These constraints probably lead to novel loop conformations and thus in an increase in paratope repertoire. Furthermore, VHHs are more prone to insertion and deletion events near or within the paratope compared to VHs. This is translated into an increase of the surface area of the hypervariable regions and contributes to the structural variation [10].

2. The therapeutic potential of extracellular and intracellular nanobodies

Several monoclonal antibodies (mAbs) have already been approved for clinical use [11], but some limitations are still present despite their success. This includes their large size, relative instability, which imposes restrictions on the administration route and their relative expense of manufacturing. The potential of nanobodies as a therapeutic agent was rapidly recognized as they overcome some of the aforementioned limitations of mAbs. The small size of nanobodies in combination with their extended CDR loops allows them to bind into clefts and cavities, whereas mAbs preferably recognize flat and concave surfaces. Many biological interactions take place in clefts, and nanobodies can target these otherwise inaccessible surfaces and thus function as neutralizing agents or antagonists of protein-protein interactions. More specifically, this property is advantageous when it comes to therapeutically targeting infectious diseases since the essential epitopes of pathogens are often hidden. When cancer has to be targeted, the small size permits a better tissue penetration and thus a significant improvement of the effective antibody concentrations that can be reached in solid tumors. Unfortunately, this advantageous property comes with a price. The small size of nanobodies results in their rapid clearance from the human body and thus in a limited in vivo half-life (a few hours). Therefore, nanobodies are often linked to a serum albumin-binding monomer to prolong serum half-life. The monomeric nature of nanobodies simplifies antibody engineering. For instance, nanobodies can be assembled into multimers, thereby increasing their potency due to avidity effects. The development of therapy resistance can also be curbed by creating bispecific nanobodies. The creation of a targeted drug delivery vehicle is also possible, since nanobodies can easily be linked with drugs [12–17]. Additionally, the outstanding stability of nanobodies under extreme conditions opens the possibility to more patient-friendly routes of administration. In general, mAbs are administered via injections, but due to the extraordinary stability of nanobodies, they can be administered orally, topically, and even via inhalation [15, 18, 19]. The cost of nanobody production lies several times below those of mAb production. The fact that nanobodies are efficiently produced in microbial systems keeps the expenses low. Considering the fact that immunotherapy involves administration of relatively high doses of antibody during prolonged periods, this is a factor that should not be underestimated [7, 8, 20]. Currently, there are no nanobody-based products approved as therapeutic agent, but several products are in the pipeline or in advanced clinical trials. Their value in treating envenoming [21], infections [22], amyloidosis [23, 24], cancer, and other pathologies [25, 26] has already been proven. The research concerning the use of nanobodies as a therapeutic agent is mainly performed on extracellular targets. Nonetheless, nanobodies can also aid in identifying intracellular targets since they directly target a resident, endogenous protein, similar to how a conventional drug acts. RNAi-based approaches rather eradicate, or at least downregulate, expression which is quite different from the mode of action of an average drug. Hence, caution is warranted when making predictions regarding the therapeutic value of a given protein target using this approach. Moreover, nanobodies retain their functionality in the reducing intracellular environment. The major stumbling block toward a successful clinical implementation however is their inability to traverse the cell membrane. For that reason, most experiments are limited to cell cultures and transgenic animals. In the following paragraph, the use of nanobodies to target intracellular proteins with possible therapeutic implications will be described.

2.1. Intracellular nanobodies and antiviral therapy

2.1.1. Hepatitis

About 500 million people worldwide are chronically infected with hepatitis B virus or hepatitis C virus (HBV or HCV). Infection induces an acute and chronic inflammatory liver disease, which puts the patient at risk of developing liver cirrhosis and possibly hepatocellular carcinoma. Currently, there is no vaccine available against HCV, and there is also no cure for most people who are already infected with HBV [27]. Initially, therapy existed of a strict and intensive treatment with ribavirin and PEGylated interferon. This regimen was however associated with severe side effects [28], emphasizing the importance of further research into the pathogenesis of the viruses and how they evade our immune systems. Extensive research led to the discovery of direct-acting antivirals (DAAs), which are small compounds targeted against viral enzymes. The second-generation DAAs are highly potent in treatment, show less side effects, and have a less intensive treatment regimen [29]. However, during infection a large number of viral variants are continuously produced, resulting in the presence of *quasi species* within the patient. This heterogeneity implies that not all therapeutic agents will be equally effective and that drug resistance may develop. Therefore, the search for other therapeutics remains useful. Sarrazin et al. mention that compounds targeting a more conserved region of viral proteins have a better chance of efficacy. Importantly, compounds targeting the active site of the viral polymerase show a high barrier to the development of resistance, due to the fact that mutations at this site often result in loss of polymerase function [30]. As stated previously, nanobodies can bind epitopes localized in clefts, like the active site of an enzyme, and thus are perfect candidates for antiviral drug development.

The potency of nanobodies for counteracting HCV infection has been evaluated. Several nonstructural HCV proteins have been targeted via nanobodies: NS5B, NS3, NS4A, and NS4B [28, 31–33]. NS5B functions as an RNA-dependent RNA polymerase. NS3 has a dual function and displays serine protease activity in its N-terminal region and helicase activity in its C-terminal region. The helicase is involved in the replication of the viral genome and is also thought to increase the translational efficiency of the polyprotein by melting highly stable secondary structures in the HCV RNA [34]. The N-terminal serine protease domain is, together with NS4A, involved in downstream processing of the HCV polyprotein with the formation of mature proteins [32]. NS4B plays a major role in HCV replication by inducing an ER membrane web on which HCV replication takes place [31]. Nanobodies against the different nonstructural proteins were obtained via screening of a VH/VHH library constructed from peripheral blood mononuclear cells of an 8-month-old naïve male dromedary. Recombinant nanobodies reduced NS5B activity by two-thirds (ELISA) [28], and NS3 helicase activity was inhibited up to 88–100% in the presence of the nanobodies, depending on the assay used [33]. Cell-based assays were performed on Huh7 cells (human hepatoma cell line) transfected with RNA (genomic replicon of heterologous HCV). The nanobodies also led to a significant reduction of HCV RNA levels in Huh7 cells transfected with the JFH1 genotype 2a strain, both inside the cells as in the culture medium, when compared to control conditions. Overall, the nanobodies were capable of eliciting responses of a magnitude similar as seen for conventional therapeutic strategies (ribavirin + PEGylated interferon or telaprevir) [28, 31–33]. Furthermore, treatment of cells with the nanobodies against NS3/NS4A and NS4B induced the expression of genes involved in the innate immune response (IRF3, IL28-B, and IFN-β). This is interesting because the innate immune response signaling is interrupted by the virus [31, 32]. In general, these studies lack a detailed insight into the molecular mechanisms behind the observed effects. The authors used computerized modeling to make an assumption about which epitopes are recognized by the nanobodies. Crystallization studies would allow a more detailed view and could help to resolve remaining questions. Even more, the crystal structures could lay the foundation for small molecule development and thus be invaluable. The nanobodies certainly have potential, but there are some remaining questions that need to be resolved before continuing with animal experiments.

As mentioned earlier, currently the biggest obstacle for using nanobodies as a therapeutic against intracellular targets is their inability to traverse cellular membranes. In the aforementioned articles, it was reported that coupling the nanobody with a cell-penetrating peptide (penetratin) seemingly promoted cellular uptake of the nanobody with efficiencies of roughly 80% [28]. However, some caution is warranted here, since the mechanisms behind the internalization of CPPs are still a matter of debate. Even more, in the highly cited article of Richard et al., it has been shown that experiments used to detect the occurrence of CPP internalization are sensitive to artifacts. It appeared that even mild fixation protocols used for fluorescence imaging can induce an artifactual redistribution of these peptides in the nucleus. Furthermore, the highly cationic nature of, for example, penetratin peptides lead to their strong binding to the overall negatively charged plasma membrane [35]. It is thus of crucial importance to remove membrane-bound peptide before analyzing cellular uptake of the construct. Initially, it was thought that CPPs allowed the delivery of biomolecules without relying on endocytosis. Adaptations of the used protocols, however, gave rise to data supporting an active process of cellular internalization involving endocytosis. Applications with CPPs and the controversial issues regarding their internalization mechanisms are elaborately reviewed and will not be discussed in detail [36, 37]. Internalization via endocytosis is however associated with a major drawback, since the delivered biomolecule needs to escape from the endosomal vesicles before it traffics back to the plasma membrane for recycling or it fuses with lysosomes. This might strongly limit the bioavailability of the compound, thus curbing its efficacy. Finally, the nonspecificity of CPP-conjugated constructs imposes a risk of drug-induced toxic effects on normal tissues [37]. In conclusion, a meticulous evaluation of intracellular uptake of the bioactive molecule and of possible toxic effects on normal tissues is warranted, before taking any further steps in its development as a therapeutic agent.

The genome of hepatitis B virus (HBV) is translated into HBV surface proteins, polymerase protein, X protein, or core and pre-core proteins [38]. Targeting the hepatitis B surface antigen (HBsAg) and the hepatitis B core antigen (HBcAg) with antiviral drugs to, respectively, reduce viral secretion and replication is a feasible strategy. HBsAg is the major component of the viral envelope. HBcAg, on the other hand, is the structural unit of the nucleocapsid that encloses the viral genome within a viral particle [38, 39].

To obtain nanobodies against the aforementioned proteins, a llama was immunized with recombinant HBcAg and HbsAg. The peripheral blood cells and cervical lymph node cells were used to construct a VHH library. Both immune and naïve libraries are good sources for retrieving antigen-specific binders. However, in general, superior binding affinities are observed for nanobodies originating from immune libraries, since they were subjected to in vivo affinity maturation. On the other hand, naïve libraries offer an elegant solution for those cases where immunization is difficult due to the lack of an antigen, low immunogenicity, or toxic antigens [39]. The nanobodies against HBsAg were cloned in frame with an ER-targeting signal and an ER retention signal. Co-transfection of these nanobodies and a HBV-expressing plasmid in HepG2 cells induced the intracellular accumulation of HBsAg and caused a reduction of HbsAg particle secretion of approximately 80–90%. The in vivo potential of the HBsAg nanobodies was examined in a SCID mouse. The mouse model for HBV infection was created using a hydrodynamics-based transfection method. Remarkably, measured HBsAg levels in the plasma decline in the presence of the nanobody, and this reduction goes hand in hand with an increase in intracellular HBsAg levels. This observation implies that less virions are secreted. The researchers assume that the observed effects are either due to the disruption of the interaction between the nucleocapsid and the S-type of viral membrane proteins or due to the prevention of the interaction between individual proteins in the ER [40].

2.1.2. HIV

The current anti-HIV treatment strategy, known as highly active antiretroviral therapy (HAART), has changed the field and has turned HIV into a chronic manageable disease. However, patients are lifelong bound to this regimen, its associated side effects, and drug-drug interactions. Sometimes, treatment fails due to multidrug resistance which warrants research for alternative drugs [41]. Nanobodies could serve as a useful purpose in the treatment of HIV infection and have been successfully raised against Rev and Nef. Rev is involved in the nuclear export of late viral mRNA to the cytoplasm. Rev multimers form a higher affinity complex with RRE (Rev-response element), and this affinity is a determining factor for the efficiency of RNA export [42, 43]. The idea of targeting Nef with antivirals came from the observation that a limited amount of patients, infected with Nef-deleted HIV, presented a lack of disease progression. The Nef protein exerts multiple functions: CD4 downregulation, major histocompatibility complex downregulation (MHC1), activation of p21-activated protein kinase (pak2), and enhancement of virion infectivity. These functions can be targeted each independently from one another since the activities are genetically separable. Interfering with Nefs' capacity to downregulate CD4 appears to be the most effective strategy [44].

Vercruysse et al. produced nanobodies against the N-terminal multimerization domain of Rev, because its ability to form multimers is essential for its function. One nanobody is capable of efficiently inhibiting Rev multimerization in cell-based assays. The nanobody induces a cytoplasmic delocalization of Rev. that is similar to that observed for Rev mutants incapable of multimerization. In addition, the nanobody is able to suppress the Rev-dependent expression of late viral mRNAs and consequently also de novo virus production [42]. Further experiments were performed to elucidate whether the nanobody displays a broad-spectrum anti-HIV activity. This was examined by infecting several cell lines, expressing the nanobody in a stable manner, with different HIV-1 subtypes. Virus replication was monitored 5 days post infection by measuring cytopathogenic effects and the presence of virus-associated p24 levels in the supernatant. The nanobody strongly reduced p24 levels for infected cells compared to a control nanobody. More specifically, p24 levels were reduced by >10 folds for subtype A, > 100 folds for subtypes C and G, and >10,000 folds for subtypes B, D, and H [45]. The cells proved to be resistant to viral replication and survived infection. These results are relevant, considering the fact that subtypes A, B, and C are the most prevalent genetic forms on a global scale [46].

Bouchet et al. picked Nef, a HIV-1 nonstructural protein, as target for antiviral therapy. Using cell-based assays and in vivo assays, it was established that the Nef-specific nanobody efficiently counteracted Nef-induced CD4 downregulation and p21-activated protein kinase (pak2) activation. The functional effects of the nanobody are thought to result from its interference with the interaction between Nef and other cellular partners [47]. Nef-induced CD4 downregulation in infected cells is important to prevent interaction between the envelope protein (Env) of the budding virion and CD4 of the host cell, since this interaction might impede the formation of fully infectious particles [44]. The nanobody is capable of reducing the rate of Nef-induced CD4 internalization back to levels measured in uninfected cells. The biological relevance of this observation was tested in a mouse model ($CD4^{+}$/HIV Nef Tg mouse) that presents a downregulation of cell surface CD4, an altered thymic CD4 T-cell development, and a profound peripheral CD4 T-cell depletion. The nanobody rescued the Nef-mediated thymic CD4+ T-cell maturation defect and reversed the downregulation of cell surface CD4 in vivo. T-cell receptor signaling normally leads to profound actin cytoskeleton rearrangements. The Nef-pak2 complex, however, halts these rearrangements by deregulating cofilin, an actin-severing factor. Actin polymerization in infected T cells is thus strongly disturbed. The nanobody disrupts the Nef-Pak2 complex and counteracts as such the inhibition of actin remodeling in a dose-dependent manner. Finally, it was also observed that the inhibition of specific Nef functions by the nanobody resulted in the reduction of virus infectivity of new progeny virions by 80% (molar ratio of 1:1) [47].

Current HAART targets four different steps in the HIV-1 replication circle: the conversion of viral genomic RNA into dsDNA, the maturation of budding viral particles, the entry of the virus into new target cells, and the insertion of viral DNA into a host cell chromosome. Although current strategy is effective, it remains important to explore novel treatment strategies. The development of compounds that inhibit less explored drug targets would be of benefit, and structural biology can aid in defining new drug targets [48]. Nanobodies targeted against both Rev. and Nef appear to have pronounced effects on pathogeny of HIV-1. Crystallization studies to elucidate the exact binding epitopes for both nanobodies are thus of paramount importance since they could aid in new small compound design.

2.2. Intracellular nanobodies as a means to suppress toxins

There exists a multitude of antimicrobial drugs, but compounds capable of neutralizing the produced toxins are often lacking. The question whether or not antibodies hold great potential as toxin-neutralizing agents has been investigated by several researchers. Examples of studies where monoclonal antibodies are used as antitoxins are listed in the review of Chow et al. [49]. Several researchers have exploited nanobodies as a means to neutralize toxins. Intrabodies have been employed to counteract following toxins: ricin, *Salmonella* SpvB protein, and botulinum neurotoxin.

2.2.1. Ricin

Ricin is a naturally occurring toxin derived from the castor bean plant and a well-known type 2 ribosome-inactivating protein. It achieves an inhibition of eukaryotic ribosomes by the depurination of a specific adenine in the 28S ribosome resulting in cell death. Exposure might be lethal, and unfortunately current treatments are mainly of a symptomatic and supportive nature [50]. Herrera et al. constructed a bispecific nanobody, named JJX12, consisting of a VHH targeted against the enzymatic subunit of ricin coupled with a VHH targeted against the galactose-binding subunit [51]. JJX12 fully protects mice against a ricin challenge (molar ratio of 4:1). The protective effects observed for the bispecific construct are superior to those observed for an equimolar mixture of the nanobodies and are the result of both extracellular and intracellular effects. JJX12 promotes aggregation of ricin in solution and makes cell-bound ricin-JJX12 complexes more resistant to dissociation as shown by ricin competition assays with lactose [51]. In the presence of these complexes, further ricin binding to the cell surface is reduced by shielding cell surface receptors for the galactose-binding subunit of ricin [52]. The presence of aggregates changes the internalization and intracellular trafficking of ricin. Internalization of the aggregates occurs via a macropinocytosis-like mechanism rather than via receptor-mediated clathrin-dependent and clathrin-independent endocytosis, which is normally observed for ricin. Furthermore, biochemical and live cell imaging techniques showed a 54% reduction of the retrograde transport of ricin to the trans-Golgi network and the accumulation of ricin in late endosomes in the presence of JJX12, which probably targets ricin for degradation [51].

2.2.2. Salmonella SpvB protein

Salmonella bacteria are Gram-negative enterobacteria associated with human enteric fever. The systemic virulence of the bacterium is largely dependent on the SpvB gene, encoding an actin ADP-ribosylating toxin that is secreted into the host cell cytosol. The toxin interferes with actin polymerization resulting in apoptotic cell death. Nanobodies targeted against the SpvB protein are capable of blocking its enzymatic and cytopathic effects. By means of in vitro radioactivity and fluorescence assays, it was demonstrated that the nanobody completely rescues actin polymerization from the inhibitory effects of the SpvB toxin at a molar ratio of 1:1. Cell-based assays, performed on RAW macrophages and Vero cells, confirmed these observations, since cells exposed to the toxin presented no signs of cell rounding or actin cytoskeleton disintegration in the presence of the nanobody [53].

2.2.3. BoNTs

Botulinum neurotoxins (BoNTs) produced by the Gram-positive bacterium *Clostridium botulinum* can cause flaccid paralysis in humans, which can last for several months. The toxins deliver their light chain, possessing a protease function, to the motor neurons. The protease cleaves SNARE proteins and as such prevents the release of acetylcholine from presynaptic nerve terminals at the neuromuscular junction causing a neuromuscular blockade [54, 55]. Two different strategies were used to suppress botulinum neurotoxin intoxication. Tremblay et al. investigated the potential of using nanobodies as a protease inhibitor per se [55], whereas Kuo et al. implemented the nanobody as a part of a targeted F-box agent to induce accelerated degradation of the protease [54]. A nanobody with nanomolar affinity (Kd ~ 1 nM) for the light chain of BoNT serotype A (A-Lc) was used for both strategies.

Serotype A is associated with the longest persistence and is thus most relevant for therapeutic intervention. The nanobody allows a near stoichiometric inhibition of BoNT-A function as shown by an in vitro FRET-based SNAP25 cleavage assay [55]. The production of cells expressing the nanobody in a stable manner could offer an elegant solution to problems associated with transient transfection techniques and was consequently implemented in the studies performed with the targeted F-box reagent.

Kuo et al. made a fusion protein between a nanobody and a truncated F-Box protein (TrCP) that is capable of associating with Skp1 and Cullin1, with the formation of the SCF complex. This complex, called targeted F-box (TFB), functions as an E3 ubiquitin ligase, thus targeting BoNT proteases for proteasomal degradation. Two constructs were made in which a nanobody targeted against either A-Lc or B-Lc was incorporated. The TFB fusion proteins reduce A-Lc and B-Lc levels with 65 and 50%, respectively (capture ELISA experiments), and decrease the half-life of the A-Lc protease (from ~3.7 to ~1.5 days). Application of MG132, a proteasome inhibitor, results in the accumulation of poly-ubiquitinylated BoNT protease and eliminates the effect of the TFB fusion proteins on its steady-state levels. This indicates that the observed effects are due to the increased degradation of the BoNT protease. Furthermore, in the presence of the TFB fusion proteins, cells are less sensitive to BoNT-A intoxication and also recover 2.5 times faster [54].

2.3. Camelid intrabodies: a ministering angel for patients suffering from protein misfolding diseases?

Proteins exert crucial roles in a variety of cellular processes. Each of these proteins has to adopt its native tridimensional structure to acquire the functional biological state and thus to act faultlessly. However, sometimes proteins fail to either fold correctly or to maintain the native state due to the presence of mutations or increased protein levels. When these proteins escape the inherent quality control systems, serious diseases can develop. These disorders can be characterized by the deposition of misfolded peptides or proteins in the nervous system or other tissues and organs resulting in pathological and insoluble aggregates.

Preventive and curative treatments are often lacking. These therapeutic approaches are feasible when using nanobodies as a tool: increasing the stability of the correctly folded proteins, neutralization of toxic protein/peptide species, and inhibiting or reversing the aggregation of misfolded proteins into oligomers or fibrils [56]. Several research groups have already exploited the use of nanobodies for targeting protein misfolding diseases [57–59]; however, most of the time, they aim at extracellular targets. We will focus on the intracellular application of nanobodies.

2.3.1. *Oculopharyngeal muscular dystrophy*

Oculopharyngeal muscular dystrophy (OPMD) is an autosomal dominant disease characterized by an extended N-terminal poly-alanine stretch of polyadenylate-binding protein nuclear 1 (PABPN1). The poly-alanine stretch is extended from 10 to 12–17 alanines. The mutant protein forms aggregates in skeletal muscles, and this phenomenon is, at least in part, responsible for the disease, although the exact pathological mechanisms are still poorly understood. PABPN1 is a multifunctional protein and is involved in pre-mRNA polyadenylation, transcription regulation, and mRNA nucleocytoplasmic transport [56].

Verheesen et al. screened a nonimmune VHH library for PABPN1-selective binders. Panning yielded six nanobodies with affinities ranging between 5 and 57 nM. Initial experiments were performed with nanobody 3F5 (Kd = 5 nM), which binds PABPN1 at its N-terminal coiled-coiled domain. Co-transfection of mutant PABPN1 and nuclear targeted 3F5 (3F5-NLS) in HeLa and COS cells showed a dose-dependent reduction in the formation of aggregates (37% → 10% in HeLa cells, $P < 0.01$). The expression of the nanobody neither induces cytotoxic effects (MTT assay) nor has any effects on mutant PABPN1 expression levels [60]. A more in-depth analysis on how the formation of intranuclear inclusions is prevented revealed that the nanobody reduces the formation of oligomers of mutant PABPN1 but not of insoluble aggregates [61]. The in vivo efficiency of the six nanobodies was tested in a *Drosophila* model of OPMD in which the expression of mutant PABN1 and the nuclear targeted nanobodies is induced with the muscle-specific driver Mhc-Gal4. Nanobody 3F5-NLS showed the best in vivo efficacy and alleviated several symptoms of OPMD in the *Drosophila* model, including prevention of degenerative effects on flight muscles and the restoration of muscle fiber ultrastructure (Z and M bands). Transcriptome analysis performed to evaluate thorax gene expression patterns demonstrated that 3F5-NLS induced a partial or complete rescue of 58% of the genes deregulated by the presence of mutant PABPN1. These effects are the strongest in the early stages (day 2 after induction) but persist during the life span [62].

2.3.2. *Gelsolin amyloidosis*

Gelsolin amyloidosis is an autosomal dominant disease for which currently only symptomatic treatment strategies exist. A point mutation in the GSN gene (G654 A/T) is responsible for the incorrect folding of the secondary domain of mutant gelsolin (D187 N/Y) that adopts a protease-sensitive conformational state. A pathological proteolytic cascade involving furin and MT1-MMP like proteases leads to the secretion of amyloidogenic 8 and 5 kDa peptides in the extracellular matrix and thus to the formation of extracellular deposits [63]. Van Overbeke et al. used gelsolin nanobodies to shield mutant plasma gelsolin (PG) from aberrant furin cleavage [24]. Furin is a membrane-associated pro-protein convertase that is ubiquitously expressed. It cleaves mutant PG as it passes through the trans-Golgi network (TGN) and generates a C-terminal 68 kDa fragment (C68) that is secreted into the extracellular matrix [63]. This initial step in the amyloidogenic cascade is targeted using a Nb that binds mutant PG near the furin cleavage site with low nanomolar affinity (10 nM, in the presence of Ca^{2+}). In vitro experiments demonstrated a dose-dependent decrease of mutant PG cleavage. The C68 signal intensity is reduced by 76% ($P < 0.001$) when a twofold molar excess of Nb is added. In cell-based assays, the nanobody drastically reduced secretion of C68 in the cell medium. The in vivo efficiency of the nanobody was further analyzed in a gelsolin amyloidosis/nanobody double-positive mouse model expressing human mutant PG. The Nb not only positively affects transgenic mutant gelsolin proteostasis in skeletal muscle tissue but also attenuates the decrease in contraction speed of the extensor digitorum longus in an 8-min fatigue protocol

[24]. Using adeno-associated virus as a vehicle, a bispecific nanobody was introduced in these mice that protects against both furin and MT1-MMP, yielding similar effects on muscle contraction speed [64, 65]. Inhibiting the enzymatic activity of furin could be an alternative strategy, and noncompetitive furin-inhibiting nanobodies have been identified although they have not been tested for treatment of gelsolin amyloidosis [66]. However, despite the involvement of furin in several pathological processes, some considerations have to be made regarding its use as a therapeutic target. Although a complete/partial cleavage redundancy of furin toward several substrates was observed in the liver of an interferon-inducible Mx-Cre/loxP, furin knockout mouse model and obvious adverse effect were absent; a complete knockout of furin in a mouse model resulted in embryonic lethality at day 11 [67, 68]. This observation probably precludes their use in chronic treatments because it is rather unlikely that the long-term inhibition of furin does not go hand in hand with severe adverse effects. Therefore, shielding mutant PG from aberrant cleavage seems to be the better strategy. Moreover, this approach is already successfully implemented in the treatment of early-stage familial amyloid polyneuropathy caused by amyloidogenic variants of transthyretin, thus highlighting its feasibility [69].

3. Camelid intrabodies: a versatile research tool

Over the years, nanobodies have earned their mark as a research tool. A variety of extracellular and intracellular applications using nanobodies exist, and the latter will be discussed here. Intrabodies are often used to unravel protein functions and to gain insight into their dynamics. The versatility of nanobodies and the ease by which they can be engineered allow researchers to use different lines of approach (**Figure 2**). Chromobodies, consisting of a nanobody fused with a fluorescent protein, allow researchers to recognize and trace endogenous proteins in living cells [70]. Since they are already well known, they will not be discussed in detail here.

3.1. Pinpointing protein functions

Nanobodies are an attractive tool for the determination of endogenous protein function. They not only complement well-known RNAi and CRISPR/Cas9 techniques but also allow a more detailed insight by pinpointing specific functions with "surgical precision" by targeting individual protein domains (rather than eliminating the entire protein altogether) and protein conformations, which cannot be achieved by expression modulation. In other words, nanobodies can be of inestimable value to deepen our knowledge of several biological pathways. Researchers have employed several strategies for assessing the functionality of proteins or protein domains, and the different options will be discussed here.

As stated earlier, nanobody cDNAs are available, and these are easily engineered. This implies that the addition of a delocalization tag is fairly straightforward. A variety of targeting sequences are available and can be used to induce the enrichment of both nanobody and its target at specific (ectopic) subcellular compartments. This strategy allows researchers to assess the interaction between the nanobody and its target in the strongly reducing intracellular environment

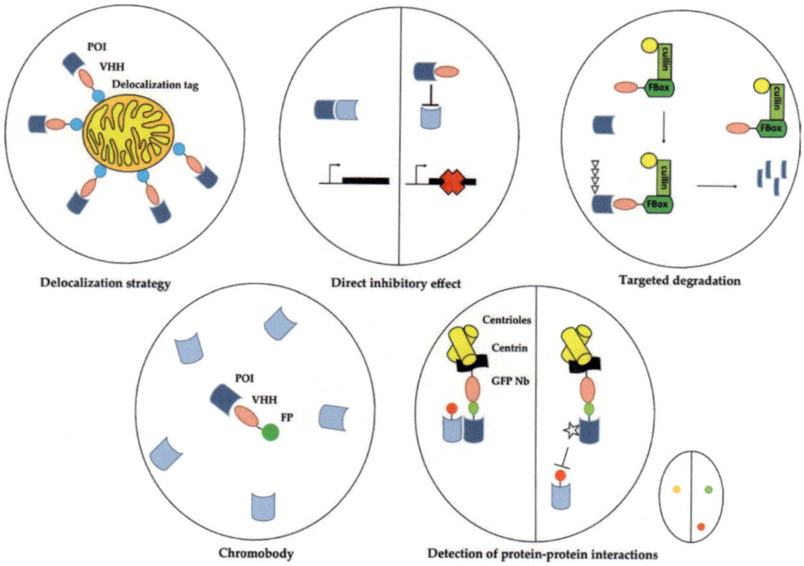

Figure 2. Schematic overview of nanobody-based applications in research. Upper panel. *Left*: Nanobodies can be equipped with a delocalization signal sequence, which allows the enrichment of a protein of interest (POI) at a specific subcellular localization, such as mitochondria. *Middle*: Nanobodies can exert a direct inhibitory effect which induces a protein knockout. *Right*: Nanobodies can be used to target a POI for proteasomal degradation. For this purpose, the nanobody is fused with a cullin-RING E3 ubiquitin ligase. Lower panel. *Left*: A chromobody, consisting of a fusion between a nanobody and a fluorescent protein (FP), allows the visualization and tracing of endogenous proteins in a background of contaminating proteins. *Right*: This nanobody-based application allows one to determine whether or not two proteins of interest interact. Both proteins are labeled with a different fluorophore. One protein, labeled with GFP, is recruited to a specific location via a GFP Nb coupled with a targeting signal. If the second protein, in this example labeled with RFP, is an interaction partner, both fluorescent signals will co-localize. When a compound interferes with a specific protein-protein interaction, the co-localization is absent.

and thus to confirm the in vivo functionality of nanobodies. Moreover, in this way, one can also disturb protein function by restricting free diffusion of the protein and limiting its availability at places where it is needed [71]. Considering that the paratope of the nanobody is located at its N-terminal end, it is safer to fuse the tag at the C-terminal end of the nanobody. Otherwise, a substantial risk at disturbing antigen binding exists [2], although there are examples where a long tag is added to the nanobody N-terminus without disturbing its functionality [72]. Beghein et al. elegantly demonstrated how effectively nanobodies can delocalize their target protein to a variety of subcellular organelles. A survivin Nb (Kd ~ 1 nM) was capable of guiding endogenous survivin in or out the nucleus (*nuclear localization sequence* tag and *nuclear export sequence* tag), capturing survivin on the outer membrane of mitochondria (*mitochondrial outer membrane* tag) and even at the intermembrane area (*mitofilin* tag) which probably required (partial) unfolding of the nanobody and possibly chaperone-assisted entry into mitochondria. This had not yet been investigated. Also, transport of survivin in the peroxisomes (PST-1 tag) was demonstrated [72]. Since interaction between the nanobody and survivin apparently did not perturb survivin functionality, the tagged nanobody is a perfect research tool for further elucidating survivin biology. This strategy also provided evidence that only actin-free gelsolin is able to migrate to the nucleus (in contrast to the actin-gelsolin complex) to potentially act as a nuclear cofactor for the androgen receptor [73], that fascin plays a role in the formation of filopodia/cell spreading and is also involved in MMP9 secretion, and that the SH3 domain of cortactin directly regulates MMP secretion [74].

Some nanobodies exert a direct inhibitory effect, resulting in a functional knockout of the protein. These nanobodies can help researchers to define the biochemical activities of proteins. For example, mechanistic insights in podosome formation were revealed by two inhibitory nanobodies targeted against L-plastin (LPL). LPL Nb5 is capable of blocking the actin-bundling activity of L-plastin, and LPL-Nb9 locks LPL in an inactive conformation. Experiments involving these nanobodies revealed the participation of L-plastin (LPL) in podosome formation and stability [75]. Furthermore, L-plastin is a component of cancer cell invadopodia and contributes to matrix degradation and cancer cell invasion. These effects are mediated by the actin-bundling activity of L-plastin and its bundling independent role in MMP9 secretion and activity, as revealed by the differential effects observed in the presence of LPL Nb5 and LPL Nb9 [76]. One can also interfere with signaling pathways by specific inhibition of the transcriptional activity of proteins, like beta-catenin and p53 [77, 78]. These nanobodies can be used to elucidate the impact of cofactors and post-translational modifications on the targeted protein and allow us to broaden our understanding of the respective signaling pathways. Insight into pathological mechanisms, which might result in the identification of druggable targets, can also be obtained. For example, nanobodies were used to investigate the role of two enzymatic domains of TcdB, a toxin produced by *Clostridium difficile*. Using specific inhibition of the effector glycosyltransferase activity or the cysteine protease, it was, among other things, established that the TcdB-cytopathic effects are mainly mediated by the glycosyltransferase activity [79].

Finally, nanobodies are known to stabilize certain protein conformations and are often used as an aid in crystallization experiments [2]. This property also comes in handy when one wants to study the mechanisms by which cellular receptors translate extracellular cues into intracellular responses. Depending on which conformation the receptor adopts after ligand binding, certain downstream signaling events can be either activated or inhibited. Staus et al. have identified nanobodies that preferentially recognize and stabilize the β2 adrenergic receptor in its active or inactive conformation resulting in a variety of functional effects [80]. These experiments indicate that nanobodies, by acting as an allosteric modulator of receptors, can help us to understand receptor biology.

3.2. Depleting endogenous proteins through proteasomal targeting

An alternative way to determine the function of a protein of interest (POI) in an in vivo setting is to selectively induce their degradation and study the resulting knockout phenotype. To achieve this goal, three different groups have exploited a combination of nanobodies and the endogenous ubiquitin proteasome pathway, a system that is responsible for selective protein degradation in eukaryotes [81–83]. Caussinus et al. were the first to use the ubiquitin pathway for targeted degradation by making adaptations of an E3 ubiquitin ligase, more specifically the cullin-RING 1 (CLR1) E3 ligase complex. For this purpose, a fusion between the F-box domain of *Slmb* and a GFP Nb (VHH GFP4) was made. *Slmb* is part of an F-box protein, responsible for substrate recognition that is expressed in *Drosophila melanogaster*. When this construct, called DeGradFP, was expressed in mammalian cells or *D. melanogaster* embryos, certain GFP-tagged proteins were depleted. DeGradFP was also capable of phenocopying specific loss of function mutations. In spite of these successful results, treatment with DeGradFP was not always followed by the degradation of the targeted protein (e.g., GFP) [81]. In addition to that, a broader application of DeGradFP is still to be demonstrated.

Just like DeGradFP, the cullin-RING E3 ubiquitin ligases were used as the framework for synthetic E3 ligase design. In an attempt to enhance the E3 activity, however, the GFP Nb was fused directly to a truncated adaptor protein instead of the substrate recognition protein. The best results were obtained with Ab-SPOP, a synthetic version of the CLR3 E3 ligase complex, displaying a 10-fold stronger signal reduction of a GFP-tagged protein compared to DeGradFP (50-fold vs. 5-fold). Importantly, the construct degrades only nuclear proteins, and possibly in the future, similar constructs may become available that degrade cytoplasmic proteins. The in vivo effectiveness of Ab-SPOP was confirmed in zebra fish embryos. Ab-SPOP-induced depletion of Hmg2a-citrine, a protein responsible for the modulation of nucleosome and chromatin structure, resulted in various early developmental defects [83]. Fulcher et al. tailored the von Hippel-Lindau (VHL) protein as an affinity-directed protein missile, called AdPROM. Under normoxic conditions, this substrate recognition protein recruits the hypoxia-inducible factor (HIF1α) to the CLR2 E3 ligase. AdPROM is composed of a fusion between the VHL protein and a GFP Nb. It was of crucial importance that the GFP Nb was positioned at the C-terminus of the VHL protein in order to obtain a proper orientation of the target proteins to the CLR2 E3 ligase complex. Since the paratope of a nanobody is localized at the N-terminal end, one should definitely check for potential detrimental effects of this fusion on the binding capacity of the nanobody itself. However, the affinity-directed protein missile was competent in inducing the specific degradation of GFP-tagged VPS34 and PAWS1 proteins in human cell lines, which was further substantiated by the observation of functional effects. Interestingly, during these experiments the researchers observed the co-degradation of UVRAG which is a regulatory component of the VPS34 kinase complex. This suggests that AdPROM has the potential of destroying protein complexes although only individual proteins are targeted [82]. Targeted degradation of proteins of interest by the use of nanobodies holds great potential and might be the perfect complement to CRISPR/Cas systems or RNAi in the elucidation of protein function. The tunability of this system is a huge benefit. Future experiments should point out whether the GFP Nb can be replaced by highly selective nanobodies targeted against specific proteins. In this way, one could investigate the functions of the protein of interest in a more direct manner, without the requirement of protein tags.

3.3. Detection of protein-protein interactions

Nanobodies can be utilized for the detection of protein-protein interactions in cell-based assays. There is a large supply of in vitro methods which can be used for the detection of protein-protein interactions. These methods are widely used and highly efficient for high-throughput screenings but are limited by the fact that they don't operate in intact mammalian cells. Screening for interaction between proteins in their native environment guarantees their proper folding and the presence of necessary cofactors or regulatory proteins. Both nanobody-based methods rely on the interaction between a GFP Nb and a GFP-tagged protein. Herce et al. covalently linked a GFP Nb with a protein that accumulates at a specific subcellular location. In mammalian cells, this protein could be, for example, laminin B1 or centrin, which results in the delocalization of the GFP Nb to the nuclear lamina or the cytoplasmic centrioles, respectively. Subsequently, a GFP-tagged protein will be recruited to a specific location. If the second protein of interest, labeled with another fluorophore, interacts with the first protein of interest, the fluorophores will co-localize at a discrete spot. This interaction can be visualized by a single-fluorescence snapshot. Interestingly, this technique also allows screening for inhibitors of protein-protein interactions [84]. Another recently developed technique uses biocompatible engineered upconversion nanoparticles (UCNPs) conjugated with GFP Nbs. Visualization of the interaction between two proteins of interest is based on the lanthanide resonance energy transfer (LRET). As a proof of concept, they probed for the indirect interaction between the mitochondrial proteins TOM20 and TOM7. The latter was expressed as a fusion protein with EGFP and the former as a fusion protein with dsRed and a Halo tag. This Halo tag was subsequently labeled with tetramethylrhodamine (TMR), while the EGFP was recognized by the GFP Nb-labeled UCNPs. Co-localization of both proteins results in the detection of LRET-sensitized TMR emission. Remarkably, TOM7 and TOM20 are spatially separated by TOM40. The capacity of this technique for reporting indirect long-distance interactions might be of interest to unravel cellular protein complexes [85].

4. Concluding remarks

Nanobodies are highly versatile tools with interesting biochemical properties, which result in their application in various fields ranging from basic research and diagnostics to therapy. In this chapter, we aim to shed light on their multifunctionality and in this way encourage other researchers to include this technology in their future projects. Since their discovery in 1993, the numbers of publications wherein nanobodies are employed are gradually increasing which indicate that their merit has been proved. Here, we have shown that nanobodies have a high therapeutic potential and form an ideal stepping stone to drug development. Despite isolated cases, nanobodies are not capable of traversing the cellular membrane, preventing their direct use as a therapeutic. The effects observed with nanobody treatment are established through multiple mechanisms. Nanobodies can act as an inhibitor of enzymatic activity, interfere with specific protein-protein interactions, and shield a protein of interest from aberrant cleavage, or they can be used as a tool to target proteins for proteasomal degradation. We believe that effects triggered by nanobodies in vitro or in vivo are a faithful representation of what to expect with conventional pharmacological drugs, since both compounds directly target the resident endogenous protein. However, since current experiments are often limited to cell-based assays, animal experiments are warranted to confirm their effectiveness. Furthermore, nanobodies have a lot to offer as a research tool. They can help researchers to elucidate protein functions and thereby gain insight in biological pathways. Several strategies are possible, ranging from subcellular delocalization to the induction of protein knockouts. Last but not least, nanobodies may represent an adequate answer to problems encountered with (conventional) antibody reproducibility

http://dx.doi.org/10.5772/intechopen.70495

[86, 87]. Indeed, particularly polyclonal antibodies run out of stock at some point in the future, making experimental verification impossible. Because nanobody cDNAs are readily obtained and researchers all over the world can use exactly the same nanobody in their experiments, problems of reproducibility can be reduced. In the future, we hope to stimulate a closer consultation within the nanobody field and by doing so taking the research to the next level.

Acknowledgements

This work was supported by grants from the Research Foundation Flanders (Fonds Wetenschappelijk Onderzoek (FWO) Vlaanderen) and Ghent University (BOF13/GOA/010). AS and LB are supported by the Agency for Innovation by Science and Technology in Flanders (IWT-Vlaanderen). We apologize to those researchers whose work could not be cited.

Author details

Anneleen Steels, Laurence Bertier and Jan Gettemans*

*Address all correspondence to: jan.gettemans@ugent.be

Department of Biochemistry, Faculty of Medicine and Health Sciences, Ghent University, Belgium

References

[1] Hamerscasterman C, Atarhouch T, Muyldermans S, Robinson G, Hamers C, Songa EB, et al. Naturally-occurring antibodies devoid of light-chains. Nature. 1993 Jun 3;**363**(6428):446-448 PubMed PMID: WOS:A1993LE93800057

[2] Muyldermans S. Nanobodies: Natural single-domain antibodies. In: Kornberg RD, editor. Annual Review of Biochemistry. 2013;**82**:775-797

[3] Famm K, Hansen L, Christ D, Winter G. Thermodynamically stable aggregation-resistant antibody domains through directed evolution. Journal of Molecular Biology. 2008;**376**(4):926-931

[4] Kim DY, To R, Kandalaft H, Ding W, van Faassen H, Luo Y, et al. Antibody light chain variable domains and their biophysically improved versions for human immunotherapy. MAbs. 2014/01/01;**6**(1):219-235

[5] Ward ES, Gussow D, Griffiths AD, Jones PT, Winter G. Binding activities of a repertoire of single immunoglobulin variable domains secreted from *Escherichia coli*. Nature. 1989;**341**(6242):544-546

[6] Zielonka S, Empting M, Grzeschik J, Konning D, Barelle CJ, Kolmar H. Structural insights and biomedical potential of IgNAR scaffolds from sharks. MAbs. 2015;**7**(1):15-25 PubMed PMID: WOS:000348463300003. English

[7] Harmsen MM, De Haard HJ. Properties, production, and applications of camelid single-domain antibody fragments. Applied Microbiology and Biotechnology. 2007 Nov;**77**(1):13-22 PubMed PMID: WOS:000250115200002. English

[8] Kolkman JA, Law DA. Nanobodies—From llamas to therapeutic proteins. Drug Discovery Today: Technologies. 2010;**7**(2):e139-ee46

[9] De Genst E, Saerens D, Muyldermans S, Conrath K. Antibody repertoire development in camelids. Developmental & Comparative Immunology. 2006;**30**(1-2):187-198

[10] Nguyen VK, Hamers R, Wyns L, Muyldermans S. Camel heavy-chain antibodies: Diverse germline VHH and specific mechanisms enlarge the antigen-binding repertoire. EMBO Journal. 2000 Mar 1;**19**(5):921-930 PubMed PMID: WOS:000085749600014

[11] Ecker DM, Jones SD, Levine HL. The therapeutic monoclonal antibody market. MAbs. 2015 Jan-Feb;**7**(1):9-14 PubMed PMID: WOS:000348463300002. English

[12] Behdani M, Zeinali S, Karimipour M, Khanahmad H, Schoonooghe S, Aslemarz A, et al. Development of VEGFR2-specific nanobody pseudomonas exotoxin a conjugated to provide efficient inhibition of tumor cell growth. New Biotechnology. 2013 Jan;**30**(2):205-209 PubMed PMID: WOS:000313786400015

[13] Fang T, Duarte JN, Ling J, Li Z, Guzman JS, Ploegh HL. Structurally defined alphaMHC-II Nanobody-drug conjugates: A therapeutic and imaging system for B-cell lymphoma. Angewandte Chemie (International Edition in English). 2016 Feb 12;**55**(7):2416-2420 PubMed PMID: 26840214. Pubmed Central PMCID: PMC4820396. Epub 2016/02/04. eng

[14] Gray MA, Tao RN, DePorter SM, Spiegel DA, BR MN. A nanobody activation immunotherapeutic that selectively destroys HER2-positive breast cancer cells. Chembiochem. 2016 Jan;**17**(2):155-158 PubMed PMID: WOS:000369963500008

[15] Riazi A, Strong PCR, Coleman R, Chen WX, Hirama T, van Faassen H, et al. Pentavalent single-domain antibodies reduce *Campylobacter jejuni* motility and colonization in chickens. PLoS One. 2013 Dec;**8**(12):1-12 PubMed PMID: WOS:000329325200145

[16] Roovers RC, Vosjan M, Laeremans T, el Khoulati R, de Bruin RCG, Ferguson KM, et al. A biparatopic anti-EGFR nanobody efficiently inhibits solid tumour growth. International Journal of Cancer. 2011 Oct;**129**(8):2013-2024 PubMed PMID: WOS:000294224300023. English

[17] Steeland S, Puimege L, Vandenbroucke RE, Van Hauwermeiren F, Haustraete J, Devoogdt N, et al. Generation and characterization of small single domain antibodies inhibiting human tumor necrosis factor receptor 1. The Journal of Biological Chemistry. 2015 Feb;**290**(7):4022-4037 PubMed PMID: WOS:000349458400015

[18] Detalle L, Stohr T, Palomo C, Piedra PA, Gilbert BE, Mas V, et al. Generation and characterization of ALX-0171, a potent novel therapeutic nanobody for the treatment of respiratory syncytial virus infection. Antimicrobial Agents and Chemotherapy. 2015 Oct 05;**60**(1):6-13 PubMed PMID: 26438495. Pubmed Central PMCID: PMC4704182. Epub 2015/10/07

[19] Vandenbroucke K, de Haard H, Beirnaert E, Dreier T, Lauwereys M, Huyck L, et al. Orally administered *L. lactis* secreting an anti-TNF nanobody demonstrate efficacy in chronic colitis. Mucosal Immunology 2010 Jan;**3**(1):49-56. PubMed PMID: 19794409. Epub 2009/10/02

[20] Wang YZ, Fan Z, Shao L, Kong XW, Hou XJ, Tian DR, et al. Nanobody-derived nanobiotechnology tool kits for diverse biomedical and biotechnology applications. International Journal of Nanomedicine. 2016;**11**:3287-3302 PubMed PMID: WOS:000380059100003. English

[21] Darvish M, Behdani M, Shokrgozar MA, Pooshang-Bagheri K, Shahbazzadeh D. Development of protective agent against *Hottentotta saulcyi* venom using camelid single-domain antibody. Molecular Immunology. 2015;**68**(2):412-420 PubMed PMID: WOS:000366767900004. English

[22] Yang ZY, Schmidt D, Liu WL, Li S, Shi LF, Sheng JL, et al. A novel multivalent, single-domain antibody targeting TcdA and TcdB prevents fulminant clostridium difficile infection in mice. The Journal of Infectious Diseases. 2014 Sep;**210**(6):964-972 PubMed PMID: WOS:000344608300015. English

[23] Lafaye P, Achour I, England P, Duyckaerts C, Rougeon F. Single-domain antibodies recognize selectively small oligomeric forms of amyloid beta, prevent a beta-induced neurotoxicity and inhibit fibril formation. Molecular Immunology. 2009 Feb;**46**(4):695-704 PubMed PMID: WOS:000263429500022. English

[24] Van Overbeke W, Wongsantichon J, Everaert I, Verhelle A, Zwaenepoel O, Loonchanta A, et al. An ER-directed gelsolin nanobody targets the first step in amyloid formation in a gelsolin amyloidosis mouse model. Human Molecular Genetics. 2015 May;**24**(9):2492-2507 PubMed PMID: WOS:000355325400007. English

[25] Ulrichts H, Silence K, Schoolmeester A, de Jaegere P, Rossenu S, Roodt J, et al. Antithrombotic drug candidate ALX-0081 shows superior preclinical efficacy and safety compared with currently marketed antiplatelet drugs. Blood. 2011 Jul;**118**(3):757-765 PubMed PMID: WOS:000292967300039. English

[26] Roovers RC, Laeremans T, Huang L, De Taeye S, Verkleij AJ, Revets H, et al. Efficient inhibition of EGFR signalling and of tumour growth by antagonistic anti-EGFR nanobodies. Cancer Immunology, Immunotherapy. 2007 Mar;**56**(3):303-317 PubMed PMID: WOS:000243186200003. English

[27] El-Serag HB. Epidemiology of viral hepatitis and hepatocellular carcinoma. Gastroenterology. 2012 May;**142**(6):1264-+. PubMed PMID: WOS:000303156300002. English

[28] Thueng-in K, Thanongsaksrikul J, Srimanote P, Bangphoomi K, Poungpair O, Maneewatch S, et al. Cell penetrable humanized-VH/VHH that inhibit RNA dependent RNA polymerase (NS5B) of HCV. PloS One. 2012 Nov;**7**(11):1-13 PubMed PMID: WOS:000312269500092. English

[29] Jothimani D, Govil S, Rela M. Management of post liver transplantation recurrent hepatitis C infection with directly acting antiviral drugs: A review. Hepatology International. 2016 Sep;**10**(5):749-761 PubMed PMID: WOS:000382659600007. English

[30] Sarrazin C, Zeuzem S. Resistance to direct antiviral agents in patients with hepatitis C virus infection. Gastroenterology. 2010;**138**(2):447-462

[31] Glab-ampai K, Malik AA, Chulanetra M, Thanongsaksrikul J, Thueng-in K, Srimanote P, et al. Inhibition of HCV replication by humanized-single domain transbodies to NS4B. Biochemical and Biophysical Research Communications. 2016 Aug;**476**(4):654-664 PubMed PMID: WOS:000379886500073. English

[32] Jittavisutthikul S, Thanongsaksrikul J, Thueng-in K, Chulanetra M, Srimanote P, Seesuay W, et al. Humanized-VHH transbodies that inhibit HCV protease and replication. Viruses-Basel. 2015 Apr;**7**(4):2030-2056 PubMed PMID: WOS:000353720400025. English

[33] Phalaphol A, Thueng-in K, Thanongsaksrikul J, Poungpair O, Bangphoomi K, Sookrung N, et al. Humanized-VH/VHH that inhibit HCV replication by interfering with the virus helicase activity. Journal of Virological Methods. 2013 Dec;**194**(1-2):289-299 PubMed PMID: WOS:000328521600044. English

[34] Kwong AD, Rao BG, Jeang KT. Viral and cellular RNA helicases as antiviral targets. Nature Reviews. Drug Discovery. 2005 Oct;**4**(10):845-853 PubMed PMID: WOS: 000232546100023. English

[35] Richard JP, Melikov K, Vives E, Ramos C, Verbeure B, Gait MJ, et al. Cell-penetrating peptides—A reevaluation of the mechanism of cellular uptake. The Journal of Biological Chemistry. 2003 Jan;**278**(1):585-590 PubMed PMID: WOS:000180255700076. English

[36] Hassane FS, Saleh AF, Abes R, Gait MJ, Lebleu B. Cell penetrating peptides: Overview and applications to the delivery of oligonucleotides. Cellular and Molecular Life Sciences. 2010 Mar;**67**(5):715-726 PubMed PMID: WOS:000274655600004. English

[37] Koren E, Torchilin VP. Cell-penetrating peptides: Breaking through to the other side. Trends in Molecular Medicine. 2012 Jul;**18**(7):385-393 PubMed PMID: WOS: 000306625900005. English

[38] Rehermann B, Nascimbeni M. Immunology of hepatitis B virus and hepatitis C virus infection. Nature Reviews. Immunology. 2005 Mar;**5**(3):215-229 PubMed PMID: WOS: 000227302400012. English

[39] Revets H, De Baetselier P, Muyldermans S. Nanobodies as novel agents for cancer therapy. Expert Opinion on Biological Therapy. 2005 Jan;**5**(1):111-124 PubMed PMID: WOS:000226398900010

[40] Serruys B, Van Houtte F, Verbrugghe P, Leroux-Roels G, Vanlandschoot P. Llama-derived single-domain intrabodies inhibit secretion of hepatitis B virions in mice. Hepatology (Baltimore, Md). 2009 Jan;**49**(1):39-49 PubMed PMID: 19085971. Epub 2008/12/17. English

[41] Desai M, Iyer G, Dikshit RK. Antiretroviral drugs: Critical issues and recent advances. Indian Journal of Pharmacology. 2012 May-Jun;**44**(3):288-298 PubMed PMID: WOS: 000304603000002. English

[42] Vercruysse T, Pardon E, Vanstreels E, Steyaert J, Daelemans D. An intrabody based on a llama single-domain antibody targeting the N-terminal alpha-helical multimerization domain of HIV-1 rev prevents viral production. The Journal of Biological Chemistry. 2010 Jul;**285**(28):21768-21780 PubMed PMID: WOS:000279516100062. English

[43] Daugherty MD, D'Orso I, Frankel AD. A solution to limited genomic capacity: Using adaptable binding surfaces to assemble the functional HIV rev oligomer on RNA. Molecular Cell. 2008 Sep 26;**31**(6):824-834 PubMed PMID: 18922466. Pubmed Central PMCID: PMC2651398. Epub 2008/10/17. English

[44] Foster JL, Garcia JV. HIV-1 Nef: At the crossroads. Retrovirology. 2008 Sep;**5**:1-13 PubMed PMID: WOS:000260010700003. English

[45] Boons E, Li GD, Vanstreels E, Vercruysse T, Pannecouque C, Vandamme AM, et al. A stably expressed llama single-domain intrabody targeting Rev displays broad-spectrum anti-HIV activity. Antiviral Research. 2014 Dec;**112**:91-102 PubMed PMID: WOS:000346943900009. English

[46] Buonaguro L, Tornesello ML, Buonaguro FM. Human immunodeficiency virus type 1 subtype distribution in the worldwide epidemic: Pathogenetic and therapeutic implications. Journal of Virology. 2007 Oct;**81**(19):10209-10219 PubMed PMID: 17634242. Pubmed Central PMCID: PMC2045484. Epub 2007/07/20. English

[47] Bouchet J, Basmaciogullari SE, Chrobak P, Stolp B, Bouchard N, Fackler OT, et al. Inhibition of the Nef regulatory protein of HIV-1 by a single-domain antibody. Blood. 2011 Mar;**117**(13):3559-3568 PubMed PMID: WOS:000288999800013. English

[48] Engelman A, Cherepanov P. The structural biology of HIV-1: Mechanistic and therapeutic insights. Nature Reviews Microbiology. 2012 Apr;**10**(4):279-290 PubMed PMID: WOS:000301780900013. English

[49] Chow S-K, Casadevall A. Monoclonal antibodies and toxins—A perspective on function and isotype. Toxins. 2012;**4**(6):430 PubMed PMID: doi:10.3390/toxins4060430

[50] Musshoff F, Madea B. Ricin poisoning and forensic toxicology. Drug Testing and Analysis. 2009 Mar-Apr;**1**(3-4):184-191 PubMed PMID: WOS:000275020300015. English

[51] Herrera C, Klokk TI, Cole R, Sandvig K, Mantis NJ. A bispecific antibody promotes aggregation of ricin toxin on cell surfaces and alters dynamics of toxin internalization and trafficking. PLoS One. 2016 Jun;**11**(6):1-18 PubMed PMID: WOS:000377822200019. English

[52] Herrera C, Tremblay JM, Shoemaker CB, Mantis NJ. Mechanisms of ricin toxin neutralization revealed through engineered homodimeric and heterodimeric camelid antibodies. The Journal of Biological Chemistry. 2015 Nov;**290**(46): 27880-+. PubMed PMID: WOS:000365757500037

[53] Alzogaray V, Danquah W, Aguirre A, Urrutia M, Berguer P, Vescovi EG, et al. Single-domain llama antibodies as specific intracellular inhibitors of SpvB, the actin ADP-ribosylating toxin of *Salmonella typhimurium*. The FASEB Journal. 2011 Feb;**25**(2):526-534 PubMed PMID: WOS:000286724800011. English

[54] Kuo CL, Oyler GA, Shoemaker CB. Accelerated neuronal cell recovery from botulinum neurotoxin intoxication by targeted ubiquitination. PLoS One. 2011 May;**6**(5):1-10 PubMed PMID: WOS:000291005800044. English

[55] Tremblay JM, Kuo CL, Abeijon C, Sepulveda J, Oyler G, Hu XB, et al. Camelid single domain antibodies (VHHs) as neuronal cell intrabody binding agents and inhibitors of Clostridium botulinum neurotoxin (BoNT) proteases. Toxicon. 2010 Nov;**56**(6):990-998 PubMed PMID: WOS:000282253900015. English

[56] Pain C, Dumont J, Dumoulin M. Camelid single-domain antibody fragments: Uses and prospects to investigate protein misfolding and aggregation, and to treat diseases associated with these phenomena. Biochimie. 2015 Apr;**111**:82-106 PubMed PMID: WOS:000353178300008

[57] Dumoulin M, Last AM, Desmyter A, Decanniere K, Canet D, Larsson G, et al. A camelid antibody fragment inhibits the formation of amyloid fibrils by human lysozyme. Nature. 2003 08/14/print;**424**(6950):783-788

[58] De Genst E, Chan P-H, Pardon E, Hsu S-TD, Kumita JR, Christodoulou J, et al. A nanobody binding to non-amyloidogenic regions of the protein human lysozyme enhances partial unfolding but inhibits amyloid fibril formation. The Journal of Physical Chemistry B. 2013;**117**(42):13245-13258

[59] David MA, Jones DR, Tayebi M. Potential candidate camelid antibodies for the treatment of protein-misfolding diseases. Journal of Neuroimmunology. 2014;**272**(1-2):76-85

[60] Verheesen P, de Kluijver A, van Koningsbruggen S, de Brij M, de Haard HJ, van Ommen GJB, et al. Prevention of oculopharyngeal muscular dystrophy-associated aggregation of nuclear poly(A)-binding protein with a single-domain intracellular antibody. Human Molecular Genetics. 2006 Jan;**15**(1):105-11. PubMed PMID: WOS:000234219000011. English.

[61] Raz V, Abraham T, van Zwet EW, Dirks RW, Tanke HJ, van der Maarel SM. Reversible aggregation of PABPN1 pre-inclusion structures. Nucleus-Austin. 2011 May-Jun;**2**(3):208-218 PubMed PMID: WOS:000208669000012. English

[62] Chartier A, Raz V, Sterrenburg E, Verrips CT, van der Maarel SM, Simonelig M. Prevention of oculopharyngeal muscular dystrophy by muscular expression of llama single-chain intrabodies in vivo. Human Molecular Genetics. 2009 May;**18**(10):1849-1859 PubMed PMID: WOS:000265525400011. English

[63] Solomon JP, Page LJ, Balch WE, Kelly JW. Gelsolin amyloidosis: Genetics, biochemistry, pathology and possible strategies for therapeutic intervention. Critical Reviews in Biochemistry and Molecular Biology. 2012 May-Jun;**47**(3):282-296 PubMed PMID: WOS:000303244100006. English

[64] Van Overbeke W, Verhelle A, Everaert I, Zwaenepoel O, Vandekerckhove J, Cuvelier C, et al. Chaperone nanobodies protect gelsolin against MT1-MMP degradation and alleviate amyloid burden in the gelsolin amyloidosis mouse model. Molecular Therapy. 2014 Oct;**22**(10):1768-1778 PubMed PMID: WOS:000342542000009. English

[65] Verhelle A, Nair N, Everaert I, Van Overbeke W, Supply L, Zwaenepoel O, et al. AAV9 delivered bispecific nanobody attenuates amyloid burden in the gelsolin amyloidosis mouse model. Human Molecular Genetics. 2017 Apr;**26**(7):1353-64 PubMed PMID: WOS: 000400911300012. English

[66] Zhu JJ, Declercq J, Roucourt B, Ghassabeh GH, Meulemans S, Kinne J, et al. Generation and characterization of non-competitive furin-inhibiting nanobodies. The Biochemical Journal. 2012 Nov;**448**:73-82 PubMed PMID: WOS:000311462600008. English

[67] Roebroek AJ, Umans L, Pauli IG, Robertson EJ, van Leuven F, Van de Ven WJ, et al. Failure of ventral closure and axial rotation in embryos lacking the proprotein convertase furin. Development. 1998 Dec;**125**(24):4863-4876 PubMed PMID: 9811571. Epub 1998/11/13. English

[68] Roebroek AJM, Taylor NA, Louagie E, Pauli I, Smeijers L, Snellinx A, et al. Limited redundancy of the proprotein convertase furin in mouse liver. The Journal of Biological Chemistry. 2004 Dec;**279**(51):53442-53450 PubMed PMID: WOS:000225680600078

[69] Bulawa CE, Connelly S, Devit M, Wang L, Weigel C, Fleming JA, et al. Tafamidis, a potent and selective transthyretin kinetic stabilizer that inhibits the amyloid cascade. Proceedings of the National Academy of Sciences of the United States of America. 2012 Jun;**109**(24):9629-9634 PubMed PMID: WOS:000305511300083. English

[70] Rothbauer U, Zolghadr K, Tillib S, Nowak D, Schermelleh L, Gahl A, et al. Targeting and tracing antigens in live cells with fluorescent nanobodies. Nature Methods. 2006 Nov;**3**(11):887-889 PubMed PMID: WOS:000241788500010. English

[71] Van Audenhove I, Van Impe K, Ruano-Gallego D, De Clercq S, De Muynck K, Vanloo B, et al. Mapping cytoskeletal protein function in cells by means of nanobodies. Cytoskeleton. 2013 Oct;**70**(10):604-622 PubMed PMID: WOS:000326150300006. English

[72] Beghein E, Van Audenhove I, Zwaenepoel O, Verhelle A, De Ganck A, Gettemans J. A new survivin tracer tracks, delocalizes and captures endogenous survivin at different subcellular locations and in distinct organelles. Scientific Reports. 2016 Aug;**6**:1-16 PubMed PMID: WOS:000381290900001. English

[73] Van den Abbeele A, De Clercq S, De Ganck A, De Corte V, Van Loo B, Soror SH, et al. A llama-derived gelsolin single-domain antibody blocks gelsolin-G-actin interaction. Cellular and Molecular Life Sciences. 2010 May;**67**(9):1519-1535 PubMed PMID: 20140750. Epub 2010/02/09. English

[74] Van Audenhove I, Boucherie C, Pieters L, Zwaenepoel O, Vanloo B, Martens E, et al. Stratifying fascin and cortactin function in invadopodium formation using inhibitory nanobodies and targeted subcellular delocalization. The FASEB Journal. 2014 Apr;**28**(4):1805-1818 PubMed PMID: WOS:000335344300026. English

[75] De Clercq S, Boucherie C, Vandekerckhove J, Gettemans J, Guillabert A. L-Plastin Nanobodies perturb matrix degradation, podosome formation, stability and lifetime in THP-1 macrophages. PloS One. 2013 Nov;**8**(11):1-16 PubMed PMID: WOS: 000327254700009. English

[76] Van Audenhove I, Denert M, Boucherie C, Pieters L, Cornelissen M, Gettemans J. Fascin rigidity and L-plastin flexibility cooperate in cancer cell invadopodia and filopodia. The Journal of Biological Chemistry. 2016 Apr;**291**(17):9148-9160 PubMed PMID: WOS:000374849000026. English

[77] Bethuyne J, De Gieter S, Zwaenepoel O, Garcia-Pino A, Durinck K, Verhelle A, et al. A nanobody modulates the p53 transcriptional program without perturbing its functional architecture. Nucleic Acids Research. 2014 Nov;**42**(20):12928-12938 PubMed PMID: WOS:000347693200052. English

[78] Newnham LE, Wright MJ, Holdsworth G, Kostarelos K, Robinson MK, Rabbitts TH, et al. Functional inhibition of b-catenin-mediated Wnt signaling by intracellular VHH antibodies. MAbs. 2015 Jan-Feb;**7**(1):180-191 PubMed PMID: WOS:000348463300018. English

[79] Li S, Shi LF, Yang ZY, Zhang YR, Perez-Cordon G, Huang TX, et al. Critical roles of clostridium difficile toxin B enzymatic activities in pathogenesis. Infection and Immunity. 2015 Feb;**83**(2):502-513 PubMed PMID: WOS:000347955700006. English

[80] Staus DP, Wingler LM, Strachan RT, Rasmussen SGF, Pardon E, Ahn S, et al. Regulation of beta(2)-adrenergic receptor function by conformationally selective single-domain intrabodies. Molecular Pharmacology. 2014 Mar;**85**(3):472-481 PubMed PMID: WOS: 000332865500009. English

[81] Caussinus E, Kanca O, Affolter M. Fluorescent fusion protein knockout mediated by anti-GFP nanobody. Nature Structural & Molecular Biology. 2012 Jan;**19**(1):117-U42 PubMed PMID: WOS:000299046000020. English

[82] Fulcher LJ, Macartney T, Bozatzi P, Hornberger A, Rojas-Fernandez A, Sapkota GP. An affinity-directed protein missile system for targeted proteolysis. Open Biology. 2016 Oct;**6**(10):1-9 PubMed PMID: 27784791. Pubmed Central PMCID: PMC5090066. Epub 2016/10/28. English

[83] Shin YJ, Park SK, Jung YJ, Kim YN, Kim KS, Park OK, et al. Nanobody-targeted E3-ubiquitin ligase complex degrades nuclear proteins. Scientific Reports. 2015 Sep;**5**: 1-11. PubMed PMID: WOS:000361293700001. English

[84] Herce HD, Deng W, Helma J, Leonhardt H, Cardoso MC. Visualization and targeted disruption of protein interactions in living cells. Nature Communications. 2013 Oct;**4**:1-8 PubMed PMID: WOS:000326473300001. English

[85] Drees C, Raj AN, Kurre R, Busch KB, Haase M, Piehler J. Engineered upconversion nanoparticles for resolving protein interactions inside living cells. Angewandte Chemie-International Edition. 2016 Sep;**55**(38):11668-11672 PubMed PMID: WOS: 000383748900068. English

[86] Baker M. Blame it on the antibodies. Nature. 2015 May 21;**521**(7552):274-276 PubMed PMID: WOS:000354816500027

[87] Bradbury A, Plueckthun A. Standardize antibodies used in research. Nature. 2015 Feb 5;**518**(7537):27-29 PubMed PMID: WOS:000349098000013

Chapter 10

Structural Diversity Problems and the Solving Method for Antibody Light Chains

Emi Hifumi, Hiroaki Taguchi, Ryuichi Kato,
Mitsue Arakawa, Yoshiki Katayama and Taizo Uda

Additional information is available at the end of the chapter

http://dx.doi.org/10.5772/intechopen.72516

Abstract

The structural diversity (heterogeneity) problem of antibodies has become a big subject along with the development of antibody drugs and catalytic antibodies. The detailed studies on the subject have not been conducted because many difficult and complex problems are existed in the phenomena. The heterogeneity problem is observed in a whole antibody as well as a catalytic antibody. The difficulty and complexity of the heterogeneity are in the generation of many isoforms caused by different charges, different molecular sizes, and/or modifications of amino acid residues. We found that the constant region domain of the antibody light chain also plays an important role in the heterogeneity. It is desirable that the antibody and/or the subunits must have a defined structure for practical use. We found interesting phenomena that copper ion can convert the multi-molecular forms of antibodies to mono-molecular forms. The ion contributed greatly to the enrichment of the dimer-form and the homogenation of the differently charged full-length and constant region domain of the light chain. The role of copper ion must be significant for preparing a single, defined, not multiple, isoform structure. Note that the big problem could be solved by using copper ion during the purification process.

Keywords: charge heterogeneity, 2D electrophoresis, antibody light chain, pI, copper ion

1. Introduction

In recent year, many monoclonal antibody drugs have been developed, and some of them are practically used in therapy [1–3]. With respect to catalytic antibodies, they have extensively been

INTECH
open science | open minds

© 2018 The Author(s). Licensee InTech. This chapter is distributed under the terms of the Creative Commons Attribution License (http://creativecommons.org/licenses/by/3.0), which permits unrestricted use, distribution, and reproduction in any medium, provided the original work is properly cited.

developed [4–14] for the last two decades from the viewpoint of both basic research and the application, where it has been proved that there are many catalytic antibodies being effective against anti-rabies virus [15], anti-influenza virus [16], anti-*Helicobacter pylori* [17], anti-HIV [7, 8, 10], anti-Alzheimer's disease [14, 18], etc. Interestingly, some of them have been advanced to the stage tested *in vivo* in this decade [15–19]. In the case of catalytic antibodies, some of them play the role as a whole structure of IgG [5, 9, 11, 13], IgA [20], or IgM [21–23]. On the other hand, in some cases, their subunits (light chain or heavy chain) exhibit unique functions [1–4, 6–8, 12]. Once the antibody subunits are separated, the structure of the light or heavy chain becomes flexible and has a tendency to possess structural diversity (or molecular heterogeneity). Regarding structural heterogeneity, it was found about 20 years ago that a whole antibody possesses the structural heterogeneity. These studies were extensively studied by Harris et al. [24] and Nebija et al. [25] using the capillary isoelectric focusing and the 2D-gel electrophoresis [26, 27].

We have also reported about the molecular heterogeneity caused by different electrical charges and different molecular size in mouse monoclonal antibody [28]. This phenomenon is not good for the preparation efficacy, high reproducibility, and practical application. In addition, the structural diversity leads us to ask what structure plays the most important role in exhibiting the catalytic antibody functions. It also provides us with another subject of how we can best make a significant structure with high reproducibility and productivity.

We have recently found a crucial method to solve the heterogeneity problem by using copper ion, which can convert the multi-molecular forms into mono-molecular forms for many recombinant human antibody light chains. In addition, the constant region domain of the light chain (CL) plays an important role in generating a mono-molecular form.

In this review, we will describe a novel method for preparing a single and defined mono-form structure in detail.

2. Structural heterogeneity of monoclonal antibodies

2.1. Examples found in natural monoclonal antibodies

We have found an interesting phenomenon in 2D-gel electrophoresis for mouse type monoclonal antibodies (mAbs), which were prepared against the hemagglutinin molecule of influenza virus [29]. In the experiment, these monoclonal antibodies showed many different spots at the same molecular size [28]. **Figure 1a** shows the results using InfA-9 mAb. In the case, the whole antibody and the subunits, heavy and light chains separated and purified from the parent whole antibody, were analyzed by 2D-gel electrophoresis. In **Figure 1a**, many spots in the whole antibody of InfA-9 are shown. The clear four spots (pI = 6.0, 6.1, 6.2 and 6.5) in the heavy chain and three spots (pI = 5.9, 6.1 and 6.5) in the light chain were detected. Except these spots, many faint spots were observed in the same molecular size (the spots observed over the heavy chain were unknown). Then, the heavy and light chains were separated from the whole antibody of InfA-9, highly purified, and submitted to 2D-gel electrophoresis. The results exhibited the similar phenomena. In the heavy chain, similar spots are seen, and clear five spots (pI = 6.1, 6.3, 6.5, 6.7 and 6.9) were detected in this case. The pI positions of the spots

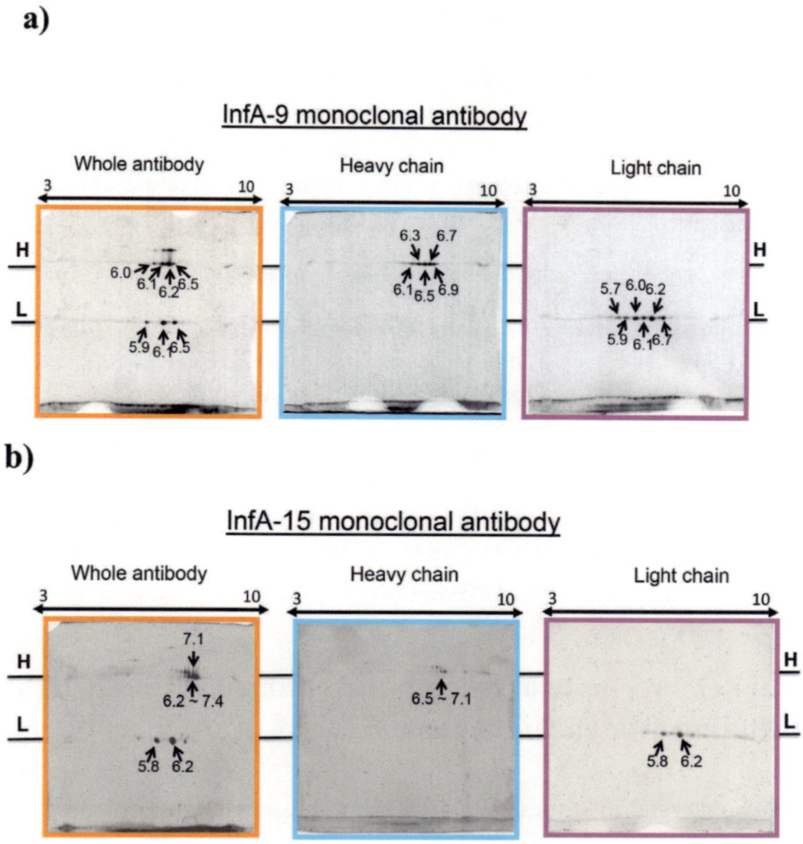

Figure 1. 2D electrophoresis for mouse type monoclonal antibodies against hemagglutinin molecule of influenza virus. SDS-PAGE; Running gel 12.5%. Strip; pH 3–10 nonlinear 7 cm. Sample; whole antibody 3.2 μg, heavy and light chain: 1.6 μg. Staining; deep purple (GE Healthcare). (a) InfA-9 monoclonal antibody. Whole antibody: many spots are seen in the whole antibody of InfA-9. The clear four spots (pI = 6.0, 6.1, 6.2 and 6.5) in the heavy chain and three spots (pI = 5.9, 6.1 and 6.5) in the light chain were detected. Heavy chain (H): clear five spots (pI = 6.1, 6.3, 6.5, 6.7 and 6.9) were detected. The pI positions of the spots were a little bit different compared to the whole antibody. Light chain (L): clear six spots (pI = 5.7, 5.9, 6.0, 6.1, 6.2 and 6.7) were detected. The number of spots increased compared with those of the whole antibody. (b) InfA-15 monoclonal antibody. For the whole antibody and the heavy and light chain, similar results showing many spots at different pI for the same molecular sizes were observed, suggesting that the molecular heterogeneity of antibodies are generally occurring events.

were a little bit different compared to the whole antibody. For the case of the light chain, clear six spots (pI = 5.7, 5.9, 6.0, 6.1, 6.2 and 6.7) were detected. The number of spots increased compared with those of the whole antibody. These phenomena are not exceptional, but general. The mAb, InfA-15, exhibited similar results. **Figure 1b** shows 2D-gel electrophoresis using InfA-15 mAb. In the results of the whole antibody and the heavy chain and the light chain, the pattern of spots were a little different from those of InfA-9 mAb, but several different pI spots were observed in all cases. Namely, different pI spots are present at the same molecular size in any mAb. Note that structural diversity (molecular heterogeneity) should be existing even in the monoclonal antibody and the subunits, while they are a single protein. In our case, it is considered that the various electrical charges of the molecule may be one of the causes.

2.2. Recombinant monoclonal antibody Herceptin

The structural diversity of antibodies has been found about 20 years ago [26, 27], suggesting that an antibody has some different structures (not a mono-form structure) caused by the various electrical charges. Regarding the charge heterogeneity, Harris et al. [24] and Nebija et al. [25, 30] have extensively studied this phenomenon with recombinant antibodies using capillary isoelectric focusing and 2D-gel electrophoresis.

The former paper [24] pointed out a deamidation of Asn residues in the protein.

The latter papers showed multiple spots of pI spreading at heavy and light chains, caused by generation of charge-related isoforms. The pI spreading pattern in 2D-gel electrophoresis [30] is similar to our cases. The effects of sugar chains are also taken into account for molecular heterogeneity.

As it is well known that an antibody light chain has no sugar chain, this can be excluded for this subunit. Thus, in our case, it is thought that the structural diversity is mostly due to the heterogeneity of the different electrical charges. In addition, the possibility of deamidation is excluded because it is hardly considered that the addition of a copper ion causes a reverse reaction of the deamidation and the heterogeneity is lost.

3. Structural heterogeneity of recombinant human antibody light chains (including catalytic light chains)

3.1. Phenomena observed in several human antibody light chains

3.1.1. Chromatograms of antibody light chain C51

In this section, we will describe the phenomena of structural diversity using full-length light chains of human antibodies. **Figure 2a** shows the amino acid sequences of human antibody kappa light chains of C51, #4 and #7. The proteins were expressed in *Escherichia coli* in accordance with the protocol described in the section of Materials and Methods in Refs. [19, 31, 32]. Methionine was adducted at the N-terminus and confirmed by amino acid sequence analysis after cloning the cDNA of the light chain into the *Nco I* site of the pET-20b vector. Leu and Glu residues were inserted by employing the *Xho I* site before a histidine–tag (His × 6) included in the vector for purification.

After the transformed *E. coli* cells were recovered by centrifugation, they were sonicated. Then, the soluble fraction was subjected to purification using Ni-NTA affinity chromatography. The result of a Ni-NTA affinity chromatography for the C51 light chain is shown in **Figure 2b**. The C51 light chain was eluted from fraction 28 (Fr.28) to Fr.44. Fr.35 showed the maximum absorbance. Fr.35 was collected and analyzed by SDS-PAGE with CBB staining, where the C51 light chain was mainly the monomer form with a slight contamination of dimer forms.

The eluted fractions from Fr.30 to Fr.40 were collected and subjected to a cation exchange chromatography. **Figure 2c** shows the chromatogram, where several peaks were observed. The SDS-PAGEs of the peaks were shown in the figure on the right side. The peaks 1, 2, and 3 were the monomer, the mixture of monomer and dimer, and the dimer, respectively.

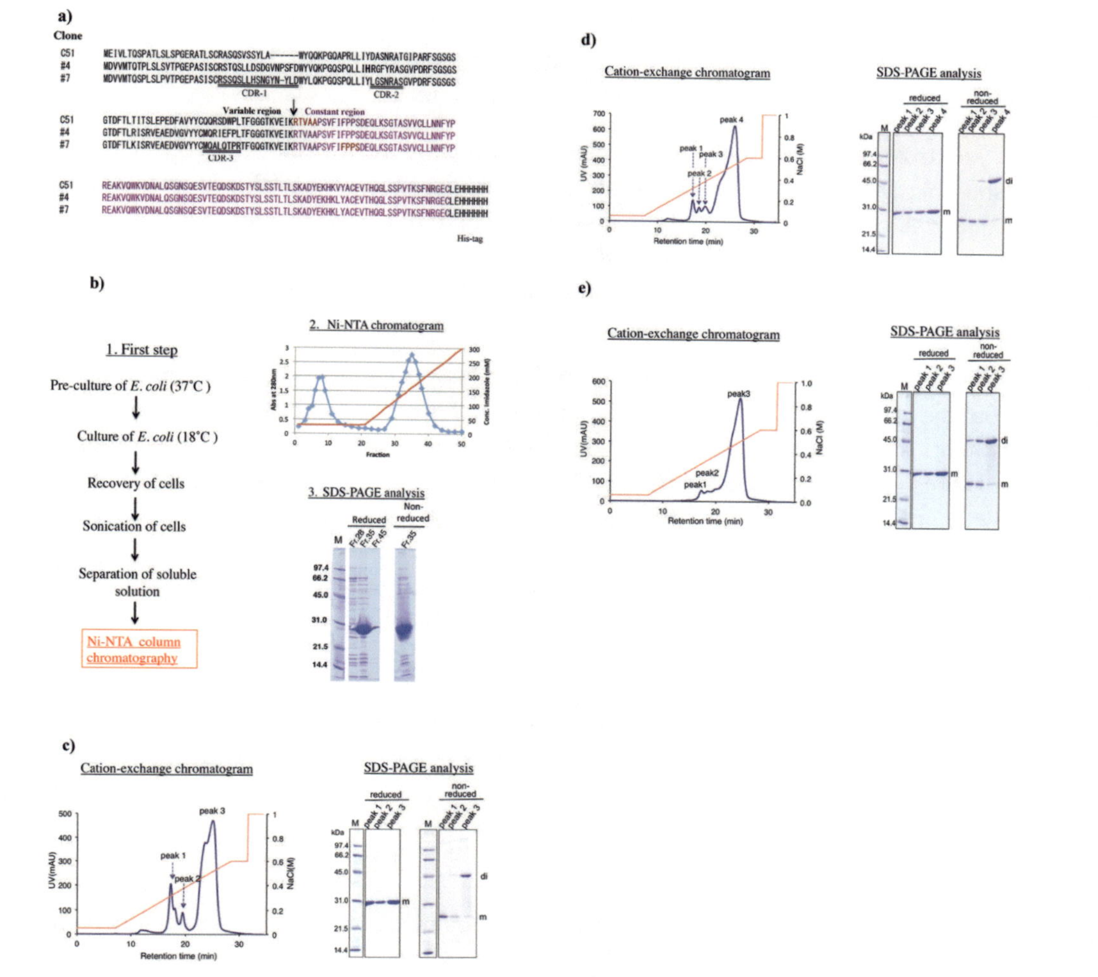

Figure 2. C51 light chain. (a) Amino acid sequences of human light chains (kappa type). (b) First-step purification of C51 light chain. (b-1) Steps from *E. coli* culture to Ni-NTA column chromatography. (b-2) Ni-NTA column chromatogram for C51 light chain. (b-3) Results of SDS-PAGE of fraction 28–45. C51 light chain was mainly the monomer form with a slight contamination of dimer forms at approximately 45 kDa. (c) Cation exchange chromatography as the second-step purification without copper ion. Several peaks were observed from 15 to 27 min. The peaks 1, 2, and 3 were the monomer, the mixture of monomer and dimer, and the dimer, respectively. (d) Cation exchange chromatography as the second-step purification with addition of 0.5 eq. copper ion in cell suspension. A main peak (peak 4) was observed at the retention time of 26 min but other peaks (1–3) were small. The SDS-PAGE gave a dimer for peak 4. (e) Cation exchange chromatography as the second-step purification with addition of 0.5 eq. copper ion in the Ni-NTA eluent. Only a main peak (peak 3) was observed at the retention time of 26 min but other peaks (1 and 2) were scarcely detected. The SDS-PAGE gave a dimer for peak 3. The addition of Cu^{2+} led to formation of dimers.

3.1.2. *Effect of copper ions*

Twenty μM of $CuCl_2$ (Cu^{2+}) was added to either the cell suspension after recovery of the cells (cell-suspension) or the eluent of Ni-NTA chromatography (Ni-NTA eluent). By the addition of Cu^{2+} to the cell suspension, the chromatogram changed to that shown in **Figure 2d**, where a main peak (peak 4) was observed at the retention time of 26 min but other peaks (1, 2 and 3) were small. The SDS-PAGE gave a dimer for peak 4. In **Figure 2e**, 20 μM of Cu^{2+} (0.5 equivalent to the light chain) was added to the Ni-NTA eluent. In this case, only a main peak (peak 3) was observed at the retention time of 26 min but other peaks (1 and 2) were scarcely detected. The SDS-PAGE gave a dimer for peak 3. The addition of Cu^{2+} led to dimer formation.

Mass spectroscopic (MS) analysis was performed for the main peaks observed above (data not shown). Briefly, a monomeric light chain was detected at 25,000 m/z and a dimer at 49,000 m/z. A small trimer and tetramer were also detected at 74,000 and 98,000 m/z, respectively. By the addition of Cu^{2+} to the cell suspension or the Ni-NTA eluent, the signal for the monomer was substantially reduced. Conclusively, the addition of Cu^{2+} was effective for the formation of the dimer.

In order to examine the pI of the light chain, 2D-gel electrophoresis was performed with and without the addition of Cu^{2+}. The results are shown in **Figure 3a** and **b**. In the case without Cu^{2+}, many spots at different pIs were observed with the same molecular size of 31 kDa (**Figure 3a**). The pI spots were widely located from 6.12 to 10.0. The strong spot was observed at pI = 6.45–6.73. In contrast, in the case with the addition of Cu^{2+}, the spots were gathered on the strongest spot at pI = 6.57, while two faint spots were detected at around pI = 6.32 and 6.90 (**Figure 3b**). It is evident that the electrical charges of the molecule became mono-form by the effect of Cu^{2+}.

3.2. #4 and #7 light chains

It must be invested whether or not the changes from multi-molecular forms to mono-molecular forms by the addition of copper ions is a general phenomenon. The following experiments were carried out.

3.2.1. Chromatograms

For the purpose of confirmation of the observed phenomena on the structural diversity, other antibody light chains such as #4 and #7 were examined. As stated above, the chromatogram in Ni-NTA purification is similar for many light chains. Thus, the following is focused on the results of cation exchange chromatography, which were very different in each light chain used. The effect of copper ions on the diversity issue will be discussed.

The cation chromatograms for #4 light chain are shown in the cases without and with Cu^{2+} as presented in **Figure 4a** and **b**, respectively. In the case without Cu^{2+}, there were several peaks. The results of SDS-PAGE (non-reduced condition) corresponding to three peaks are also shown. The observed peaks were a mixture of monomers and dimers. Namely, several structurally different light chains caused by different electrical charges are coexisting in the solution. However, when 20 μM of Cu^{2+} (0.5 equivalent to the light chain) was added to the Ni-NTA eluent, the several peaks in **Figure 4a** surprisingly became a single peak (**Figure 4b**), which was mainly the dimer.

In the case of the chromatography for #7 light chain, huge three peaks were observed in the case without Cu^{2+} as shown in **Figure 5a**. The peak of the retention time at 9 min was the monomer. The peak at 13 min was a mixture of monomer and dimer. The peak at 22 min was also a mixture. Note that light chains possess different molecular sizes and electrical charges in solution.

http://dx.doi.org/10.5772/intechopen.72516

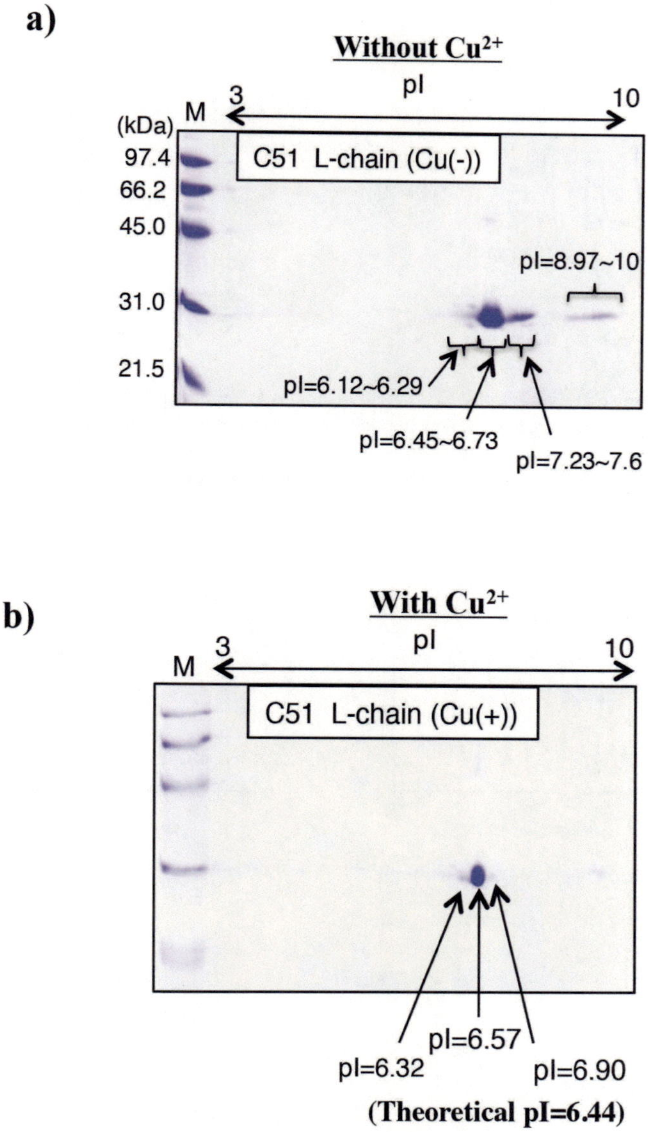

Figure 3. 2D-gel electrophoresis for C51 light chain. (a) Without copper ion. The pI spots were widely located from 6.12 to 10.0. (b) With copper ion. The spots were gathered on the strongest spot at pI = 6.57, although two faint spots were detected at around pI = 6.32 and 6.90.

When 15 μM of Cu^{2+} (0.38 eq.) was added to the Ni-NTA eluent, two peaks at 12 min and 23 min of retention time were observed in the chromatography. The results of SDS-PAGE analysis (**Figure 5b**) indicated that both peak A and peak B were dimers. It is interesting that two kinds of dimers with different electrical charges were coexisting. When 40 μM of Cu^{2+} (1.0 eq.) was added to the same eluent, only peak C, which corresponds to peak A in **Figure 5b**, was observed at 12 min and peak B was not detected (**Figure 5c**). It is thought that peak B moved to peak A in **Figure 5b**. Conclusively, the dimeric light chains possessing two kinds of electrical charges became one kind of state possessing a unique electrical charge by the addition of 40 μM of Cu^{2+}.

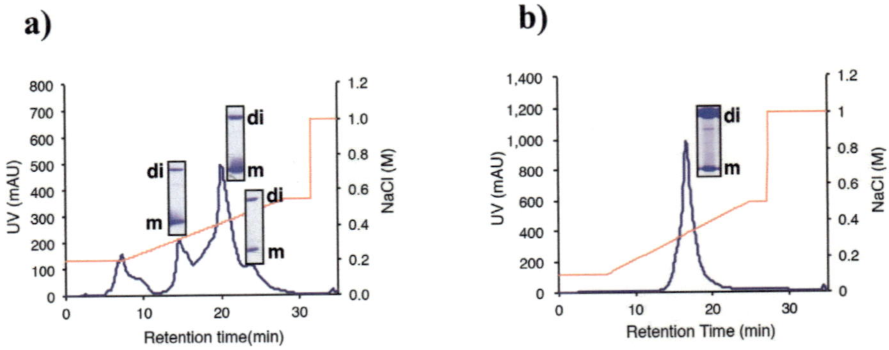

Figure 4. Cation exchange chromatography for #4 light chain. (a) Without copper ion. There were mainly three peaks, which were a mixture of monomers and dimers. Namely, several structurally different light chains caused by different electrical charges are coexisting in the solution. (b) With copper ion of 0.5 eq. When 0.5 equivalent to the light chain was added to the Ni-NTA eluent, the several peaks became a single peak of mainly the dimer.

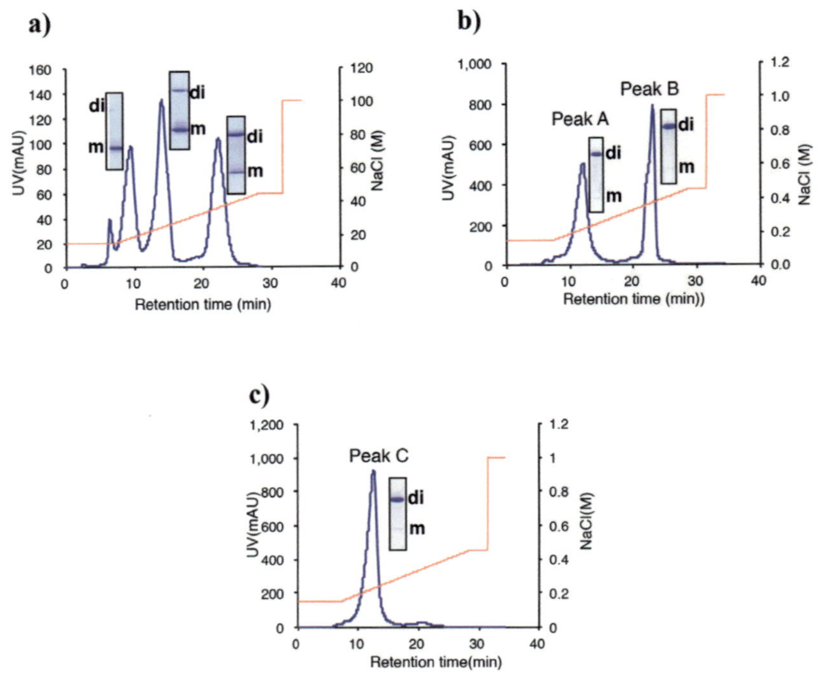

Figure 5. Cation exchange chromatography for #7 light chain. (a) Without copper ion. Huge three peaks were observed. The peak of the retention time at 9 min was the monomer, peak at 13 min was the mixture of monomers and dimers, and peak at 22 min was a mixture. In this case, the light chains possess different molecular sizes and electrical charges in solution. (b) With copper ion of 0.38 eq. Two peaks at 12 min and 23 min retention time were observed and both peak A and peak B were dimers. (c) With copper ion of 1.0 eq. Only peak C, which corresponds to peak A in (b), was observed at 12 min as the dimer form.

A chemical analysis of Cu^{2+} gave interesting results. The ratio of Cu to light chain (Cu/light chain) is 0.48, 0.03, and 0.64 for peaks A, B and C, respectively. When the ratio of Cu/light chain was 0.48 in **Figure 5b** and 0.64 in **Figure 5c**, the dimer was eluted at 12 min. In contrast, at a ratio of 0.03, the retention time was 23 min. These results suggest that whenever enough Cu^{2+} is present in the solution, an electrically homogeneous light chain could be observed at a retention time of 12 min.

UV/VIS spectroscopy for these peaks was also conducted. The results are shown in **Figure 6**. We could see the absorbance around 560 nm, which is assigned to the absorbance of the interaction of cupper with the amino acids for peak A and peak C, but not for peak B, whose spectrum was very similar without copper ion.

3.2.2. AFM analysis

In order to investigate the morphology of antibody light chains, we conducted atomic force microscopy (AFM) analysis. The peaks of A, B, and C were collected and subjected to AFM analysis as shown in **Figure 7a–c**. **Figure 7a** shows the AFM image for peak A. The images for peak B and C are shown in **Figure 7b** and **c**, respectively. The red circle represents the clear image of the dimeric light chain. The size of the dimer was roughly estimated at an

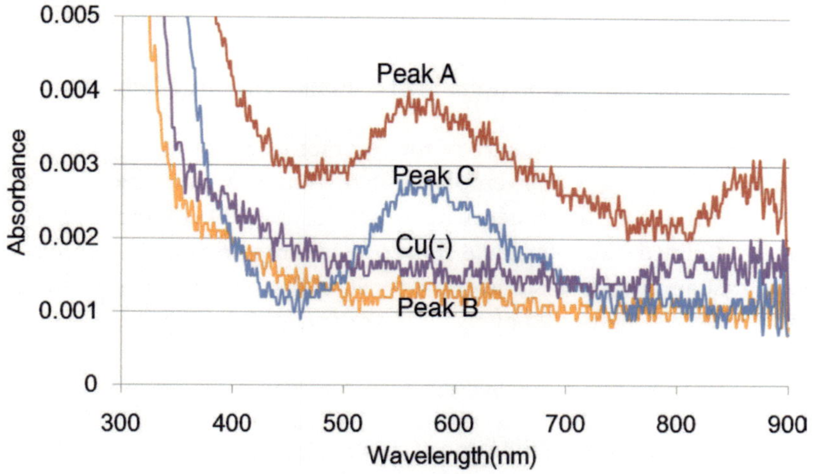

Figure 6. UV/VIS spectroscopy. The absorbance around 560 nm, which is assigned to the absorbance of the interaction of a copper ion with the amino acids, was observed for peak A and peak C, but not for peak B. It is obvious that peak B has no copper ion.

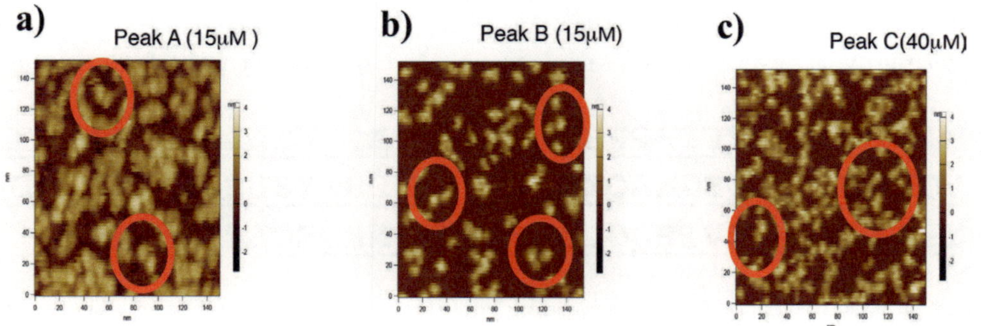

Figure 7. AFM analysis. The peaks of A, B, and C were collected and subjected to AFM analysis. The red circle represents the clear image of the dimeric light chain. (a) Peak A included Cu^{2+} with the ratio of Cu/#7 light chain = 0.48. (b) Peak B did not include Cu^{2+} (Cu/#7 light chain = 0.03). (c) Peak C included Cu^{2+} with the ratio of Cu/#7 light chain = 0.64. The size of the dimer was roughly estimated at an approximate length of 20 nm, the width of 10 nm, and the height of 4 nm.

approximate length of 20 nm, the width of 10 nm, and the height of 4 nm. The lateral and height length are comparable with the AFM image of IgG by Querghi et al. [33]. We could not identify the position of the copper ion residing in the light chain from this AFM analysis.

4. Structural heterogeneity of the constant region domains of light chains (CLs)

In the previous section, we focused on a full-length light chain, which is consisted of the variable and the constant domain. It is noteworthy to study which domain, the former or latter, causes the structural diversity problem. Although there are many studies on the role of the constant domains (especially for a Fc region) of the heavy chain of the antibody, the reports on the role of the constant region domain of the light chain are scarcely seen. From this point of view, we investigated the role of the constant domain as described in the following.

4.1. Sequence of the constant region domain of a human antibody light chain

Figure 8 shows the amino acid sequence of the recombinant constant region domain (kappa type) of a human antibody light chain employed in this study. Methionine (M) and alanine (A) at position nos. 1 and 2 of the aa sequence have been inserted by cloning using the restriction enzyme *Nco I*. Underlined is the sequence of the constant region domain. Arginine (R) at position no. 3 is the first amino acid residue of the constant region. Leucine (L) and glutamic acid (E) before His × 6 were also inserted by using the restriction enzyme (*Xho I*).

4.1.1. Chromatography and SDS-PAGE analysis

The expression and purification of the kappa type constant domain were similarly conducted as made in the full-length light chain. Ni-NTA chromatography was also performed to purify the recovered constant region domain. The result was also similar with that obtained in the case of full-length light chain except for the molecular size. The SDS-PAGE analysis for the collected fraction in the Ni-NTA chromatography is shown in **Figure 9**. Under non-reduced condition, a strong band was detected in the monomeric form at 15 kDa as well as a weak band in the dimeric form at 30 kDa. Under reduced condition, only the monomeric form was observed and the purity was over 95%. This sample was applied to cation exchange chromatography.

MARTVAAPSVFIFPPSDEQLKSGTASVVCLLNNFYPREAK
VQWKVDNALQSGNSQESVTEQDSKDSTYSLSSTLTLSKAD
YEKHKVYACEVTHQGLSSPVTKSFNRGECLEHHHHHH

Figure 8. Amino acid sequence of the constant region domain of a human antibody light chain (kappa type). Underlined is the aa sequence of the constant region domain of the kappa light chain. Methionine (M) and alanine (A) of the aa sequence at the first and second position were inserted by cloning using the restriction enzyme *Nco I*. Arginine (R) at the third position is the first amino acid residue of the constant region. Leucine (L) and glutamic acid (E) before His × 6 were also inserted by cloning using the restriction enzyme *Xho I*.

http://dx.doi.org/10.5772/intechopen.72516

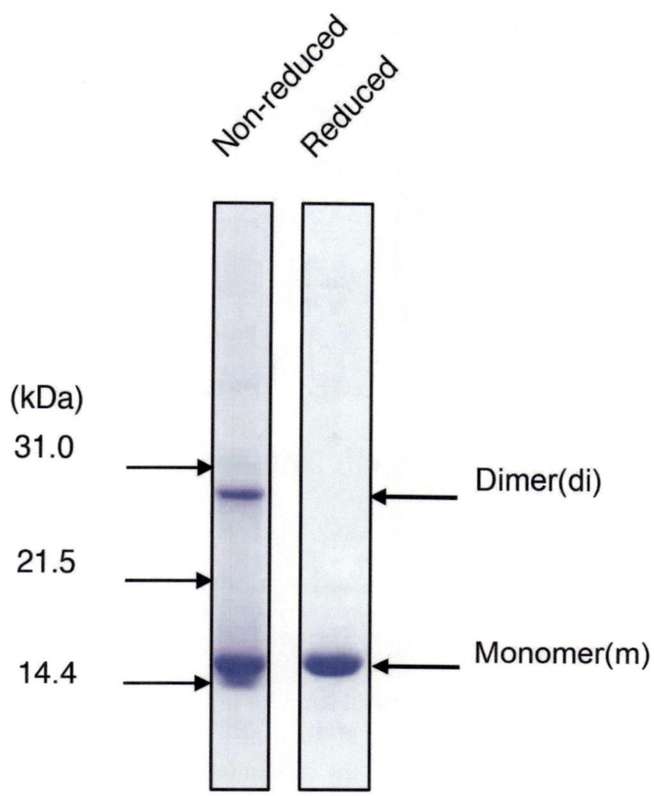

Figure 9. SDS-PAGE of the constant region domain after Ni-NTA chromatography. Under non-reduced condition, a strong band was detected in the monomeric form at 15 kDa as well as a weak band in the dimeric form at 30 kDa. Under reduced condition, only the monomeric form was observed and the purity was over 95%.

The results are shown in **Figure 10** along with the SDS-PAGE analysis under non-reduced condition. Several peaks were observed at retention times from 5 to 25 min while it was a single material of the constant domain. In **Figure 10**, peak 1 appearing at the retention time of 7.5 min is a monomer, and peaks 2, 3, and 4 appearing at 14–17 min contain mainly monomers. The dimers or/and trimer were detected for peaks 2 and 4. Peaks 5 and 6 appearing at 21–23 min are the dimer. These results mean that differently charged molecules of the constant region domain as well as differently sized molecules coexisted in solution at the same time. It is obvious that a constant region molecule shows molecular heterogeneity (structural diversity) from the viewpoint of both electrical charge and molecular size, which are very similar with those observed in the full-length light chain.

4.2. Effect of copper ions

As stated previously, copper ion (Cu^{2+}) hugely influenced the structural diversity of the full-length light chain. The same experiment was performed with the constant region domain molecule. The results are summarized in **Figure 11a–f**. In the case of 0.1 eq. addition of Cu^{2+} for the constant region domain molecule, we observed a small peak 7 and one main peak

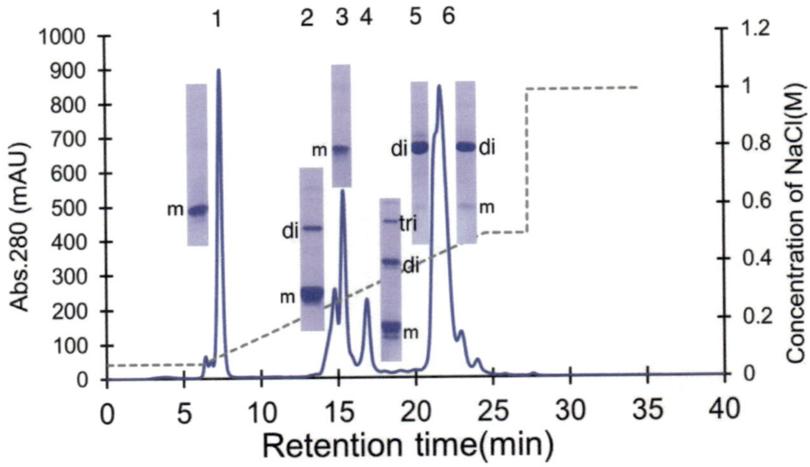

Figure 10. Cation exchange chromatography for the constant region domain molecule of the light chain (CL). Peak 1 appearing at the retention time of 7.5 min is a monomer and peaks 2, 3, and 4 appeared at 14–17 min contain mainly monomers. The dimers or/and trimer were detected for peaks 2 and 4. Peaks 5 and 6 appearing at 21–23 min are the dimer. These results mean that differently charged molecules of the constant region domain as well as differently sized molecules coexisted in solution at the same time. This result was very similar with that observed with the full-length light chain.

8, which were eluted at the retention time around 16 and 22 min, respectively (**Figure 11a**). Peak 8 was the dimer by the SDS-PAGE analysis under non-reduced condition (peak 7 was not analyzed because of the small peak). In the case of 0.2 eq. addition of copper, mainly two peaks (9 and 10) were obtained (**Figure 11b**). The elution times of peaks 9 and 10 were identical with those of peaks 7 and 8, respectively. Peak 9 included mainly the dimer with a very slight amount of the monomer. Peak 10 was the dimer. For these two peaks, UV/VIS spectroscopy was performed. The results are presented in **Figure 12**. Peak 9 showed an absorbance of around 580 nm, which was based on the interaction of Cu^{2+} and amino acids of the constant region domain molecule. On the other hand, no absorbance was detected for peak 10. Namely, protein of peak 9 bound to Cu^{2+} but peak 10 did not. Though the peaks are dimeric forms of the constant region domain, they were separated by the cation exchange column chromatography whether or not the peak contains Cu^{2+}. For the case of 0.3 eq. addition, the main peak was peak 11 observed at the retention time of 16 min, which included the dimer along with a slight monomer and trimer forms (**Figure 11c**). In the case of 0.4 eq. addition, a clear single peak of the dimer form was detected at the retention time of 16 min (**Figure 11d**). In **Figure 11e** and **f**, peaks 13 and 14 were observed as single peak at the retention time of 16 min. And they were the dimer. It seems that enough content of added copper ion was 0.4 eq. to induce mono-form formation from the multi-forms of the constant region domain molecule.

The amount of Cu^{2+} bound to the constant region domain molecule was also quantified using a commercially available copper detection kit (Copper, Low Concentration, Assay Kit, AKJ, CU21M, Metallogenics Co., Ltd., Chiba, Japan). For the peak appearing at the retention time of 16 min and containing Cu^{2+}, the ratio of Cu^{2+}: constant region domain was around 0.55. This result agreed with those of the UV/VIS spectroscopy, suggesting that two constant region domain molecules bind one copper ion.

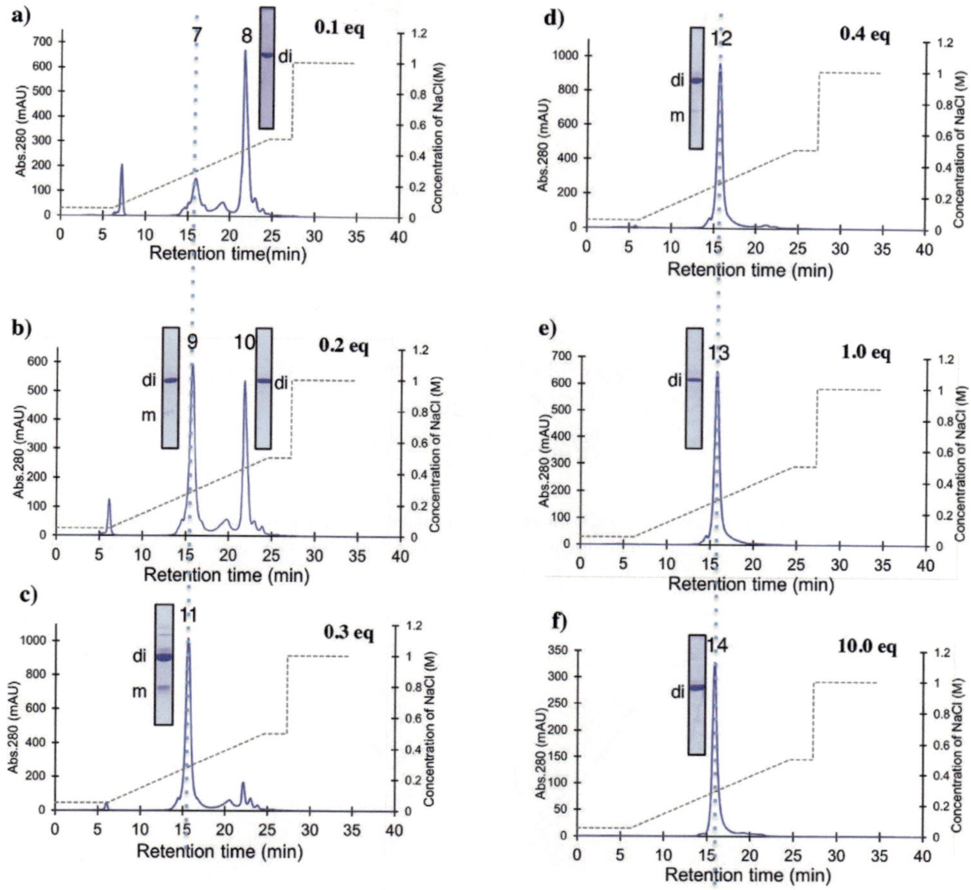

Figure 11. Effect of copper ions. (a) 0.1 eq. addition of Cu^{2+}: a small peak 7 and one main peak 8 were observed at the retention time around 16 and 22 min, respectively. Peak 8 was the dimer. (b) 0.2 eq. addition of Cu^{2+}: the eluted times of peaks 9 and 10 were identical with those of peaks 7 and 8, respectively. Peak 9 included mainly the dimer with a very slight contamination of the monomer. Peak 10 was the dimer. (c) 0.3 eq. addition of Cu^{2+}: peak 11 was observed as the main peak at the retention time of 16 min. (d) 0.4 eq. addition of Cu^{2+}: A clear single peak of the dimer form was detected at the retention time of 16 min. (e) 1.0 eq. addition of Cu^{2+}: only peak 13 was observed at the retention time of 16 min. It was the dimer. (f) 10.0 eq. addition of Cu^{2+}: only peak 14 was observed at the retention time of 16 min. It was also the dimer. It seems that the amount of 0.4 eq. added copper ions is sufficient to induce the mono-molecular form from the multi-molecular forms of the constant region domain molecule.

4.3. Binding affinity of copper ions

The UV/VIS spectrum changed as different concentrations of Cu^{2+} was added to the Ni-NTA elution after the samples were dialyzed against PBS. The results are presented in **Figure 13**. The absorbance of 580 nm became larger along with an increase in the amount of added Cu^{2+}, as showing a slight red shift. In **Figure 14**, the values for the concentration of added Cu^{2+} were plotted vs. the maximum absorbance, which is the absorption isotherm curve for Cu^{2+} binding to constant region domain molecules. The Langmuir plot is shown in the inset of **Figure 14**, indicating a good linear relationship. The binding constant was estimated to be 48.0 μM^{-1}.

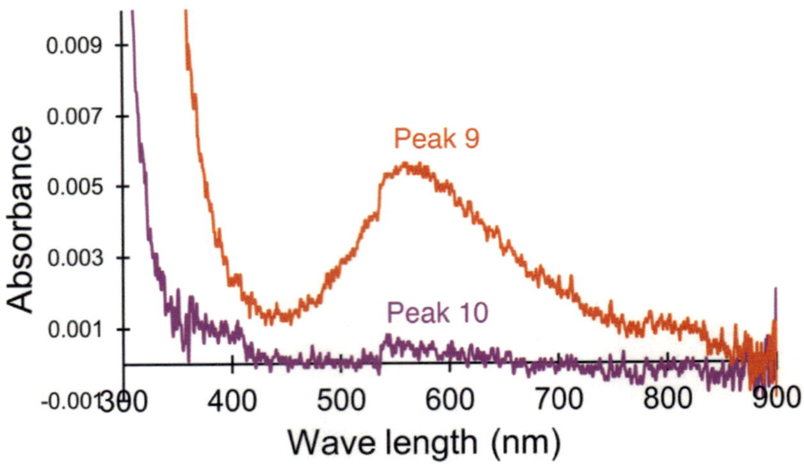

Figure 12. UV/VIS spectra. Peak 9 showed the absorbance of around 580 nm, which was based on the interaction of Cu^{2+} and amino acids of the constant region domain molecule. On the other hand, no absorbance was detected for peak 10.

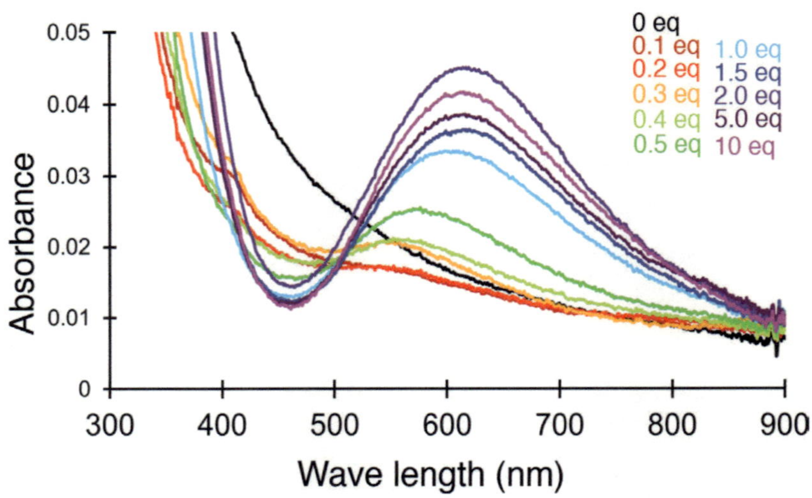

Figure 13. Spectrum changes with the concentration of added Cu^{2+}. Along with an increase of the concentration of added Cu^{2+}, the absorbance at around 580 nm became larger.

The binding affinity from several proteins incorporating divalent metal ions was investigated. The values (K) are presented in **Table 1**. Hemocyanin and metallothionein have very strong affinity to bind Cu^{2+}. Carbonic anhydrase-binding Zn^{2+} shows a strong affinity. Aminopeptidase III binding Co^{2+} possesses a weak affinity. In the case of CL, the value (48.0 μM^{-1}) seems to be intermediate among those metalloproteins.

In order to further investigate the molecular heterogeneity of the constant region domain molecule, two-dimensional (2D) electrophoresis was performed using samples with or without Cu^{2+}. **Figure 15a** and **b** shows the results for the cases without and with the addition of Cu^{2+}

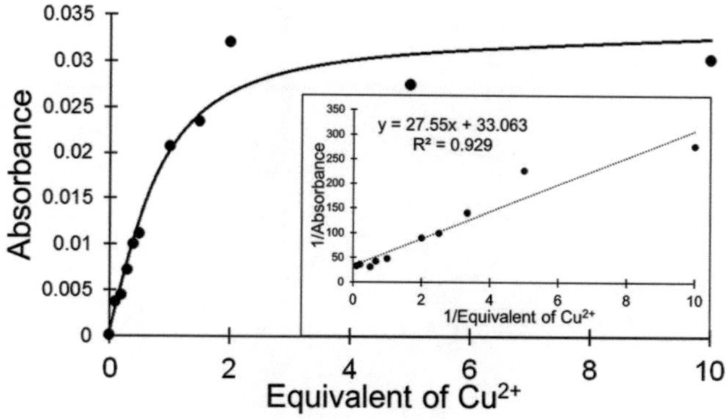

Figure 14. Kinetic analysis. The values for the concentration of added Cu^{2+} were plotted vs. the absorbance at 580 nm, which is the isothermal curve for copper binding to the CL protein. The Langmuir plot is presented in the inset of the graph, indicating a good linear relationship. The binding constant was estimated to be 48.0 μM^{-1}.

Proteins (metal ion)	K (M^{-1})	Affinity
Hemocyanin (Cu^{2+})	10^{17}–10^{19}	Very strong
Metallothionein (Cu^{2+})	10^{17}–10^{19}	Very strong
Carbonic anhydrase (Zn^{2+})	~10^{12}	Strong
Aminopeptidase III (Co^{2+})	2×10^4	Weak
CL (Cu^{2+})	4.8×10^7	Medium

Table 1. Comparison of the binding affinities of some proteins with metal ions.

under non-reduced conditions, respectively. In the former case, many spots were observed: two spots at pI = 6.9 for the dimer and three spots at pI = 6.2, 6.5, and 6.9 for the monomer. In contrast, one strong spot was observed at pI = 6.9 for the dimer in the case with the addition of Cu^{2+}, while very faint spots were detected in the positions of the monomer. Note that Cu^{2+} can facilitate changes from the multimeric form to the monomeric form as well as from different electrical charges to a single electrical charge.

4.4. Other metal ions

About 1.0 eq. of a metal ion such as Ca^{2+}, Mg^{2+}, Ni^{2+}, and $Zn^{2+}$was added in each Ni-NTA elution and incubated overnight. **Figure 16** shows the results of the cation exchange chromatography and SDS-PAGE (non-reduced) for peaks P3 and P5. For the cases of Ca^{2+}, Mg^{2+}, and Ni^{2+} (**Figure 16a–c**, respectively), a large peak P3 was observed at 17 min along with a small peak P5 at 23 min. Interestingly, a large peak P3 was observed and peak P5 became very small in the case of Zn^{2+} (**Figure 16d**). The chromatogram resembled the case of Cu^{2+} (**Figure 16e**). From the results of the SDS-PAGE, the peak P3 was mostly in a monomeric form for all the cases of Ca^{2+}, Mg^{2+}, Ni^{2+}, and Zn^{2+}. On the other hand, P3 of Cu^{2+} was the dimer. The molecular form (size) of P3 in the case of Ca^{2+}, Mg^{2+}, Ni^{2+}, and Zn^{2+} was quite different from that of

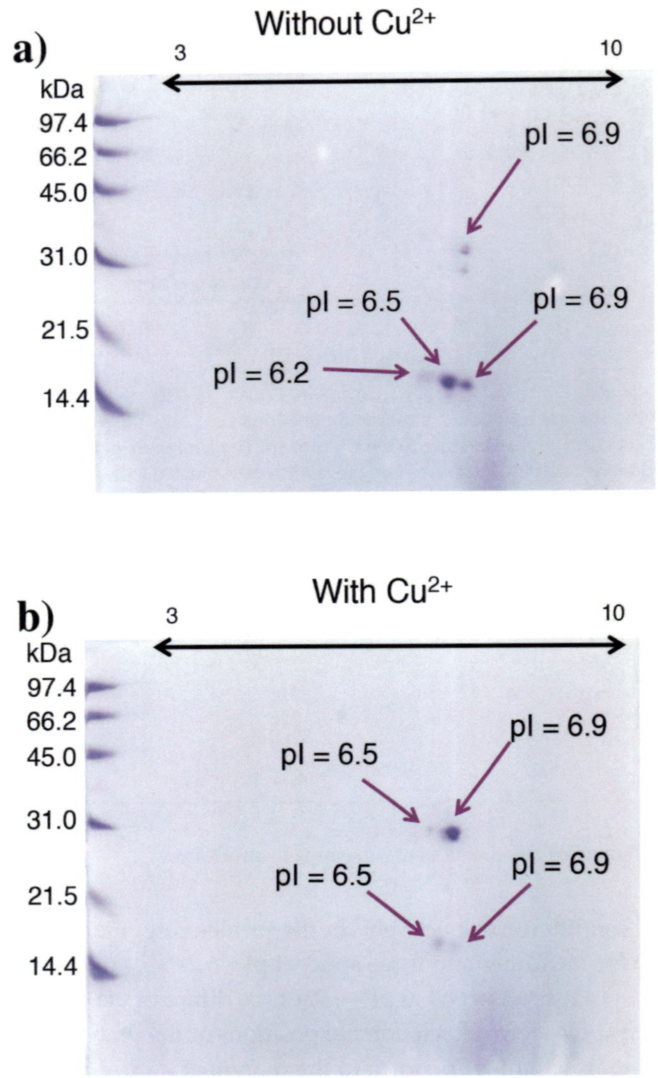

Figure 15. 2D electrophoresis for the constant region domain (CL). (a) Without Cu^{2+}: two spots at pI = 6.9 for the dimer and three spots at pI = 6.2, 6.5, and 6.9 for the monomer were found. (b) With Cu^{2+}: one strong spot was observed at pI = 6.9 for the dimer. It is revealed that copper ion accelerates both dimerization and generation of a mono-molecular form of the light chain.

Cu^{2+}. It must be considered that the Zn^{2+} could not accelerate the dimerization of the constant region domain molecule, while the ion decreased the peak P5 and showed a large peak P3. Zn^{2+} could have some ability to unify the structural diversity, but the effect is different from that of copper.

Zn^{2+} did not accelerate the dimerization of the constant region domain molecule but has some functions that may contribute to solve the heterogeneity problem. Out of the several metals analyzed, Zn^{2+} exhibited an interesting behavior, which must be a characteristic feature

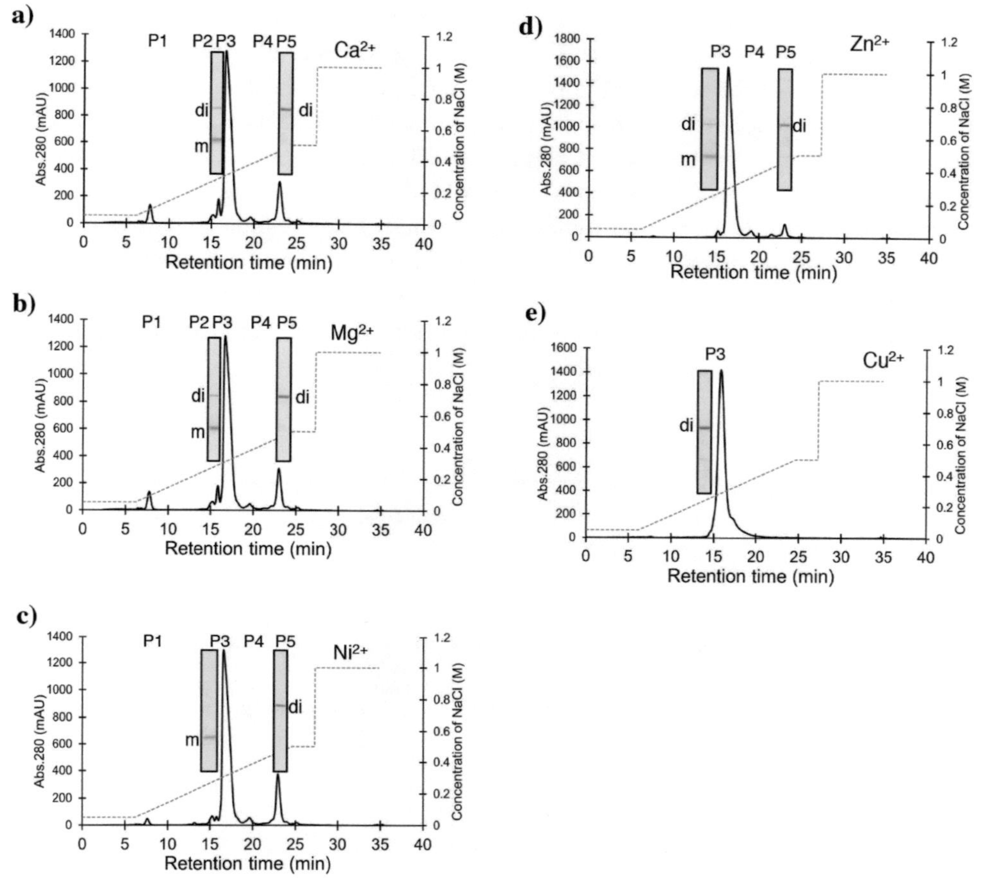

Figure 16. Other metal ions. In all cases, 1.0 eq. metal ion was added. Cation exchange chromatograms are presented with the results of SDS-PAGE (under non-reduced condition). m: monomer; di: dimer. (a) Addition of Ca^{2+}. (b) Addition of Mg^{2+}. (c) Addition of Ni^{2+}. (d) Addition of Zn^{2+}. (e) Addition of Cu^{2+}. Peak P3 was mostly in a monomeric form for all the cases of Ca^{2+}, Mg^{2+}, Ni^{2+} and Zn^{2+}. In the cases of addition of Ca^{2+}, Mg^{2+}, and Ni^{2+} (**Figure 16a–c**, respectively), a large peak, P3, was observed at 17 min along with a small peak, P5, at 23 min. In the case of Zn^{2+} (**Figure 16d**), a large peak P3 was observed and peak P5 became very small. The chromatogram seemed to be like the case of Cu^{2+}.

of Zn^{2+}. Although there are several reports on the relationship between metal ions and the enzymatic activity of catalytic antibodies, details of the contributions of metal ions to the molecular structure of catalytic antibodies are unclear at present [20, 34]. Paul et al. reported an interesting function regarding Zn^{2+}, which was essential for exhibiting the catalytic function of the antibody light chain to cleave beta-amyloid peptides, while the ion will not affect the catalytic site [14].

4.5. Consideration about unstable forms and a stable form of CL

For the reason why the addition of copper hugely effects the formation of a mono-form structure of the constant light chain domain, we postulated one of the situations from the viewpoint of potential energy and the wall height as illustrated in **Figure 17**. It is likely that the energy potential of each molecular form is at a comparable level after the preparation of the molecule (CL) without Cu^{2+}, as shown in **Figure 17a**. In this case, transfer of the potential well A to B (or C) is easy because the walls of the potential energies of the wells are low (**Figure 17b**). However, the energy potential is drastically changed when copper ions are added. The multi-molecular forms of the constant region domain, which are sitting in each potential well, drop in one deep potential energy level, as shown in **Figure 17c**, resulting in the formation of a mono-molecular form from the multi-molecular forms. Once the molecule dropped into the deep potential well, the form would be no longer able to transfer to other forms. As a consequence, the monomolecular form of the constant region domain molecule became stable. This situation can be achieved by the presence of copper ion in a ratio of more than 0.5 eq. of Cu^{2+} to the constant region domain molecule.

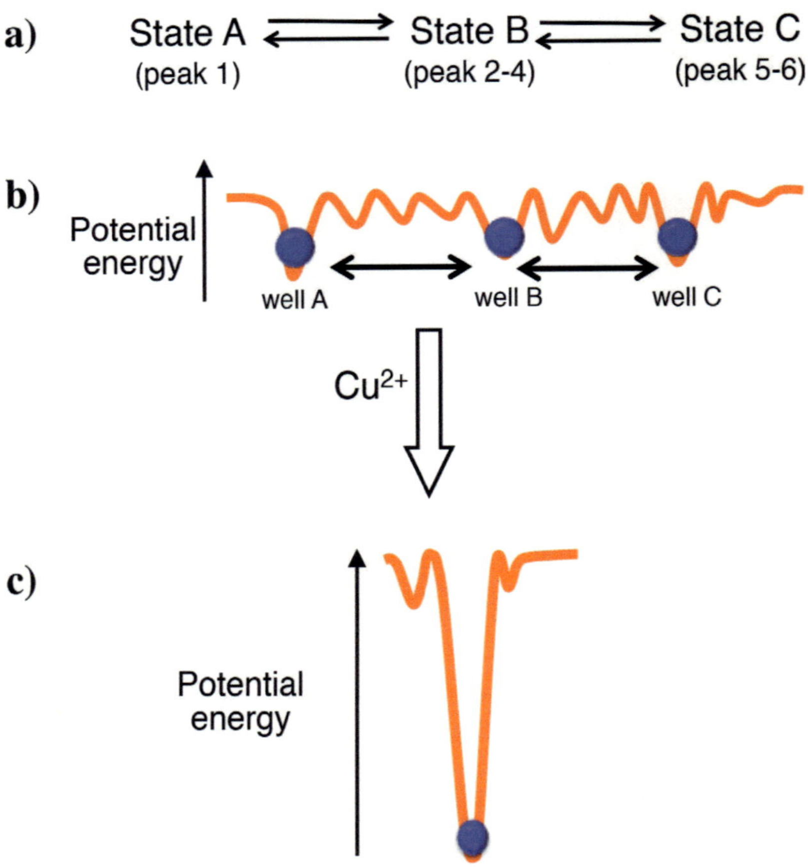

Figure 17. Consideration about conversion of unstable forms to a stable form of CL. (a) State A (corresponding to peak 1 in **Figure 10**), State B (corresponding to peaks 2, 3, and 4 in **Figure 10**), and State C (corresponding to peaks 5 and 6 in **Figure 10**) may stay in a chemical equilibrium. (b) Assumed situation in potential energy for the case without Cu^{2+}: each potential energy level for the case without Cu^{2+} may be comparable in wells of A, B, and C. The walls among the potential energy wells are not high. (c) Assumed situation of potential energy for the case with Cu^{2+}: when Cu^{2+} is incorporated, a deep potential level can be generated, and all molecules showing a different heterogeneity may drop into the well and exist as a stable form.

5. Binding of copper ions in the constant region domain

5.1. Preparation of mutants and their uptake of copper ions

In order to clarify the copper-binding site, two mutants were prepared from the C51 light chain, because the light chain has no histidine residues in the variable region compared to the sequence of the constant region domain comprising 2 His residues (**Figure 8**). Both histidine and cysteine residues are considered as the most plausible candidates for the binding site. Therefore, the residues of His195, His204, and Cys220 present in the constant region domain of the C51 light chain were mutated to Ala. As the consequence, two mutants were made. One is Cys220Ala (C220A: mono-mutant) and another is His195Ala, His204Ala, and Cys220Ala (H195A/H204A/C220A: triple-mutant; **Figure 18a**). The locations of the mutated residues are shown in **Figure 18b**.

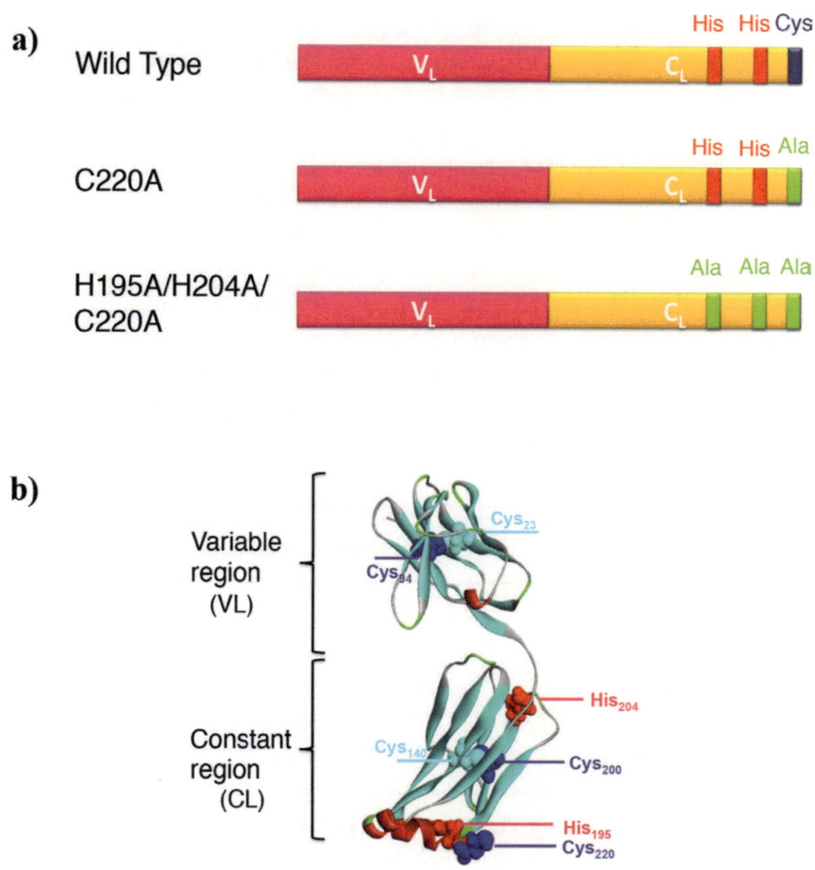

Figure 18. C51 mutants and locations of His and Cys residues. There are no histidine residues in the variable region of the C51 light chain. (a) Location of Cys220, His195 and His204 in wild type. The mutated positions, C220A and H195A/H204A/C220A, are also indicated with green colored character. (b) Three-dimensional structure of the C51 light chain. Light blue is sheet structure and red is helix structure.

These mutants were similarly expressed and purified as stated in the previous experiments. Fifty μM of Cu^{2+} (1.25 eq.) was added to both the cell suspension and the Ni-NTA eluent, where all light chains gave a single peak in the cation exchange chromatography. The copper uptake by the wild type and each mutant was chemically analyzed and the results are presented in **Table 2**. The wild type possessed 0.75 atoms of Cu^{2+} per one C51 light chain of full length. That of the C220A and H195A/H204A/C220A mutant was 0.54 and 0.25, respectively.

As stated in the above section, the value in the case of the constant region domain was 0.55. Taking together this finding and the full-length cases into account, it is considered that the variable region domain uptakes 0.20 atom (0.75–0.55 = 0.20). Therefore, the mono-mutant C220A is supposed to bind with 0.34 atom-Cu (0.54–0.20 = 0.34) and the triple-mutant H195A/H204A/C220A 0.05 atom-Cu (0.25–0.20 = 0.05). These facts are strongly implying that histidine residues at positions 195th and 204th as well as cysteine at position 220th are responsible for the copper-binding site.

5.2. Possibility of a zinc finger in the constant region domain

It is not well known that there is a zinc finger-like motif in the constant region of the antibody light chain. Interestingly, Radulescu pointed out that the motif is a type of Cys-X_3-His [35]. The sequence Cys-X_3-His-X_{15}-Cys-X_3-His is a complete motif of a zinc finger. The aa sequence of the constant region domain used in this article is presented in **Figure 8**. The sequence from positions 190th–224th of the constant region domain is CEVTHQGLSSPVTKSFNRGECLEHH. The sequence of LEHH was adducted as a His-tag was introduced. The underlined amino acids agree with those of the zinc finger motif, Cys-X_3-His-X_{15}-Cys-X_3-His, in which His224 is a part of the His-tag. This motif can uptake a metal ion such as Zn^{2+}, which is a divalent metal ion. As Cu^{2+} is also a divalent metal ion, it can bound to the motif. Based on the results of the chemical analysis of copper ions in mutants, those histidine and cysteine residues must be responsible to uptake the copper ion. It is plausible that a copper ion is able to bind to the zinc finger motif instead of a zinc ion. As seen in the investigation of divalent metal ions on the structural diversity, zinc ions showed some effect. This maybe ascribed to the presence

Clone name of C51	Cu / full length	Cu / CL	Contribution* By VL
Wild Type	0.75*	0.55*	0.20**
C220A	0.54*	0.34**	0.20***
H195A/H204A/C220A	0.25*	0.05**	0.20***

*Result: The ratio of full length of C51 vs Cu and the constant region domain of the light chain (CL) vs Cu was 0.75 and 0.55, respectively. This result suggests that the contribution of the variable domain of the light chain (VL) should be 0.20 atom. (0.75-0.55)=0.20)

**: calculation

***: assumption

Table 2. Copper uptake by each light chain and constant region domain (CL).

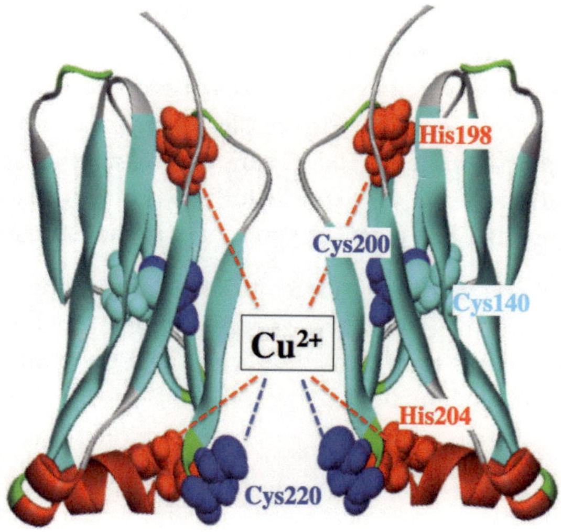

Figure 19. Assumed binding site for copper ion. A zinc finger motif, Cys-X_3-His-X_{15}-Cys-X_3-His, from positions 190th to 224th (His224 is a part of a His-tag) is existing in the constant region domain of the light chain (CL). As Cu^{2+} is also a divalent metal ion, it can be bound with the motif instead of a zinc ion, unless the ion is present in the solution. By the addition of copper ions, the CL is easily becoming the dimer form. Considering the chemical analysis of copper ions, one copper atom binds with two CL molecules (CL1 and CL2) via His and Cys residues.

of a zinc finger motif in the constant domain in the light chain (note that the zinc finger motif is conserved in both human and mouse antibody light chain (kappa type)). In addition, the similar motif composed of the same amino acids exists in the CH1 domain of the heavy chain.

As well known, a zinc finger can function as a transcription factor influencing gene regulation and protein expression. Few studies on the relationship between antibody and zinc finger have been made so far. From the viewpoint that one protein can have dual or multi-functions in case, the chemical and biochemical functions of each domain of an antibody should be investigated in detail.

5.3. Assumed binding site of a copper ion

Taking those facts mentioned above and discussed, the binding site of copper is assumed as illustrated in **Figure 19**. Cu^{2+} must be coordinated with histidine and cysteine residues of dimeric CL molecules. In this situation, the copper ion mediates the CL molecule placing the lowest potential energy level.

6. Molecular forms

6.1. AFM analysis

AFM analysis was performed using the #4 light chain as shown in **Figure 20a–g**. **Figure 20a, c,** and **e** demonstrates the wild type of the #4 light chain. The results obtained with the mutant (C220A) of the #4 light chain are shown in **Figure 20f** and **g**. The red circles in the figures represent the clear image of the AFM.

In the case of the #4 wild type, two kinds of form were observed. One is the dimer circled with #1 red color (**Figure 20a**). This seems to be a *cis* form, whose molecular conformation corresponds to that of **Figure 20b**. A variable region faces to another variable region. On the other hand, the dimer circled with #2 red color (**Figure 20c**) seems *trans* form, whose molecular conformation corresponds to that of **Figure 20d. Figure 20e** was another spot, where *cis* and *trans* forms were observed. In contrast, a very simple form was observed in the case of #4 mutant C220A, as shown in **Figure 20f** and **g.** In any spots, only monomeric forms were observed.

If copper ion is incorporated into the zinc finger motif residing in the constant region domain, the dimeric form observed in the #4 wild type is easily formed. On the other hand, the mutant C220A exists as the monomeric form, which indicates that the cysteine locating at position 220th is a crucial amino acid to bind to a copper ion.

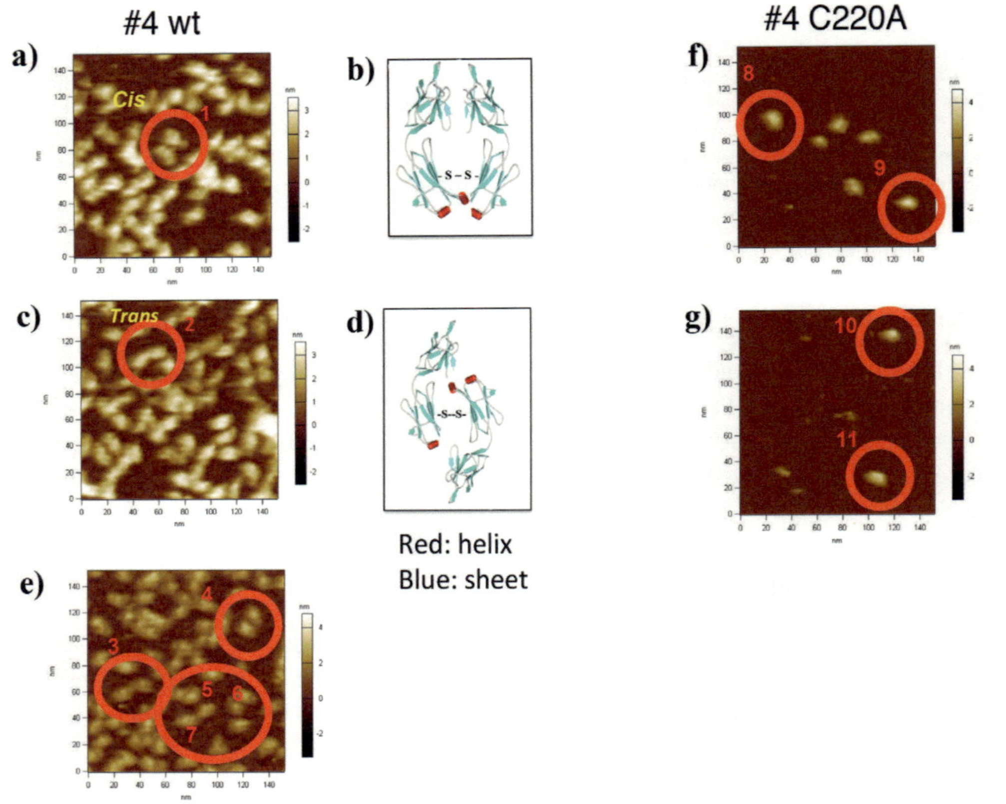

Figure 20. AFM analysis for #4 light chains. These AFM images were taken under the same condition as in **Figure 7**. (a) #4 wild type (*cis form*). (b) Molecular modeling for *cis form.* (c) #4 wild type (*trans form*). (d) Molecular modeling for *trans form.* (e) Mixture of *cis and trans forms.* In the case of the #4 wild type, two kinds of forms were observed. One is the dimer circled with #1 red color (a). This seems to be a *cis* form, whose molecular conformation corresponds to that of (b). A variable region faces to another variable region. The dimer circled with #2 red color (c) seems to be a *trans* form, whose molecular conformation corresponds to that of (d). **Figure 20e** was another view, where *cis* and *trans* forms were observed. (f) #4 mutant (C220A). (g) #4 mutant (C220A) (another spot). For #4 mutant (C220A), one simple form was observed. In any views, only monomeric forms were observed.

6.2. X-ray diffraction analysis

We are trying to determine the detailed steric conformation of a catalytic light chain. At present, the structure of the main chain of the #4 mutant C220A was clarified as a preliminary experiment. **Figure 21a** shows a single crystal of the #4 mutant C220A formed in the experiment. By using the single crystal, X-ray diffraction analysis was performed. The result is presented in **Figure 21b**, where a 3.1 Å resolution was attained. Interestingly, there are eight molecules of the #4 mutant in one lattice mediated by hydrophobic interaction.

a)

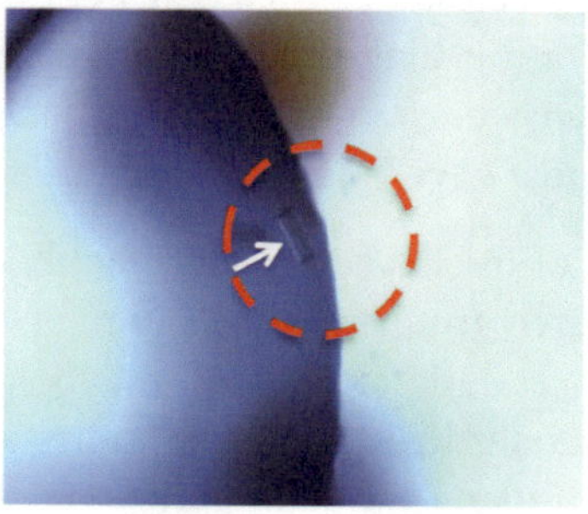

b)

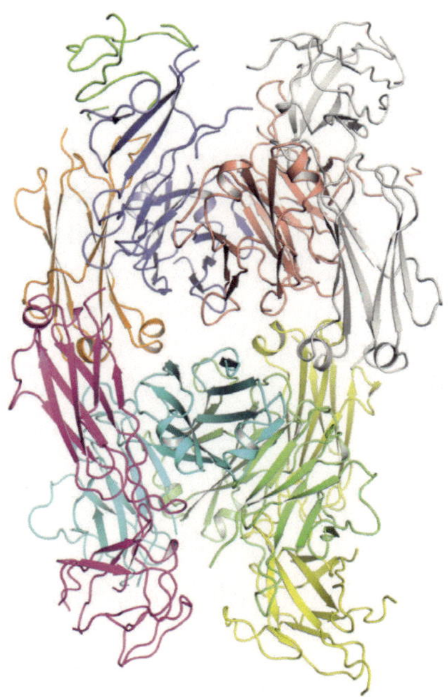

Figure 21. X-ray diffraction analysis for #4 C220A. (a) crystallization: a single crystal (like a small pillar) of the #4 mutant C220A is seen in a red dotted circle. (b) Conformation of the main chain: As the preliminary experiment, the conformation of the main chain for the #4 mutant 220A was determined. Each #4 mutant molecule is indicated with each color such as red, yellow, green, blue, etc. Eight molecules of the mutant were packed in one lattice, indicating that the mutant molecules may interact with each other by hydrophobic interaction.

In the case of the AFM analysis, the #4 mutant C220A was a monomer. This is ascribed that the mica as the supporting material firmly interacts with the #4 mutant molecule. In solution, the #4 mutant may interact with each other with a strong Van der Waals force.

7. Perspectives and conclusions

As stated in the abstract and introduction, the issue of structural diversity (heterogeneity) of antibodies has become a big subject along with the development of antibody drugs and catalytic antibodies. This subject has not been solved for a long period, because many difficult and complex problems were existing. For this long-period unsolved problem, copper ion showed a drastic effect and gave one of the answers for solving the structural diversity issue. Note that the antibody and/or the subunits must have a defined structure for practical use.

In recent years, many possibilities of the development of antibody drugs and catalytic antibodies have been reported by research groups throughout the world. This article offers huge insights into the development of catalytic antibodies, maybe, as well as antibody drugs. Because the preparation can be standardized, many scientists and engineers will easily be able to produce the defined structure and the same functional antibody under any circumstances and anywhere in the world.

Acknowledgements

This study was supported by the Japan Science and Technology Agency (CREST/"Establishment of Innovative Manufacturing Technology Based on Nanoscience"); "Super Highway": the accelerated research to bridge university IPs and practical use; and Grants-in-Aid for Scientific Research from the Ministry of Education, Culture, Sports, Science and Technology of Japan (24350085 and 16H02282). The authors thank Oxford Instruments KK (Dr. H. Sugasawa), Dr. Y. Nishikawa (High Energy Accelerator Research Organization), Dr. H. Makio (High Energy Accelerator Research Organization), and Ms. Y. Akiyoshi (Oita University) for the assistance with this study.

Author details

Emi Hifumi[1], Hiroaki Taguchi[2], Ryuichi Kato[3], Mitsue Arakawa[4], Yoshiki Katayama[5] and Taizo Uda[6,7*]

*Address all correspondence to: uda@oita-u.ac.jp

1 Research Promotion Institute, Oita University, Oita-shi, Oita, Japan

2 Faculty of Pharmaceutical Sciences, Suzuka University of Medical Science, Suzuka, Mie, Japan

3 High Energy Accelerator Research Organization, Tsukuba, Japan

http://dx.doi.org/10.5772/intechopen.72516

4 Tottori College of Nursing, Kurayoshi-shi, Tottori, Japan

5 Graduate School of System Life Science, Kyushu University, Nishi-ku, Fukuoka, Japan

6 Department of Applied Chemistry, Faculty of Engineering, Oita University, Oita-shi, Oita, Japan

7 Nanotechnology Laboratory, Institute of Systems, Information Technologies and Nanotechnologies (ISIT), Fukuoka, Japan

References

[1] Hortobagyi NG. Trastuzumab in the treatment of breast cancer. The New England Journal of Medicine. 2005;**353**:1734-1736

[2] Glassy CM, Hagiwara H. Summary analysis of the pre-clinical and clinical results of brain tumor patients treated with pritumumab. Human Antibodies. 2009;**18**:127-137

[3] Meza-Junco J, Au H-J, Sawyer BS. Critical appraisal of trastuzumab in treatment of advanced stomach cancer. Cancer Management and Research. 2011;**3**:57-64

[4] Matsuura K, Ikoma S, Yoshida K, Shinohara H. DNA hydrolyzing activity of Bence Jones proteins. Biochemical and Biophysical Research Communications. 1998;**243**:719-721

[5] Lacroix-Desmazes S, Sooryanarayana MA, Bonnemain C, Stieltjes N, Pashov A, Sultan Y, Hoebeke J, Kazatchkine MD, Kaveri SV. Catalytic activity of antibodies against factor VIII in patients with hemophilia A. Nature Medicine. 1999;**5**:1044-1047

[6] Hifumi E, Mitsuda Y, Ohara K, Uda T. Targeted destruction of the HIV-1 coat protein gp41 by a catalytic antibody light chain. Journal of Immunological Methods. 2002;**269**:283-298

[7] Paul S, Karle S, Planque S, Taguchi H, Nishiyama Y, Handy B, Salas M, Edmundson A, Hanson A. Naturally occurring proteolytic antibodies selective immunoglobulin M-catalyzed hydrolysis of HIV gp120. The Journal of Biological Chemistry. 2004;**279**: 39611-39619

[8] Planque S, Nishiyama Y, Taguchi H, Salas M, Hanson C, Paul S. Catalytic antibodies to HIV: Physiological role and potential clinical utility. Autoimmunity Reviews. 2008;**7**:473-479

[9] Wootla B, Mahendra A, Dimitrov J-D, Friboulet A, Borel-Derlon A, Rao D-N, Uda T, Borg J-Y, Bayry J, Kaveri S-V, Lacroix-Desmazes S. Factor VIII-hydrolyzing IgG in acquired and congenital hemophilia. FEBS Letters. 2009;**583**:2565-2572

[10] Durova OM, Vorobiev II, Smirnov IV, Reshetnyak AV, Telegin GB, Shamborant OG, Orlova NA, Genkin DD, Bacon A, Ponomarenko NA, Friboulet A, Gabibov AG. Strategies for induction of catalytic antibodies toward HIV-1 glycoprotein gp120 in autoimmune prone mice. Molecular Immunology. 2009;**47**:87-95

[11] Parkhomenko TA, Buneva VN, Tyshkevich OB, Generalov II, Doronin BM, Nevinsky GA. DNA-hydrolyzing activity of IgG antibodies from the sera of patients with tick-borne encephalitis. Biochimie. 2010;**92**:545-554

[12] Hifumi E, Higashi K, Uda T. Catalytic digestion of human tumor necrosis factor-α by antibody heavy chain. The FEBS Journal. 2010;**277**:3823-3832

[13] Smirnov I, Carletti E, Kurkova I, Nachon F, Nicolet Y, Mitkevich VA, Débat H, Avalle B, Belogurov AA Jr, Kuznetsov N, Reshetnyak A, Masson P, Tonevitsky AG, Ponomarenko N, Makarov AA, Friboulet A, Tramontano A, Gabibov A. Reactibodies generated by kinetic selection couple chemical reactivity with favorable protein dynamics. Proceedings of the National Academy of Sciences of the United States of America. 2011;**108**:15954-15959

[14] Nishiyama Y, Taguchi H, Hara M, Planque SA, Mitsuda Y, Paul S. Metal-dependent amyloid β-degrading catalytic antibody construct. Journal of biotechnology. 2014;**180**:17-22

[15] Hifumi E, Honjo E, Fujimoto N, Arakawa M, Nishizono A, Uda T. Highly efficient method of preparing human catalytic antibody light chains and their biological characteristics. The FASEB Journal. 2012;**26**:1607-1615

[16] Hifumi E, Fujimoto N, Arakawa M, Saito E, Matsumoto S, Kobayashi N, Uda T. Biochemical features of a catalytic antibody light chain, 22F6, prepared from human lymphocytes. The Journal of Biological Chemistry. 2013;**288**:19558-19568

[17] Hifumi E, Morihara F, Hatiuchi K, Okuda T, Nishizono A, Uda T. Catalytic features and eradication ability of antibody light-chain UA15-L against *Helicobacter pylori*. The Journal of Biological Chemistry. 2008;**283**:899-907

[18] Kou J, Yang J, Lim J-E, Pattanayak A, Song M, Planque S, Paul S, Fukuchi K-I. Catalytic immunoglobulin gene delivery in a mouse model of Alzheimer's disease: Prophylactic and therapeutic applications. Molecular Neurobiology. 2014;**51**:43-56

[19] Hifumi E, Arakawa M, Matsumoto S, Yamamoto T, Katayama Y, Uda T. Biochemical features and anti-viral activity of a monomeric catalytic antibody light chain 23D4 against influenza A virus. The FASEB Journal. 2015;**29**:2347-2358

[20] Odintsova E-S, Zaksas N-P, Buneva V-N, Nevinsky G-A. Metal dependent hydrolysis of β-casein by sIgA antibodies from human milk. Journal of Molecular Recognition. 2010;**24**:45-59

[21] Buneva VN, Kanyshkova TG, Vlassov AV, Semenov DV, Khlimankov D, Breusova LR, Nevinsky GA. Catalytic DNA- and RNA-hydrolyzing antibodies from milk of healthy human mothers. Applied Biochemistry and Biotechnology. 1998;**75**:63-76

[22] Saveliev AN, Ivanen DR, Kulminskaya AA, Ershova NA, Kanyshkova TG, Buneva VN, Mogelnitskii AS, Doronin BM, Favorova OO, Nevinsky GA, Neustroev KN. Amylolytic activity of IgM and IgG antibodies from patients with multiple sclerosis. Immunology Letters. 2003;**86**(3):291-297

[23] Ramsland RA, Terzyan SS, Cloud G, Bourne CR, Farrugia W, Tribbick G, Geysen HM, Moomaw CR, Slaughter CA, Edundson AB. Crystal structure of a glycosylated Fab from

an IgM cryoglobulin with properties of a natural proteolytic antibody. The Biochemical Journal. 2006;**396**:473-481

[24] Harris RJ, Kabakoff B, Macchi FD, Shen FJ, Kwong M, Andya JD, Shire SJ, Bjork N. Identification of multiple sources of charge heterogeneity in a recombinant antibody. Journal of Chromatography B. 2001;**752**:233-245

[25] Nebija D, Noe CR, Urban E, Lachmann B. Quality control and stability studies with the monoclonal antibody, trastuzumab: Application of 1D- *vs.* 2D-gel electrophoresis. International Journal of Molecular Sciences. 2014;**15**:6399-6411

[26] Stevens FJ, Westholm FA, Solomon A, Schiffer M. Dual conformations of an immunoglobulin light-chain dimer: Heterogeneity of antigen specificity and idiotope profile may result from multiple variable-domain interaction mechanisms. Proceedings of the National Academy of Sciences of the United States of America. 1988;**85**:6895-6899

[27] Hunt G, Moorhouse KG, Chen AB. Capillary isoelectric focusing and sodium dodecyl sulfate capillary gel electrophoresis of recombinant humanized monoclonal; antibody HER2. Journal of Chromatography. A. 1996;**744**:295-301

[28] Fujimoto N, Hifumi E, Uda T. Biochemical features of monoclonal antibodies (InfA series) against hemagglutinin molecule of influenza virus. Proceedings (J1-52) of Annual Meeting of the Chemical Society of Japan. 2009

[29] Hifumi E, Fujimoto N, Ishida K, Kawawaki H, andT. Uda, T. Characteristic features of InfA-15 monoclonal antibody recognizing H1, H3 and H5 subtypes of hemagglutinin of influenza virus A type. Journal of Bioscience and Bioengineering. 2010;**109**:598-608

[30] Nebija D, Kopelent-Frank H, Urban E, Noe CR, Lachmann B. Comparison of two-dimensional gel electrophoresis patterns and MALDI-TOF MS analysis of therapeutic recombinant monoclonal antibodies trastuzumab and rituximab. Journal of Pharmaceutical and Biomedical Analysis. 2011;**56**:684-691

[31] Hifumi E, Matsumoto S, Nakashima H, Itonaga S, Arakawa M, Katayama Y, Kato R, Uda T. A novel method of preparing the mono-form structure of catalytic antibody light chain. FASEB Journal. 2016;**30**:895-908

[32] Hifumi E, Taguchi H, Kato R, Uda T. Role of the constant region domain in the structural diversity of human antibody light chains. FASEB Journal. 2017;**31**:1668-1677

[33] Ouerghi O, Touhami A, Othmane A, Ouada HB, Martelet C, Fretigny C, Jaffrezic-Renault N. Investigating antibody–antigen binding with atomic force microscopy. Sensors and Actuators B: Chemical. 2002;**84**(2-3):67-175

[34] Bezuglova AM, Konenkova LP, Doronin BM, Buneva VN, Nevinsky GA. Affinity and catalytic heterogeneity and metal-dependence of polyclonal myelin basic protein-hydrolyzing IgGs from sera of patients with systemic lupus erythematosus. Journal of Molecular Recognition. 2011;**24**:960-974

[35] Radulescu RT. Antibody constant region: Potential to bind metal and nucleic acid. Medical Hypotheses. 1995;**44**:137-145

Chapter 11

Immune-Mediated Skin Reactions Induced by Recombinant Antibodies and Other TNF-Alpha Inhibitors

Karolína Vorčáková, Péč Juraj, Péčová Tatiana and Martinásková Klára

Additional information is available at the end of the chapter

http://dx.doi.org/10.5772/intechopen.72449

Abstract

Biologic agents that act by inhibiting tumour necrosis factor alpha (TNF-alpha) have become a breakthrough treatment for chronic inflammatory diseases. This highly effective treatment has surprisingly brought us new adverse effects that we had not encountered before the age of biologics. Immune-mediated reactions are a group of adverse effects with not clearly understood etiopathogenesis. It turns out that TNF-alpha inhibitors are able to disrupt the cytokine cascade in genetically predisposed individuals. Some of the theories assume a cross reaction and overproduction of interferon (INF) alpha, while others put an emphasis on dysregulation of cytokines, in particular interleukin (IL)-17. Similarly, debatable is the role of the reactions mentioned in the etiopathogenesis, the production of antibodies against biologics and the production of antinuclear antibodies. The most common immune-mediated skin reactions are psoriasis and psoriasiform reactions, lupus-like syndrome, sarcoidosis, alopecia areata, vasculitis and lichenoid reactions. Less common reactions described in our paper include pyoderma gangrenosum and morphea. Most of these reactions belong to the so-called paradoxical reactions. Paradoxical psoriasis is an adverse effect, represented by occurrence of a disease caused by the therapeutic class of drugs normally used to cure or improve symptoms of such disease.

Keywords: TNF-alpha inhibitors, psoriasiform reaction, paradoxical reaction, antibodies, Th17

1. Introduction

Immune-mediated adverse reactions are a new group of diseases developing during anti-TNF-alpha treatment. Their clear etiopathogenesis is not known. Most authors assume that there

INTECH
open science | open minds

© 2018 The Author(s). Licensee InTech. This chapter is distributed under the terms of the Creative Commons Attribution License (http://creativecommons.org/licenses/by/3.0), which permits unrestricted use, distribution, and reproduction in any medium, provided the original work is properly cited.

is a link to possible significant interference of the anti-TNF-alpha therapy with the immune system, which subsequently induces the above-mentioned responses. Others associate the diseases with the production of antibodies against the biologic agents and include the symptoms among hypersensitivity reactions. However, the individual genetic predisposition, which may be essential in detecting of immune-mediated reactions, must not be overlooked. The reactions include a broad variety of diseases such as lupus-like syndrome, autoimmune arthralgia, psoriasis, sarcoidosis, dermatomyositis, hepatitis, vasculitis, neurological demyelinating diseases and the like. In this chapter, we will briefly characterise the most common skin immune-mediated reactions induced by TNF-alpha inhibitors.

TNF is produced as a transmembrane protein (tmTNF), which is later cleaved by an enzyme metalloproteinase to its soluble form, sTNF [1]. Both TNFR1 and TNFR2 receptors signal through pathways that are proinflammatory and anti-apoptotic. Moreover, TNFR1 can signal directly through death domain caspase-dependent pathways that lead to apoptosis [2]. TNFR1 plays a role in response to bacterial infection [3] and TNFR2 may downregulate inflammatory signals driven by TNF [4].

Currently, five complete recombinant antibodies—infliximab, etanercept, adalimumab, golimumab and certolizumab pegol—are available TNF-α inhibitors. They are biotechnologically produced and administered as systemic drugs modifying the biological response and signalisation on the molecular level. The structural differences are key to different risk for adverse effects such as granulomatous infections, with TNF antibodies associated with higher risk compared to soluble receptor, possibly due to binding to tmTNF receptor on the activated cells [5].

Infliximab is a recombinant chimeric monoclonal antibody containing human IgG1 Fc and variable murine regions, which forms complexes with both sTNF and tmTNF. It induces the lysis of macrophages and monocytes by cytotoxicity dependent on complement and antibodies [6]. The intravenous administration is applied by a weight-dependent dose. Drug-mediated apoptosis and monocytopenia are linked to infliximab as well as its ability to bind more avidly to different forms of TNF-α [7]. Adalimumab is a humanised monoclonal antibody containing human IgG1 Fc and human variable regions that bind sTNF as well as tmTNF. The other available humanised monoclonal antibody, cetrolizumab pegol is a pegylated monoclonal Fab fragment with polyethylene glycol binding to soluble and membrane-bound TNF-α, inhibiting the proinflammatory actions of this cytokine. Unlike other TNF inhibitors, owing to its lack of the Fc component, it is incapable of fixing complement or binding to Fc receptors. Golimumab is a human anti-TNF monoclonal antibody containing the IgG1 constant region.

The other group of TNF inhibitors consists solely of etanercept, which is soluble TNF receptor containing the human IgG1 Fc portion fused to the extracellular portion of human TNFRp75. It creates less stable complexes with tmTNF and firmly binds to trimeric forms of soluble TNF.

2. Psoriasis

TNF-alpha inhibitors have become a revolutionary medication in the treatment of chronic psoriasis in recent years. Conversely, psoriasis or psoriasiform reaction is one of the most common immune-mediated reactions. Therefore, the formation of TNF alpha-induced psoriasis is also called a paradoxical reaction. All of the mentioned TNF-alpha antagonists can induce psoriasis. Cases have been reported from all indications where anti-TNF-alpha treatment is given. According to the literature, the incidence of paradoxical psoriasis is 1.04–3.0 cases per 1000 patient-years, the percentages varying widely from 0.6 to 5.3% [8]. The incidence of the manifestation is not age and gender related; some studies also show other controversial data. Manifestation may occur in any period of time during the treatment, from weeks, months, up to the years. The average time of developing psoriasis is 10 months [9, 10]. Concomitant treatment with another immunosuppressant does not appear to prevent paradoxical psoriasis, although combined suppression is used in the treatment of immune-mediated reactions.

The clinical manifestation of paradoxical psoriasis may be variable in nature. Paradoxical psoriasis includes not only newly developed psoriasis but also a radical worsening of already existing psoriasis. The disease is most commonly manifested in the area of palms and soles in the form of palmoplantar pustulosis, which is reported in 56% of cases, other most common forms include chronic plaque psoriasis in 50% of the patients and guttate manifestations, which affect 12% of the patients. Patients may also suffer from multiple forms of disease simultaneously (15%) [11]. Other manifestations include scalp or nail involvement. There are also cases of alopecia areata and paradoxical psoriasis. Some authors assume that monoclonal antibodies are associated with development of de novo-induced psoriasis, while the etanercept fusion protein causes a worsening of pre-existing psoriasis [12] (**Figure 1**).

The exact etiopathogenesis of paradoxical psoriasis is not clear, and there are several opinions and theories. The first of them states that the manifestations are a hypersensitive reaction to a drug, not a newly developed classical disease. There are papers that due to the increased production of antibodies against biologics describe manifestations of induced generalised pustulosis that could fit into the spectrum of hypersensitivity reactions. Other papers disprove this theory on the basis of skin biopsy of the patients with TNF-alpha-induced psoriasis. The incidence of palmoplantar pustulous psoriasis in the common psoriatic population is significantly lower, representing 1.7% compared to 46.2% in patients with paradoxical reaction. This fact supports the theory that it should not be a new classical form of psoriasis [13].

The most widespread theory links the relationship between TNF-alpha and type 1 interferon alpha. TNF-alpha inhibits the maturation of plasma dendritic cells that produce IFN-alpha.

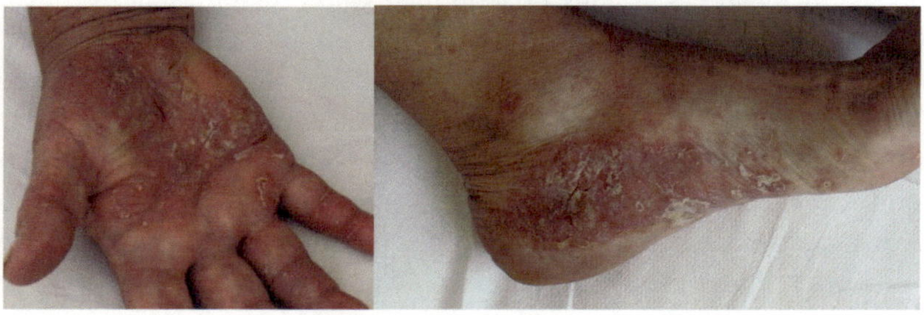

Figure 1. Patient with severe palmoplantar pustular psoriasis induced after 4 weeks of using adalimumab, this severe reaction lead to discontinuation of adalimumab.

The central role of INF-alpha in the etiopathogenesis of paradoxical psoriasiform reaction consists of cross-regulation between TNF-alpha and IFN-alpha. TNF-alpha blockers can lead to overproduction of INF-alpha. In papers that confirm this theory, increased expression of interferon alpha was demonstrated in skin biopsy compared to common psoriatic findings [14]. It is also believed that the expression of CXCL9 and CXCR3 chemokine receptors is increased, which promote the migration of lymphocytes into psoriatic dermis resulting in skin damage. IFN-alpha induces the expression of chemokine receptors on T lymphocytes [15].

One of the latest theories involves the Th17 pathway. In recent years, the Th17 signalling pathway is considered to be the major pathway of psoriasis etiopathogenesis. TNF-alpha may cause dysregulation in the immune system, which may cause the following changes. Activation of the IL-12/IL-23 pathway activates the Th17 signalling pathway followed by the production of IL-1b, IL-17, IL-21 and IL-22 together with an increased production of IL-17A and IL-22, hyperactivation of the Th17 and Th1 pathway and reduction of Treg activity [8, 15].

The genetic predisposition in patients with paradoxical reactions is not fully elucidated. Comorbidities are diseases that occur simultaneously with primary disease in higher prevalence compared to general population. Psoriasis comorbidities include a large group of diseases that are treated with anti-TNF-alpha therapies. It is believed that the genetic predisposition of an individual should also be essential for the development of immune-mediated reactions. There is a large group of "susceptibility" genes that are characteristic of several diseases and encode common inflammatory pathways. Polymorphisms of these genes are the subject of scientific research. Cabaleiro et al. presented the first paper studying 25 patients who developed paradoxical psoriasis genotyped for 173 single-nucleotide polymorphisms (SNPs) using the Illumina Veracode genotyping platform. Multivariate logistic regression revealed that five SNPs (rs11209026 in IL23R, rs10782001 in FBXL19, rs3087243 in CTLA4, rs651630 in SLC12A8 and rs1800453 in TAP1) were associated with paradoxical reactions [16].

Recently, we presented a study where we analysed antinuclear antibodies (ANA) and anti-double stranded DNA (dsDNA) antibodies in 10 patients with anti-TNF-alpha treatment induced psoriasis. ANA and anti-dsDNA antibodies were detected by ELISA. ANA serum samples were positive in 10% patients and anti-dsDNA antibody samples in 70% patients. The mechanism driving the formation of ANA and anti-dsDNA antibodies is poorly understood and their clinical significance is unknown [17]. In the literature, the frequency of ANA and anti-dsDNA antibodies in the patients after anti-TNF-alpha treatment varies extremely, possibly due to different methods of detection used. Pink et al. in their study, suggest that the development of ANA and anti-dsDNA antibodies on anti-TNF treatment may act as a marker of forthcoming treatment failure. In anti-TNF-alpha-induced lupus erythematosus, ANA and anti-dsDNA antibodies are well established and quite common (ANA, 90%; anti-dsDNA, 70–90%), but we have limited data about other immunological mediated adverse reactions [18]. Our data suggest that paradoxical psoriasis induced by anti-TNF inhibitors is associated with production of anti-dsDNA autoantibodies, but not with production of ANA antibodies. Further prospective research is necessary before general recommendations for daily practice can be announced. Genetic predisposition, clinical manifestation and production of anti-dsDNA antibodies seem to be fundamental in differentiation between adverse effects of anti-TNF-alpha treatment and associated disease comorbidity.

The therapeutic approach for anti-TNF-alpha-induced psoriasis is individual in each patient. A very important factor is the condition of the underlying disease, for which the treatment was indicated. In case of a serious condition that was stabilised with the treatment, we try to keep the biologic agent as long as possible. Equally important is what other therapeutic options are available. While in rheumatology we have a wide variety of biological medications for most diseases, including some others than anti-TNF-alpha inhibitors, the situation in patients with inflammatory bowel diseases (IBD) is much more complex.

Literature sources mention the following procedures: if the skin psoriatic manifestations involve up to 5% of the body surface, the first-line therapy should be topical (corticosteroid therapy, keratolytic therapy, treatment with vitamin D derivatives) followed by phototherapy and, in case of resistance, introducing methotrexate to the patient's therapy. In case that more than 5% of the body surface is involved, the recommended first-line therapy consists of topical corticosteroids and phototherapy, followed by methotrexate, cyclosporine and retinoids [11]. When setting up the combined suppression, the patient's comorbidities are very important. Most patients with underlying rheumatologic disease were treated with methotrexate in the past. For IBD patients, it is important to use the injection form of methotrexate, otherwise the drug may not be resorbed. In case of refractory manifestations and contraindications of combined systemic therapy, we consider discontinuing the anti-TNF-alpha agent. Interdisciplinary cooperation, consideration of the underlying disease and reassessment of further therapeutic procedure are all very important.

3. Sarcoidosis

One of the so-called paradoxical reactions is also newly developed sarcoidosis during the anti-TNF-alpha therapy. The anti-TNF-alpha therapy was described as a possible successful therapeutic modality in severe sarcoidosis manifestations. On the other hand, there is a growing number of cases that are caused by the treatment. More than 50 cases of TNF-alpha-induced sarcoidosis have been reported in the literature. Treatment with etanercept induced nearly 2/3 of the cases, and others were caused equally by infliximab and adalimumab. In most patients, the symptoms appeared after several months (1–69). Concomitant diseases include rheumatoid arthritis (in 60%), ankylosing spondylitis (in 20%), as well as psoriasis, Juvenile idiopathic arthritis (JIA) and IBD. In the clinical picture of anti-TNF-alpha-induced sarcoidosis, the pulmonary and cutaneous forms of the disease were dominant. In an aggregate paper including 38 patients, 74% of the patients suffered from the pulmonary form and 29% from the skin manifestations. The skin symptoms were manifested as erythema nodosum, pigmented scars and nodular lesions [19]. Literature data indicate a possible occurrence of sarcoidosis in 0.04% of the patients treated with TNF-alpha inhibitors [20]. Differential diagnosis of symptoms along with histological examination is important.

The role of anti-TNF on granuloma [21] and the different behaviour of antibodies and soluble anti-TNF alpha receptor in granulomatous diseases, with a greater tendency of etanercept to induce granulomatous reactions, may account for the occurrence of lesions. Monoclonal antibodies may induce apoptosis in activated monocytes and T cells. Sarcoidosis-like lesions may develop during the anti-TNF-alpha treatment. The anti-TNF-alpha treatment increases the IL-17 and IFN-ϒ expression and disturbs the balance between Th17 and Treg in favour of Th17. These two factors may result in the development of sarcoidosis [22].

4. Lupus-like syndrome

Systemic lupus erythematosus (SLE) is a common autoimmune disease, with 10% of SLE cases being drug-induced. The autoimmune drug-induced response is idiosyncratic, influenced by multiple factors, such as genetics, comorbidities, interactions with other medicinal products and external environmental factors [23]. Drug-induced lupus erythematosus (DILE) is defined as a lupus-like disease that is temporally related to drug exposure (from 1 month after the commencement of drug application but sometimes even more than 10 years) [24].

DILE may not meet all the SLE criteria. The most common manifestations are arthritis, serositis, the presence of ANA antibodies and anti-histone antibodies. The most important criterion is that the symptoms cease after discontinuing application of the suspected drug [25].

DILE induced by TNF-alpha inhibitors appears to be a separate DILE group with different signs compared to classical DILE. Women are more often affected than men, with an average age between 46.2 and 50.9 years. The average time to the manifestation of symptoms is 40.6 weeks from the commencement of drug treatment. Skin manifestations occur more frequently than in classical DILE and include butterfly erythema, photosensitivity and other skin manifestations of systemic and sub-acute lupus. The exact mechanism of DILE formation during anti-TNF-alpha treatment is unknown. Post-marketing follow-ups have demonstrated that DILE induced by TNF-alpha inhibitors may occur across all anti-TNF-alpha inhibitors. However, it is more often reported with the use of infliximab (0.19–0.22%) and etanercept (0.18%) compared to adalimumab (0.10%). An increase in ANA or anti-DNA antibodies in patients treated with anti-TNF-alpha therapy is known and relatively common [26]. The frequency of elevated ANA antibodies was higher in a greater number of patients treated with infliximab compared to a group of patients treated with etanercept [27]. Anti-dsDNA antibodies as well as ENAs (extractable nuclear antibodies) and low complement levels have been described more often than in case of classical DILE. Particularly, anti-histone antibodies have been more common in DILE induced by anti-TNF-alpha treatment [28, 29] (**Figure 2**).

The basic therapeutic procedure is the discontinuation of the treatment with the drug that induced the symptoms. In more severe conditions, it is necessary to add suppressors—corticosteroids, azathioprine, cyclosporine and methotrexate. Treatment selection is also based on the status of the underlying disease and comorbidities of the patient. In psoriasis, it is recommended to avoid systemic corticosteroids for a possible rebound phenomenon after discontinuation. There is no need to discontinue the treatment of anti-TNF-alpha in the case of ANA positivity or in very mild DILE manifestations [26]. Only limited data are available in the literature describing a switch of the treatment to another anti-TNF-alpha agent. Some authors claim that a similar reaction can be caused by any of the agents from the group of anti-TNF-alpha inhibitors [30]. As stated by Lomicova et al., an alternative treatment for chronic

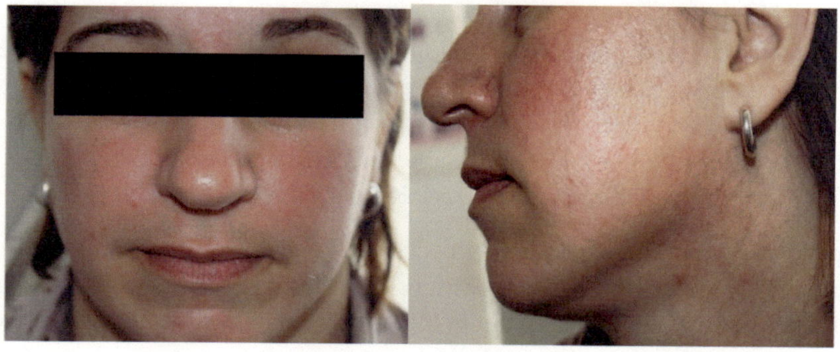

Figure 2. Significant facial erythema, total weakness and laboratory elevated ANA antibodies were observed. After discontinuation of the treatment, gradual regression of skin manifestations and neutralisation of ANA antibodies took place. Manifestations were assessed as DILE after infliximab.

plaque psoriasis is ustekinumab. Ustekinumab is also a good alternative in the treatment of inflammatory bowel disease and in the treatment of spondylarthritis or psoriatic arthritis [31]. However, the literature contains also cases of an ustekinumab-induced DILE. Biologics with a different mechanism of action are alternative treatments, but it cannot be said whether other mechanisms of action (anti-IL13/23, anti-IL-17, anti-IL 6) will be a potential threat to DILE induction in genetically predisposed individuals.

5. Vasculitis

The manifestations of vasculitis are another disease that is associated with the anti-TNF-alpha treatment. Several case reports and patient groups have been described in the literature. In almost half of the cases, leukocytoclastic vasculitis was histologically described, while the other patients included cases of necrotising vasculitis, lymphocytic vasculitis and urticarial vasculitis [32].

An aggregate paper of 118 cases of vasculitis newly formed during the anti-TNF-alpha treatment (99 cases of rheumatoid arthritis, 8 Crohn's disease, 5 juvenile rheumatoid arthritis, 3 ankylosing spondylitis, 3 psoriasis) presented skin manifestations in 86% of patients. The anti-TNF agent administered was etanercept in 60 (51%) cases, infliximab in 51 (43%), adalimumab in 5 (4%) and other agents in 2 (2%). Purpura was manifested in 63% of the patients, whereas others had other skin manifestations of vasculitis, such as ulcerations, nodosities, maculopapular manifestations, etc. Systemic involvement was observed in 24% of patients. Immunological examinations showed that the antinuclear antibodies (ANAs) were positive in 27 patients and antineutrophil cytoplasmic antibodies (ANCAs) in 11 patients (pANCA in 5 patients and cANCA in 1 patient). Treatment in the form of anti-TNF-alpha discontinuation was used in 11 patients, 71 of whom completely recovered (41% of them had additional immunosuppressive therapy) [33]. Mohan et al. describe in an aggregate paper including 50 patients that almost 63% of patients experienced a complete recovery of the manifestations after discontinuation of the anti-TNF-alpha treatment [34].

Vasculitis manifestations in patients with severe seropositive rheumatoid arthritis are debatable, because the manifestations may be evaluated as rheumatic vasculitis, which is an extra-articular manifestation of rheumatoid arthritis and not drug-induced vasculitis. In such cases, some authors recommend discontinuation of the anti-TNF-alpha treatment with possible re-exposure to the given treatment [32]. The same situation applies also to patients with IBD, where leukocytoclastic vasculitis can be associated with the disease itself [35].

The pathogenesis of vasculitis associated with anti-TNF treatment is not completely explained. An immune complex-mediated hypersensitivity vasculitis may be related to the development of antibodies against anti-TNF agents, but in this hypothesis, the cases with etanercept should be less frequent since the treatment with the soluble receptor induces less antibody formation than monoclonal antibodies. Overexpression of type I interferon secondary to imbalance between Th1 and Th2 cytokine production under TNF inhibition may favour induction of autoimmune disorders such as vasculitis [15].

6. Pyoderma gangrenosum

Pyoderma gangrenosum (PG) is a rare neutrophilic dermatosis. PG is manifested by severe painful non-infectious pustules, nodules and necrotising ulcerations. The defects are sharply demarcated, round, with distinctly dark red undermined edges. The manifestations occur mostly on the shins, but they can also be found on the torso and other body parts. The manifestations of PG can be divided into several clinical forms, namely pustulous, bullous, a vegetative form of the disease and a separate peristomic form [36]. The peristomic form is a sign of pyoderma gangrenosum with pathergy; any trauma and injury of skin cover can cause new manifestations of the disease. The peristomic form may develop from 2 weeks to 3 years after the initial creation of the stoma [37]. Key factors in the etiopathogenesis of the disease are IL1B, IL-17, TNF-alpha and other chemokines that activate neutrophils for their activity. Genetic examinations point to several autoinflammatory genes, including pyrin innate immunity regulator (MEFV) and proline-serine-threonine phosphatase interacting protein-1 (PSTPIP1) [38]. About 50% of PG cases are associated with underlying diseases, such as inflammatory bowel disease, rheumatoid arthritis, myelodysplastic syndrome and haematological malignancies [39, 40]. Several papers indicate that refractory forms of PG are well responsive to the treatment with TNF-alpha inhibitors. One of the latest summary papers on drug-induced manifestations of pyoderma gangrenosum describes five case reports of pyoderma gangrenosum induced by an anti-TNF-alpha therapy. Three patients had manifestations induced by infliximab, one case of PG was induced by etanercept and one by adalimumab. Etiopathogenesis of PG induced by TNF-alpha inhibitors may represent paradoxical reaction due to a shift towards Th-17 polarisation [41].

7. Alopecia areata

Pathogenesis of alopecia areata is associated with TNF-alpha, which, as demonstrated in *in vitro* studies, inhibits hair follicle growth. However, in clinical trials with etanercept, the efficacy of

http://dx.doi.org/10.5772/intechopen.72449

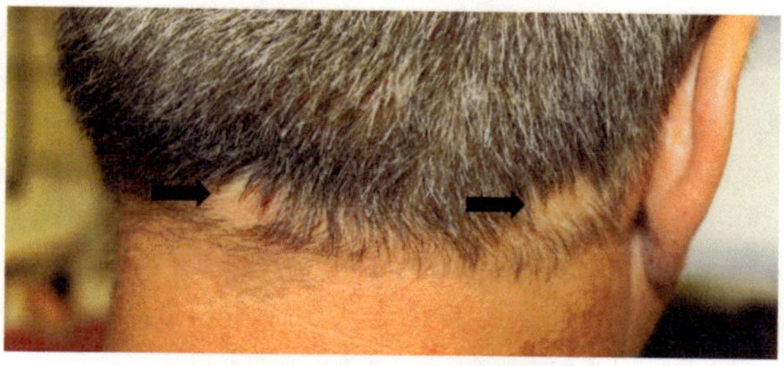

Figure 3. Adalimumab induced alopecia areata, spontaneous complete disappearance of the symptoms after 10 months without the drug discontinuation.

anti-TNF-alpha therapy for the alopecia areata was not confirmed. In the literature, however, there are cases of newly developed manifestations of alopecia areata, total and universal alopecia during anti-TNF-alpha treatment [42, 43].

French authors present data from a multicentre prospective study of patients who received anti-TNF-alpha treatment due to dermatological (11 patients), rheumatological (11 patients) and gastroenterological indications (7 patients). From these patients, 10 were treated with infliximab, 11 with adalimumab and the following 8 with etanercept. In the population, a total of 29 patients were diagnosed with alopecia areata, which was confirmed by a dermatologist. The manifestations of alopecia areata were in the area of scalp and chin in 79% of the patients. There were interesting findings related to concomitantly associated immune-mediated diseases, namely the occurrence of vitiligo, psoriasis or psoriasis-like manifestations and autoimmune thyroiditis. In the study group, nine patients had a positive family history of alopecia areata or vitiligo. A total of 14 patients discontinued the anti-TNF-alpha treatment and 15 patients continued the treatment. From patients who discontinued treatment, four were treated with infliximab, six with adalimumab and four with etanercept. Improvement up to complete disappearance of the symptoms was observed in 76% of the patients, while there was no difference between the groups in which the treatment discontinued or continued [44] (**Figure 3**).

Etiopathogenesis of alopecia areata is not clear. Some authors explain the occurrence of alopecia areata similar to TNF-alpha-induced psoriasis. Inhibition of TNF-alpha results in dysregulation of cytokines and subsequent production of IFN-alpha, which results in a pathological process [43]. However, further research is needed to better understand the occurrence of alopecia areata during anti-TNF-alpha therapy.

8. Lichen ruber planus and lichen planus-like reaction

Several cases of lichen planus and lichen planus-like paradoxically incurred lesions induced by anti-TNF-alpha therapy were reported in the literature. The manifestations have different clinical variability, including mucosal signs, but histologically they have signs of lichen planus.

The clear cause of lichenoid reactions in the treatment of anti-TNF-alpha is not known. Lichen is T-cells and dendritic cells mediated dermatosis. As with other immune-mediated diseases, pro-inflammatory cytokines and TNF-alpha play a key role [45]. Studies point to increased TNF-alpha levels in saliva and plasma in the patients with lichen planus [46, 47]. Papers indicating good therapeutic effect of TNF-alpha inhibitors on lichenoid lesions were also published. Some authors describe a similar theory of etiopathogenesis of lichen planus as in paradoxical psoriasis. As we have already mentioned in case of other immune-mediated reactions, the model in which anti-TNF-alpha induces IFN-alpha may also be valid for lichen and lichenoid reactions. Other studies indicate that type 1 IFN including IFN-alpha can induce lichen planus through the activation of cytotoxic CD8 + T cells [45].

9. Morphea-like reactions

Morphea, also called localised scleroderma, is manifested by thickening of the skin and subcutaneous tissue due to the deposition of excessive amounts of collagen. There are only a few cases of morphea induced by TNF-alpha reported in the literature. Morphea may be induced by mechanical effects or by medications. The exact etiopathogenesis of TNF-alpha-induced morphea is not known, although there are several theories of possible etiopathogenesis. TNF inhibitors can act on tumour growth factor beta (TGF beta 1), a profibrotic cytokine that effects the growth and accumulation of extracellular matrix by the action of fibroblasts and endothelial cells. An increase in Th1 and Th17 proinflammatory cytokines has been demonstrated in the early stage of localised scleroderma. Th2 lymphocytes correlate with the severity of the disease and the extent of fibrosis. Inhibition of Th1 response induced by TNF-alpha inhibitors may lead to the prevalence of Th2 lymphocytes, which may be the cause of morphea [48].

10. Vitiligo

Vitiligo is one of the other rare skin disorders that can occur with anti-TNF-alpha treatment. The role of anti-TNF-alpha inhibition in the development of vitiligo is complex and controversial. As with other paradoxical immune-mediated reactions, there are case studies where vitiligo has been significantly improved in anti-TNF-alpha therapy in vitiligo patients. The therapeutic effect of anti-TNF-alpha treatment on vitiligo is believed to be blocking the physiological effect of TNF-alpha on melanogenesis. According to the literature, TNF-alpha reduces tyrosinase levels. The melanocytic effect of TNF-alpha on vitiligo has also been demonstrated [49].

11. Other skin manifestations

Cases of newly developed dermatomyositis and polymyositis have been described in a number of papers. Most of the patients belonged to the group of patients treated for rheumatic disease. The authors predict a possible association between the presence of myositis-specific anti-Jo-1 autoantibodies and anti-TNF-alpha treatment in relation to newly developed dermatomyositis and polymyositis in patients with rheumatoid arthritis [50].

12. Discussion

TNF-alpha inhibitors are biotechnologically produced medicinal products that differ from conventional drugs in their properties, size and structure. These large molecules, even with the same mechanism of action in the form of inhibiting TNF-alpha, may act differently and they may have other adverse effects. Therefore, each biological agent is unique. Pre-clinical studies did not foreseen that TNF-alpha inhibitors will disrupt and change immunological pathways. In 2004, the first case of TNF-alpha-induced psoriasis [51] was described, and since then a number of papers have been published with immune-mediated skin reactions induced by TNF-alpha inhibitors. Their clinical spectrum is still widening; although in some cases, there are just a few case reports worldwide. Paradoxical psoriasis is the most researched and most common skin immune-mediated adverse effect. Its exact etiopathogenesis is still unclear. Development in the area of psoriasis etiopathogenesis is significantly moving forward; the Th17 pathway, which is now considered to be crucial, was discovered only a few years ago, and now we are using anti-IL17 inhibitors in clinical practice.

In conventional systemic therapy, the emergence of immune-mediated reactions is considered a comorbidity of the disease. Comorbidities are diseases that occur more frequently with the primary disease than in the general population [52]. It is assumed that the diseases have a common genetic predisposition that encodes certain inflammatory pathways. A very good example is the IL23 receptor gene, which explains the increased incidence of psoriasis in patients with ankylosing spondylitis, Crohn's disease and ulcerative colitis [52]. The literature contains only very little data about gene polymorphisms in paradoxical psoriasis. One study of gene polymorphisms that might be responsible for the above-mentioned reactions was published in 2015 by Cabaleiro et al., who observed in a group of 161 patients with psoriasis that 25 patients experienced a change in the morphology of psoriasis and 88% of the patients in the group had guttate psoriasis [16]. From a clinical point of view, it is debatable whether the monitored group had a real paradoxical psoriasis or whether it was just a worsening of the clinical condition, which is manifested in guttate form. The definition of a paradoxical psoriasiform reaction is newly induced or markedly clinically worsened psoriasis. As mentioned earlier, Collmar et al. reported that the most common clinical manifestations were palmoplantar pustulosis and chronic plaque psoriasis. Guttate forms are found in only 12% of the patients [11]. The problem of determining whether it is an adverse effect or not is encountered also with other immune-mediated reactions.

Wang et al. highlight in their paper the importance of properly diagnosing the adverse effect. The Naranjo Adverse Drug Reaction Probability Scale is used for determining the adverse effects. Based on this scoring system, it is possible to calculate the likelihood if it is an adverse drug reaction or not [41]. A very difficult situation is when determining the adverse effects in patients with IBD. More than 40% of the patients with chronic inflammatory bowel disease have extraintestinal manifestations. They are more common in the case of Crohn's disease (CD) than in patients with ulcerative colitis (UC). The most common manifestations are peripheral arthritis, aphthous stomatitis, uveitis and erythema nodosum and pyoderma gangrenosum. Skin is the most frequently affected organ in extraintestinal manifestations [53]. Therefore, if the above-mentioned manifestations of anti-TNF-alpha treatment occur, we first need to think of possible extraintestinal manifestations. Erythema nodosum (EN) is the most common skin manifestation of IBD, affecting 4–15% of the patients with CD and 3–10% of the patients with UC. EN is a reactive manifestation and correlates with the severity of the intestinal disease; it is aggravated in the case of colitis attacks [54].

Conversely, erythema nodosum may also be the first manifestation of paradoxically induced sarcoidosis. Pyoderma gangrenosum is also problematic. Pyoderma gangrenosum (PG) is the second most common, most serious and most debilitating skin manifestation in IBD. Unlike EN, the manifestations are more frequent in UC (5–12%) than in CD (1–2%) [55]. As we have already stated, pyoderma gangrenosum may also be a paradoxical response to anti-TNF-alpha treatment. The issue of comorbidity or paradoxical reaction is also in the case of vasculitis present in IBD, as well as with inflammatory rheumatic diseases. As we have stated in the previous section, only discontinuation of the biologically medicinal product and spontaneous disappearance of skin manifestations is evidence of the adverse drug reaction. Acquiring a unified view of immune-mediated adverse effects requires thorough pharmacovigilance, reporting of adverse effects, long-term monitoring of safety registry data and complementing the polymorphism research. Each biological agent is original, and even the batches do not have to be absolutely identical. By introducing biological similar molecules (biosimilars), the situation can get even more complicated. The biosimilar does not need to have the same immunogenicity as the original molecule.

Today, we know that antibodies against biologic agents are more likely to play a role in drug efficacy and hypersensitivity reactions, but some of the theories of pathogenesis of immune-mediated reactions are also associated with their production. An important fact is that there are cases where a number of immune-mediated reactions have occurred in one patient [44]. We assume that in susceptible individuals, each new biological agent may interfere with a new mechanism of action with natural physiological processes and induce still new immune-mediated adverse effects. Therefore, there is a tendency to apply one biological agent as long as possible to prevent further intervention in the cytokine cascade. We also know that the clinical response to the second and other biological agent is weaker than in treatment-naive patients, and the production of antibodies against biological medicinal products is more pronounced. The question of whether immune-mediated reactions are associated with the formation of antinuclear antibodies is also unclear. The literature describes cases of monitoring the efficacy of a biological medicinal product and the formation of antinuclear antibodies [17]. However, firm data have not yet been established; similarly, we only assume that some type of immune-mediated reactions may be associated with anti-dsDNA formation and lupus-like reactions may be induced by TNF-alpha treatment with the formation of ANA.

Our work draws attention to the issue of adverse effects that occur due to the disruption of natural mechanisms—by dysregulation of the immune system and by starting various inflammatory pathways in genetically susceptible individuals. Some of the above-mentioned reactions have a common hypothesis of formation, such as the theory of interferon induction. This knowledge may lead to the assumption that one biological agent can cause two reactions simultaneously in one patient, e.g. alopecia areata and psoriasis.

http://dx.doi.org/10.5772/intechopen.72449

Author details

Karolína Vorčáková[1]*, Péč Juraj[1], Péčová Tatiana[1] and Martinásková Klára[2]

*Address all correspondence to: karolina.vorcakova@gmail.com

1 Department of Dermatology, Comenius University in Bratislava, Jessenius Faculty of Medicine in Martin, Slovakia

2 Department of Dermatovenerology, University Hospital JA Reiman Prešov, Slovakia

References

[1] Rauch CT, Kozlosky CJ, Peschon JJ, Slack JL, Wolfson MF, Castner BJ, Stocking KL, Reddy P, Srinivasan S, Nelson N, Boiani N, Schooley KA, Gerhart M, Davis R, Fitzner JN, Johnson RS, Paxton RJ, March CJ, Cerretti DP. A metalloproteinase disintegrin that releases tumour-necrosis factor-alpha from cells. Nature. 1997;**385**:729-733

[2] Baud D, Karin M. Signal transduction by tumor necrosis factor and its relatives. Trends in Cell Biology. 2001;**11**:372-377

[3] Pfeffer K, Matsuyama T, Kündig TM, Wakeham A, Kishihara K, Shahinian A, Wiegmann K, Ohashi PS, Krönke M, Mak TW. Mice deficient for the 55 kD tumor necrosis factor receptor are resistant to endotoxic shock, yet succumb to *L monocytogenes* infection. Cell. 1993; **73**:45-67

[4] Peschon JJ, Torrance DS, Stocking KL, Glaccum MB, Otten C, Willis CR, Charrier K, Morrissey PJ, Ware CB, Mohler KM. TNF receptor-deficient mice reveal divergent roles for p55 and p75 in several models of infmammation. Journal of Immunology. 1998;**160**:943-952

[5] Wallis RS. Tumour necrosis factor antagonists: Structure, function, and tuberculosis risks. The Lancet Infectious Diseases. 2008;**8**:601-611

[6] Scallon BJ, Moore MA, Trinh H, Knight DM, Ghrayeb J. Chimeric anti-TNF-alpha monoclonal antibody cA2 binds recombinant transmembrane TNF-alpha and activates immune effector functions. Cytokine. 1995;**7**:251-259

[7] Gardam MA, Keystone EC, Menzies R, Manners S, Skamene E, Long R, Vinh DC. Anti-tumour necrosis factor agents and tuberculosis risk: Mechanisms of action and clinical management. The Lancet Infectious Diseases 2003;**3**:148-155

[8] Ciccarelli F, De Martinis M, Sirufo MM, Ginaldi L. Psoriasis induced by anti-tumor necrosis factor alpha agents: A comprehensive review of the literature. Acta Dermatovenerologica Croatica. 2016;**24**(3):169-174

[9] Wollina U, Hansel G, Koch A, Schonlebe J, Kostler E, Haroske G. Tumor necrosis factor-alpha inhibitor-induced psoriasis or psoriasiform exanthemata: First 120 cases from the

literature including a series of six new patients. American Journal of Clinical Dermatology. 2008;**9**:1-14

[10] Ko JM, Gottlieb AB, Kerbleski JF. Induction and exacerbation of psoriasis with TNF-blockade therapy: A review and analysis of 127 cases. The Journal of Dermatological Treatment. 2009;**20**:100-108

[11] Collamer AN, Battafarano DF. Psoriatic skin lesions induced by tumor necrosis factor antagonist therapy: Clinical features and possible immunopathogenesis. Seminars in Arthritis and Rheumatism. 2010;**40**:233-240

[12] Fiorentino DF. The yin and Yang of TNF-α inhibition. Archives of Dermatology. 2007;**143**: 233-236. DOI: 10.1001/archderm.143.2.233

[13] Joyau C, Veyrac G, Dixneuf V, Jolliet P. Anti-tumour necrosis factor alpha therapy and increased risk of de novo psoriasis: Is it really a paradoxical side effect? Clinical and Experimental Rheumatology. 2012;**30**(5):700-706

[14] de Gannes GC, Ghoreishi M, Pope J, Russell A, Bell D, Adams S, Shojania K, Martinka M, Dutz JP. Psoriasis and pustular dermatitis triggered by TNF-{alpha} inhibitors in patients with rheumatologic conditions. Archives of Dermatology. 2007;**143**:223-231

[15] Wendling D, Prati C. Paradoxical effects of anti-TNF-a agents in inflammatory diseases. Expert Review of Clinical Immunology. 2014;**10**(1):159-169. DOI: 10.1586/1744666X.2014.866038

[16] Cabaleiro T, Prieto-Pérez R, Navarro R, Solano G, Román M, Ochoa D, Abad-Santos F, Daudén E. Paradoxical psoriasiform reactions to anti-TNFα drugs are associated with genetic polymorphisms in patients with psoriasis. The Pharmacogenomics Journal. 2016;**16**(4):336-340. DOI: 10.1038/tpj.2015.53. Epub 2015 Jul 21

[17] Pink AE, Fonia A, Allen MH, Smith CH, Barker JN. Antinuclear antibodies associate with loss of response to antitumour necrosis factor-alpha therapy in psoriasis: A retrospective, observational study. The British Journal of Dermatology. 2010;**162**(4):780-785

[18] Dalle Vedove C, Simon JC, Girolomoni G. Drug-induced lupus erythematosus with emphasis on skin manifestations and the role of anti-TNFα agents. Journal der Deutschen Dermatologischen Gesellschaft. 2012;**10**(12):889-897

[19] Javot L, Tala S, Scala-Bertola J, Massy N, Trenque T, Baldin B, Andréjak M, Gillet P, Petitpain N; le réseau français des Centres Régionaux de Pharmacovigilance. Sarcoïdosis and anti-TNF: A paradoxical class effect? Analysis of the French pharmacovigilance system database and literature review. Thérapie. 2011;**66**(2):149-154

[20] Daïen CI, Monnier A, Claudepierre P, Constantin A, Eschard JP, Houvenagel E, Samimi M, Pavy S, Pertuiset E, Toussirot E, Combe B, Morel J, Club Rhumatismes et Inflammation (CRI). Sarcoid-like granulomatosis in patients treated with tumor necrosis factor blockers: 10 cases. Rheumatology. 2009;**48**:883-886

[21] Furst DE, Wallis R, Broder M, Beenhouwer DO. Tumor necrosis factor antagonists: Different kinetics and/or mechanisms of action may explain differences in the risk for developing granulomatous infection. Seminars in Arthritis and Rheumatism. 2006;**36**(3):159-167

[22] Vigne C, Tebib JG, Pacheco Y, Coury F. Sarcoidosis: An underestimated and potentially severe side effect of anti-TNF-alpha therapy. Joint, Bone, Spine. 2013;**80**(1):104-107

[23] Chang C, Gershwin ME. Drug-induced lupus erythematosus. Incidence, management and prevention. Drug Safety. 2011;**34**:357-374

[24] Marzano AV, Vezzoli P, Crosti C. Drug induced lupus: An update on its dermatological aspects. Lupus. 2009;**18**:935-940

[25] Antonov D, Kazandjieva J, Etugov D, Gospodinov D, Tsankov N. Drug-induced lupus erythematosus. Clinics in Dermatology. 2004;**22**:157-166

[26] Vedove CD, Simon JC, Girolomoni G. Drug-induced lupus erythematosus with emphasis on skin manifestations and the role of anti-TNFa agents. Journal der Deutschen Dermatologischen Gesellschaft. 2012;**10**:889-897

[27] Atzeni F, Turiel M, Capsoni F, Doria A, Meroni P, Sarzi-Puttini P. Autoimmunity and anti-TNF-a agents. Annals of the New York Academy of Sciences. 2005;**1051**:559-569

[28] Costa MF, Said NR, Zimmermann B. Drug induced lupus due to anti-tumor necrosis factor alpha agents. Seminars in Arthritis and Rheumatism. 2008;**37**:381-387

[29] Williams EL, Gadola S, Edwards CJ. Anti-TNF-induced lupus. Rheumatology. 2009; **48**:716-720

[30] Williams VL, Cohen PR. TNF alpha antagonist-induced lupus-like syndrome: Report and review of the literature with implications for treatment with alternative TNF alpha antagonists. International Journal of Dermatology. 2011;**50**:619-625

[31] Lomicová I, Suchý D, Pizinger K, Cetkovská P. A case of lupus-like syndrome in a patient receiving adalimumab and a brief review of the literature on drug-induced lupus erythematosus. Journal of Clinical Pharmacy and Therapeutics. 2017;**42**(3):363-366. DOI: 10.1111/jcpt.12506

[32] Marcoux BS, De Bandt M. Vasculitides induced by TNFα antagonists: A study in 39 patients in France. Joint, Bone, Spine. 2006;**73**:710-713

[33] Ramos-Casals M, Brito-Zerón P, Soto MJ, Cuadrado MJ, Khamashta MA. Autoimmune diseases induced by TNF-targeted therapies. Autoimmunity reviews. Best Practice & Research. Clinical Rheumatology. 2008;**22**(5):847-861. DOI: 10.1016/j.berh.2008.09.008

[34] Mohan N, Edwards ET, Cupps TR, Slifman N, Lee JH, Siegel JN, Braun MM. Leukocytoclastic vasculitis associated with tumor necrosis factor-alpha blocking agents. J Rheumatol. 2004;**31**:1955-1958

[35] Tsiamoulos Z, Karamanolis G, Polymeros D, Triantafyllou K, Oikonomopoulos T. Leuko cytoclastic vasculitis as an onset symptom of Crohn's disease. Case Reports in Gastroenterology. 2008;**2**:410-414

[36] Georgiou G, Pasmatzi E, Monastirli A, Tsambaos D. Cutaneous manifestations of inflammatory bowel disease. Hospital Chronicles. 2006;**1**:158-168

[37] Callen JP. Pyoderma gangrenosum. Lancet. 1998;**351**:581-585

[38] Marzano AV, Damiani G, Ceccherini I, Berti E, Gattorno M, Cungo M. Autoinflammation in pyoderma gangrenosum and its syndromic form (pyoderma gangrenosum, acne and suppurative hidradenitis). The British Journal of Dermatology 2016;**176**(6):1588-1598. DOI: 10.1111/bjd.15226

[39] Crowson AN, Mihm MC Jr, Magro C. Pyoderma gangrenosum: A review. Journal of Cutaneous Pathology. 2003;**30**(2):97-107

[40] Wollina U. Pyoderma gangrenosum—A review. Orphanet Journal of Rare Diseases. 2007; **15**(2):19

[41] Wang JY, French LE, Shear NH, Amiri A, Alavi A. Drug-induced Pyoderma gangrenosum: A review. American Journal of Clinical Dermatology. 2017 Jun 17. DOI: 10.1007/s40257-017-0308-7. [Epub ahead of print]

[42] Beccastrini E, Squatrito D, Emmi G, Fabbri P, Emmi L. Alopecia areata universalis during off-label treatment with infliximab in a patient with Behçet disease. Dermatology Online Journal. 2010;**16**(9):15

[43] Hernández MV, Meineri M, Sanmartí R. Skin lesions and treatment with tumor necrosis factor alpha antagonists. Reumatología Clinica. 2013;**9**(1):53-61

[44] Schmutz JL. Alopecia areata occurring during anti-TNF-α therapy: A French prospective multicentre study. Annales de Dermatologie et de Vénéréologie. 2015;**142**(5):386-387. DOI: 10.1016/j.annder.2015.02.003

[45] Asarch A, Gottlieb AB, Lee J, Masterpol KS, Scheinman PL, Stadecker MJ, Massarotti EM, Bush ML. Lichen planus-like eruptions: An emerging side effect of tumor necrosis factor-alpha antagonists. Journal of the American Academy of Dermatology. 2009;**61**(1):104-111. DOI: 10.1016/j.jaad.2008.09.032

[46] Erdem MT, Gulec AI, Kiziltunc A, Yildirim A, Atasoy M. Increased serum levels of tumor necrosis factor alpha in lichen planus. Dermatology. 2003;**207**:367-370

[47] Pezelj-Ribaric S, Prso IB, Abram M, Glazar I, Brumini G, Simunovic-Soskic M. Salivary levels of tumor necrosis factor-alpha in oral lichen planus. Mediators of Inflammation. 2004;**13**:131-133

[48] Ramírez J, Hernández MV, Galve J, Cañete JD, Sanmartí R. Morphea associated with the use of adalimumab: A case report and review of the literature. Modern Rheumatology. 2012;**22**(4):602-604. DOI: 10.1007/s10165-011-0550-4

[49] Jung JM, Lee YJ, Won CH, Chang SE, Lee MW, Choi JH, Moon KC. Development of vitiligo during treatment with adalimumab: A plausible or paradoxical response? Annals of Dermatology. 2015;**27**(5):620-621. DOI: 10.5021/ad.2015.27.5.620. Epub 2015 Oct 2

[50] Ishikawa Y, Yukawa N, Ohmura K, Hosono Y, Imura Y, Kawabata D, Nojima T, Fujii T, Usui T, Mimori T. Etanercept-induced anti-Jo-1-antibody-positive polymyositis in a patient with rheumatoid arthritis: A case report and review of the literature. Clinical Rheumatology. 2010;**29**:563-566

[51] Verea MM, Del Pozo J, Yebra-Pimentel MT, Porta A, Fonseca E. Psoriasiform eruption induced by infliximab. The Annals of Pharmacotherapy. 2004;**38**:54-57

[52] Duffin KC, Woodcock J, Krueger GG. Genetic variations asociated with psoriasis and arthritis found by genome-wide association. Dermatologic Therapy. 2010;**23**(2):101-113

[53] Vavricka SR, Brun L, Ballabeni P, Pittet V, Prinz Vavricka BM, Zeitz J, Rogler G, Schoepfer AM. Frequency and risk factors for extraintestinal manifestations in the Swiss inflammatory bowel disease cohort. The American Journal of Gastroenterology. 2011;**106**:110-119. DOI: 10.1111/j.1529-8019.2010.01303.x

[54] Timani S, Mutasim DF. Skin manifestations of inflammatory bowel disease. Clinics in Dermatology. 2008;**26**:265-273

[55] Danese S, Semeraro S, Papa A, Roberto I, Scaldaferri F, Fedeli G, Gasbarrini G, Gasbarrini A. Extraintestinal manifestations in inflammatory bowel disease. World Journal of Gastroenterology. 2005;**11**:7227-7236

Chapter 12

Bioinformatics as a Tool to Identify Infectious Disease Pathogen Peptide Sequences as Targets for Antibody Engineering

Lavanya Suneetha, Prasanna Marsakatla,
Rachel Supriya Suneetha and Sujai Suneetha

Additional information is available at the end of the chapter

http://dx.doi.org/10.5772/intechopen.71011

Abstract

Bioinformatics is an interdisciplinary field of information technology for understanding biological data from genome to protein. It includes a combination of fields of science, computer science, statistics, mathematics, and engineering to analyze, interpret and derive biological data. This chapter describes how to use Bioinformatics to identify pathogen virulence factor peptide sequence similarities in human nerve tissue proteins and for evaluation as antibody engineering target peptides.

Keywords: bioinformatics, infectious diseases, peptide, recombinant antibody

1. Introduction

Bioinformatics is the application of techniques derived from disciplines such as applied mathematics, computer science, and statistics to analyze and interpret biological data. In this chapter, you will learn how to use bioinformatic techniques to identify pathogen virulence factor (VF) peptide sequence similarities to human nerve tissue proteins and then how to identify target peptides that could form the basis for engineering recombinant antibodies. Also, wet experiments could be conducted on the identified overlapping sequences to help us to single out target antibodies to be tested for tissue culture studies [1, 2]. The most ideal targeted peptide sequences for antibody engineering are those physiologically relevant, easy to access, and comprise amino acid sequence regions which have high specificity in pathogenic steps and reduced amino acid string length.

INTECH
open science | open minds

© 2018 The Author(s). Licensee InTech. This chapter is distributed under the terms of the Creative Commons Attribution License (http://creativecommons.org/licenses/by/3.0), which permits unrestricted use, distribution, and reproduction in any medium, provided the original work is properly cited. (cc) BY

1.1. Bioinformatics and its role in peptide discovery

The accessibility to the extensive genomic and proteomic databases and the availability of tools to compare and evaluate the information have given rise to a new interdisciplinary field that combines biology and computer science [3]. Bioinformatics conceptualizes physical and chemical biology in terms of macromolecules and then applies "informatics" techniques (derived from disciplines such as applied mathematics, computer science, and statistics) to assimilate and organize the information associated with these molecules, on a large scale [4]. Bioinformatics is an exciting and exploratory method for peptide discovery in antibody engineering and development of antimicrobial therapies and vaccination strategies [5].

There is significantly growing evidence that a number of neurodegenerative diseases are a result of the association of host cell proteins with viral and bacterial infectious agents [6]. When pathogenic micro organisms such as bacteria, viruses, parasites, or fungi cause an infectious disease, there are many molecular interactions between the host-pathogen proteins and host peptides [7] through all the stages of the disease whether incubation, prodromal illness, decline, and convalescence. There is much experimental evidence identifying the virulence factors (VF) of pathogen and host components such as receptors and tissue-specific proteins [8, 9]. Though the pathogenic pathway of the infectious agent in various host tissues is unknown, many of these processes are suspected to be attributable to the yet undiscovered role of molecular mimics identified in pathogenic microorganisms and its corresponding host tissue proteins. The sequence and structural similarities between the pathogenic VF protein and nerve peptides could impact either directly or indirectly the pathogenesis of the infectious disease [10–12]. It could contribute to molecular mimicry, steric hindrance, receptor binding, cell signaling, and autoantibody production events (involved in neuro degeneration) in the host.

Leprosy patients with peripheral nerve damage develop autoimmunity to myelin P0 (nerve protein). The above conclusion was drawn by gathering known scientific evidence that are as follows: (1) labeling and binding studies found that *Mycobacterium leprae* (bacterium causing leprosy) binds to myelin P0 [13]; (2) clinical studies confirmed the production of autoantibodies as a response of the bacterium to interact with myelin P0 [14, 15]; and (3) bioinformatics searches identified sequences and structural similarities between *M. leprae* and the immunoglobulin regions of myelin P0 [16].

Identification of molecular mimics in pathogen-host peptide sequences is one approach to identify target peptides for antibody engineering. There are about 180 extensive biological databases to retrieve information on sequence and functional aspects of biological molecules. The updated list is available in Nucleic Acids Research [17].

1.2. The use of bioinformatics in identifying sequence similarities

This section teaches you how to conduct a search for proteins present in a target host, how to obtain its amino acid sequence/s from the existing databases, how to compare the sequence/s of the host protein to that of the pathogen protein, and finally how to interpret the results based on existing evidential data. In our case study, we identify the virulence factor peptide

http://dx.doi.org/10.5772/intechopen.71011

sequence similarities of a few selected infectious agents with human nerve tissue proteins for selecting peptides to engineer antipeptide antibodies which recognizes corresponding host/viral proteins.

1.2.1. Selection of nerve proteins

63 proteins were extracted from the Human Protein Atlas Database that were enriched and enhanced in the nervous tissue as observed by immunehistochemistry (**Figure 1**).

To conduct a search for human proteins in the nervous tissue, access the website (www.proteinatlas.org), enter the tissue of study (e.g. nervous tissue) into the search box provided and click on search.

Manual protein selection was carried out based on their tissue expression (enriched and enhanced) and also on immunohistochemistry evidence (**Figure 2**).

The list of selected proteins are as follows: agrin (AGRN_HUMAN, O00468), calbindin (CALB1_HUMAN, P05937), n-chimaerin (CHIN_HUMAN, P15882), secretogranin-2 (SCG2_HUMAN, P13521), neuromodulin (NEUM_HUMAN, P17677), kinesin (KIFC1_HUMAN, Q9BW19), tau (TAU_HUMAN, P10636), 2′,3′-cyclic-nucleotide 3′-phosphodiesterase (CN37_HUMAN, P09543), myelin-associated glycoprotein (MAG_HUMAN, P20916), myelin P0 (MYP0_HUMAN, P25189), myelin P2 (MYP2_HUMAN, P02689), oligodendrocyte-myelin

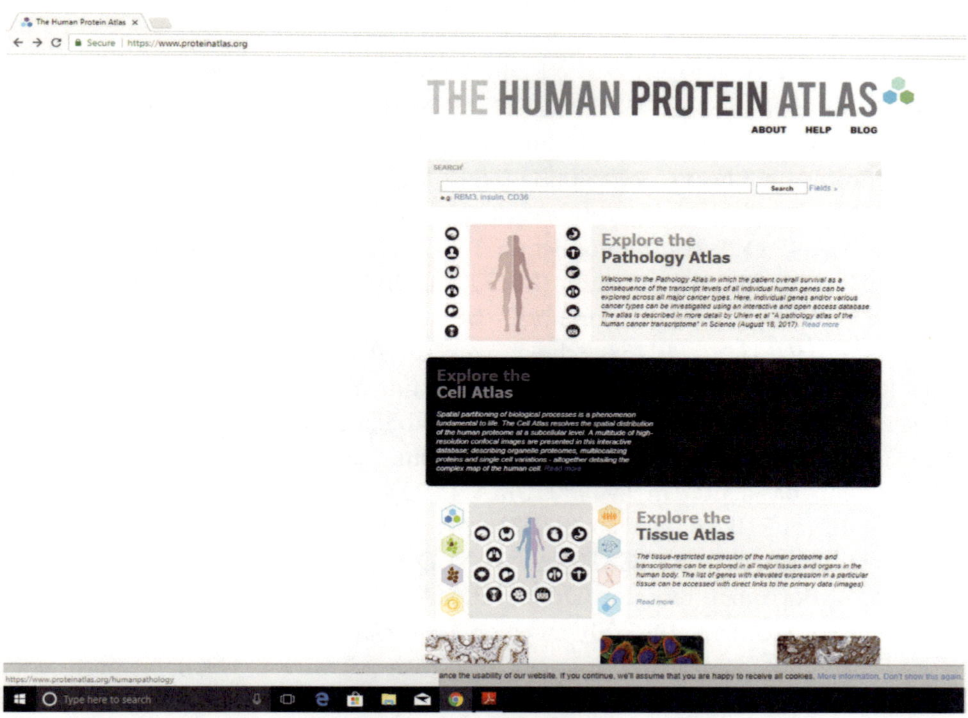

Figure 1. Conducting a search on the Human Protein Atlas Database.

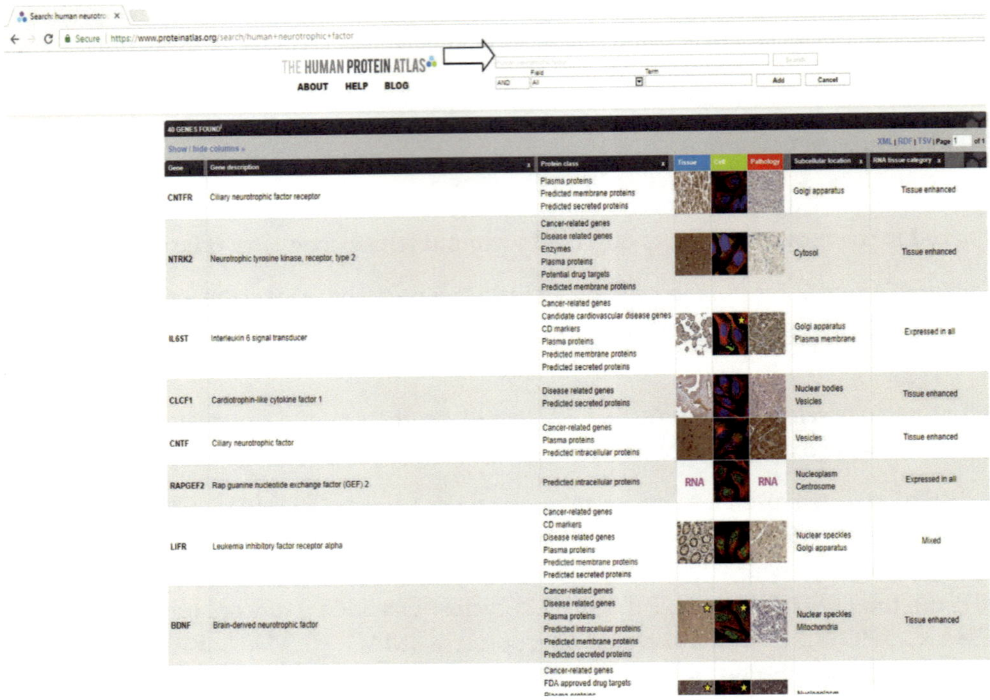

Figure 2. Conducting an advanced search on the Human Protein Atlas Database.

glycoprotein (OMGP_HUMAN, P23515), brain-derived neurotrophic factor (BDNF_HUMAN, P23560), ciliary neurotrophic factor (CNTF_HUMAN, P26441), neurotrophin-3 (NTF3_HUMAN, P20783), beta-nerve growth factor (NGF_HUMAN, P01138), nestin (NEST_HUMAN, P48681), neurofilament heavy polypeptide (NFH_HUMAN, P12036), neurogranin (NEUG_HUMAN, Q92686), voltage-dependent T-type calcium channel subunit alpha-1G (CAC1G_HUMAN, O43497), hippocalcin (HPCL1_HUMAN, P37235), neurocalcin-delta (NCALD_HUMAN, P61601), recoverin (RECO_HUMAN, P35243), bombesin receptor subtype-3 (BRS3_HUMAN, P32247), kininogen-1/bradykinin (KNG1_HUMAN, P01042), calcitonin (CALC_HUMAN, P01258), cholecystokinin (CCKN_HUMAN, P06307), galanin peptides (GALA_HUMAN, P22466), pro-neuropeptide Y (NPY_HUMAN, P01303), neurotensin/neuromedin N (NEUT_HUMAN, P30990), protein S100-B (S100B_HUMAN, P04271), synapsin-1 (SYN1_HUMAN, P17600), probable tubulin polyglutamylase (TTLL1_HUMAN, O95922), myelin basic protein (MBP_HUMAN, P02686), protein phosphatase 1 regulatory subunit 1B (PPR1B_HUMAN, Q9UD71), Arf-GAP with GTPase, ANK repeat and PH domain-containing protein 2 (AGAP2_HUMAN, Q99490), cathepsin L2 (CATL2_HUMAN, O60911), D(1A) dopamine receptor (DRD1_HUMAN, P21728), BDNF/NT-3 growth factors receptor (NTRK2_HUMAN, Q16620), melanoma-associated antigen E1 (MAGE1_HUMAN, Q9HCI5), microtubule-associated protein 6 (MAP6_HUMAN, Q96JE9), protocadherin alpha-12 (PCDAC_HUMAN, Q9UN75), carboxypeptidase E (CBPE_HUMAN, P16870), Down syndrome cell adhesion molecule (DSCAM_HUMAN, O60469), dyslexia-associated protein KIAA0319 (K0319_HUMAN, Q5VV43), uncharacterized protein KIAA1211-like (K121L_HUMAN, Q6NV74), microtubule-associated protein 1B (MAP1B_HUMAN, P46821), neuronal calcium sensor 1 (NCS1_HUMAN, P62166), neurofilament light polypeptide (NFL_HUMAN, P07196), receptor expression-enhancing protein 2 (REEP2_HUMAN, Q9BRK0), secretogranin-3 (SCG3_HUMAN, Q8WXD2), ubiquitin carboxyl-terminal hydrolase isozyme L1 (UCHL_HUMAN, P09936), galactosylgalactosylxylosylprotein 3-beta-glucuronosyltransferase 1 (B3GA1_HUMAN, Q9P2W7), beta-1,4 N-acetylgalactosaminyltransferase 1 (B4GN1_HUMAN, Q00973), caprin-2 (CAPR2_HUMAN, Q6IMN6), dopamine beta-hydroxylase (DOPO_HUMAN, P09172), FAM81A (FA81A_HUMAN, Q8TBF8), mitogen-activated protein kinase 10 (MK10_HUMAN, P53779), N-terminal EF-hand calcium-binding protein 1 (NECA1_HUMAN, Q8N987), neuroligin-3 (NLGN3_HUMAN, Q9NZ94), protein kinase C and casein kinase substrate in neurons protein 1 (PACN1_HUMAN, Q9BY11), sodium channel protein type 7 subunit alpha (SCN7A_HUMAN, Q01118), and clathrin coat assembly AP180 (AP180_HUMAN, O60641). The biological accepts of the proteins have been derived from the information presented in UniProt database for each protein [18–20].

1.2.2. Retrieving FASTA formats

FASTA formats for each of the above proteins were retrieved from NCBI PubMed. The FASTA format is a text-based format obtained from the PubMed search and represents either nucleotide sequences or peptide sequences (**Figure 3**).

Upon accessing the website, select the database in which the search is to be conducted (e.g. Protein). Type the name of the protein and its species in brackets into the search text box provided (e.g. Agrin (*Homo sapiens*)) and click on the search button.

The protein with the highest number of amino acids is chosen. Click on the hyperlinked protein to access its gene bank. Upon reaching the gene bank of the selected protein, click on the hyperlinked *FASTA* (**Figures 4**, **5** and **6**).

Obtain the FASTA format by copying all the information (Starting from the > symbol).

1.2.3. Arranging the FASTA formats

All the FASTA formats of the human proteins are saved in a sequence on Microsoft Notepad (**Figure 7**).

1.2.4. Running the BLAST

Pathogen-protein mimics, nerve protein sequences were BLAST (Basic Local Alignment Search Tool; Version 2.7.1; e-value ≤0.01) [21] against a pathogen genome (**Figure 8**).

Access the BLAST website at https://blast.ncbi.nlm.nih.gov/Blast.cgi and click on Protein (Protein~Protein) BLAST. The FASTA formats of 63 nerve proteins were copied and pasted from the notepad into the text box provided. Enter the species of the organism against which the blast has to be performed/the sequence comparison has to be carried out specifying its Tax ID (**Figure 8**).

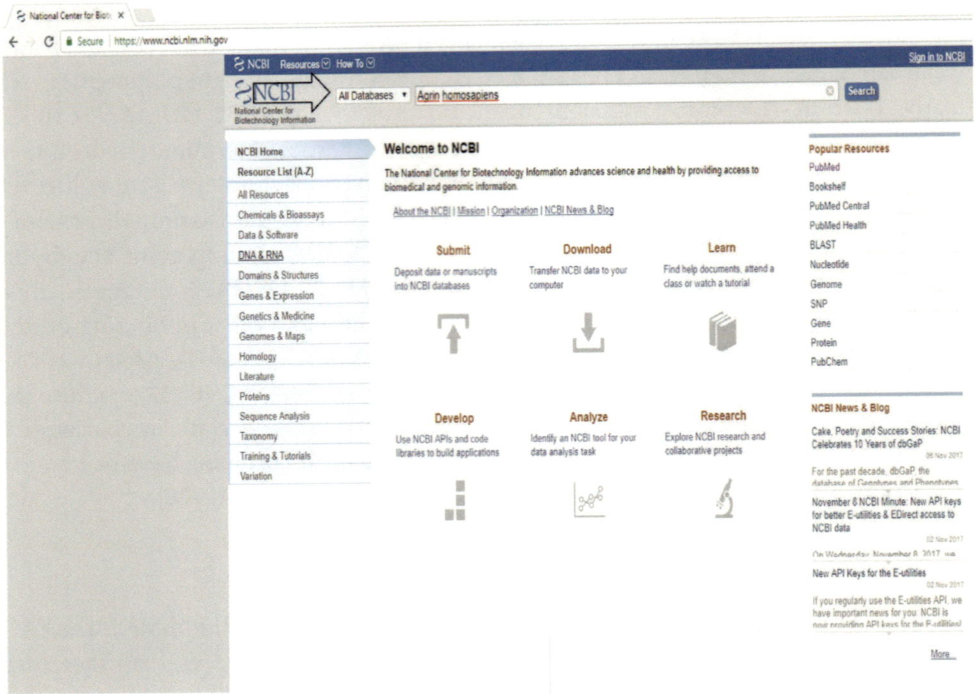

Figure 3. Conducting a search on the PubMed database.

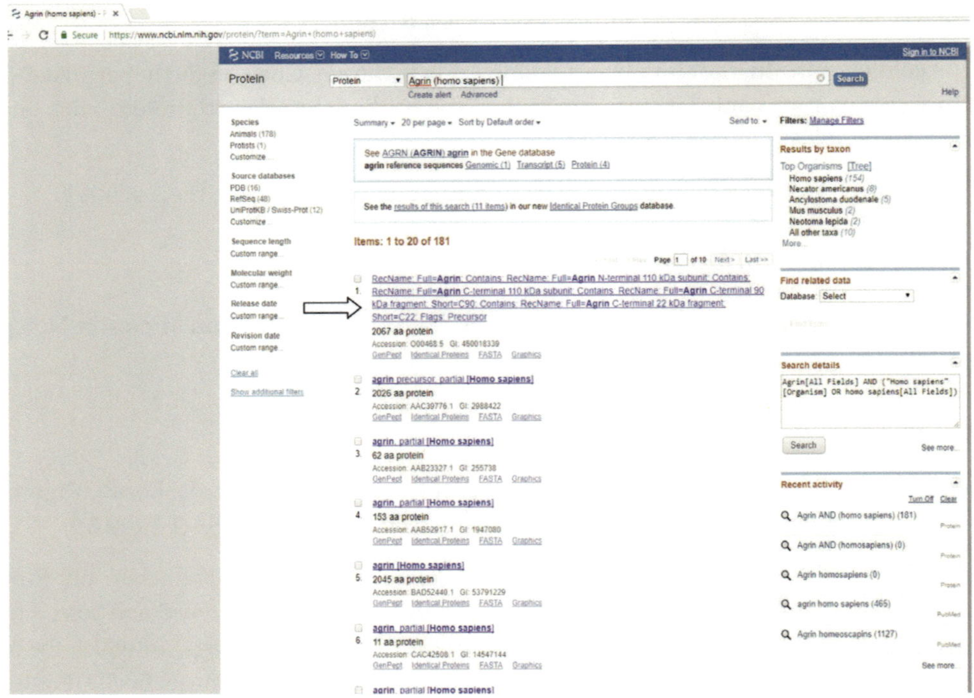

Figure 4. List of available sequenced protein information.

http://dx.doi.org/10.5772/intechopen.71011

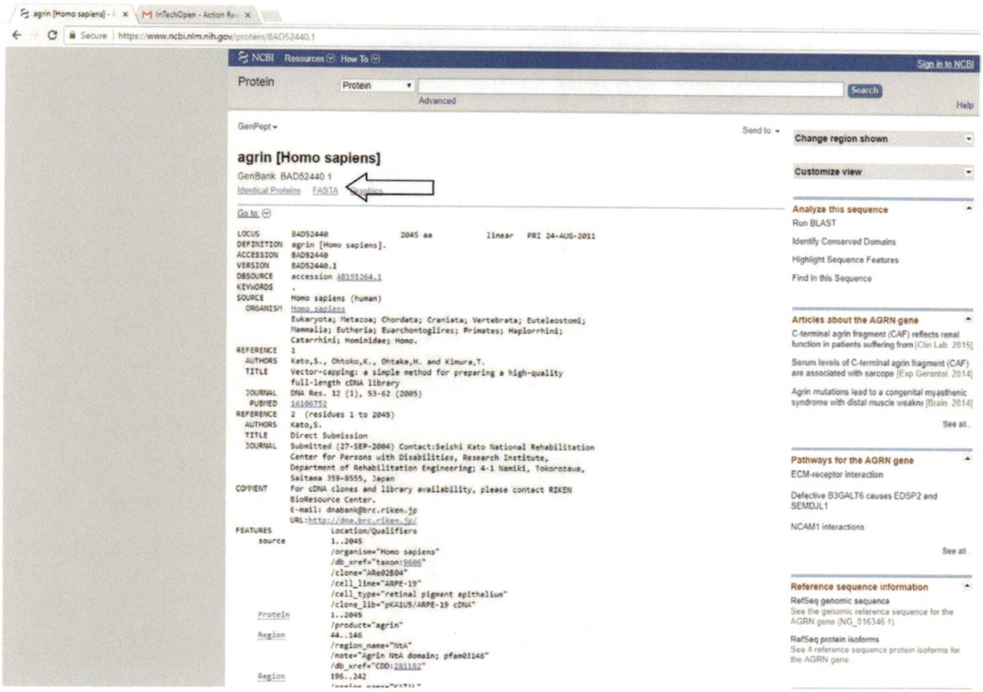

Figure 5. Gene information of agrin.

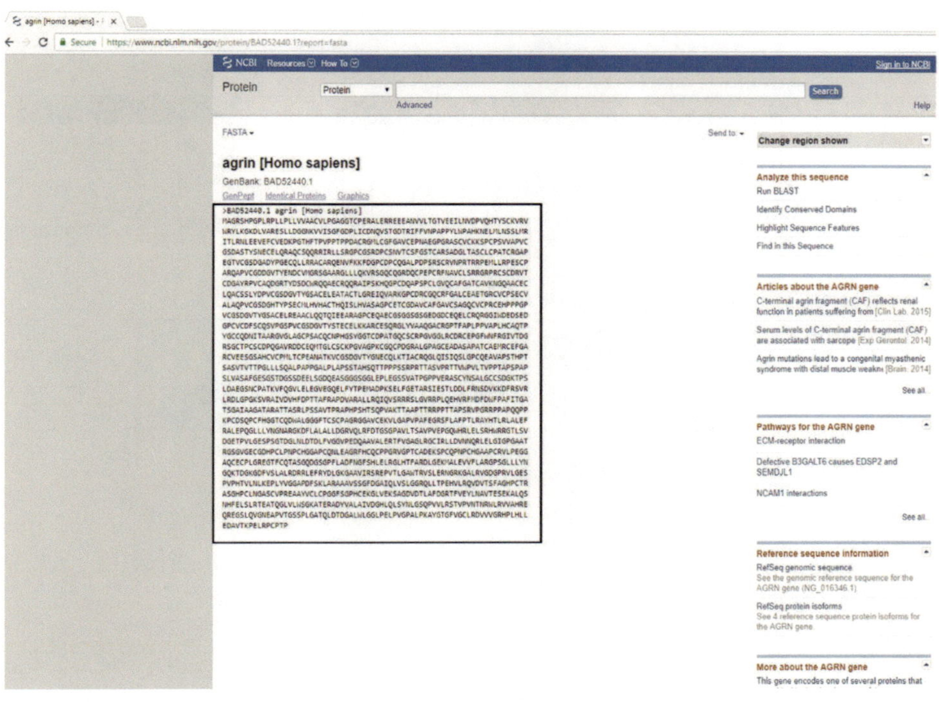

Figure 6. FASTA format of agrin.

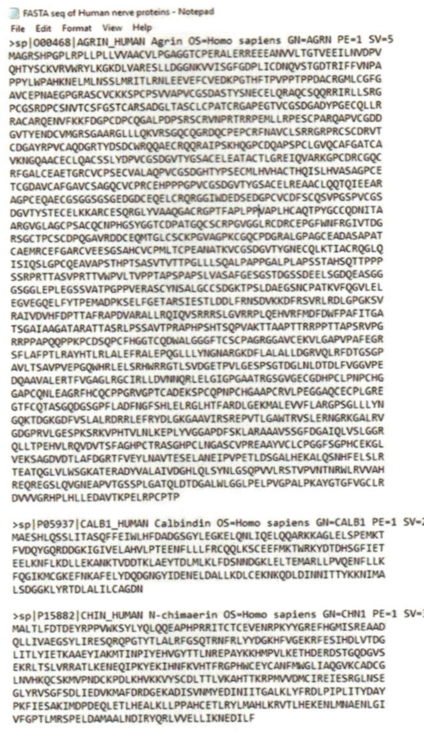

Figure 7. FASTA formats of the 63 proteins in sequence.

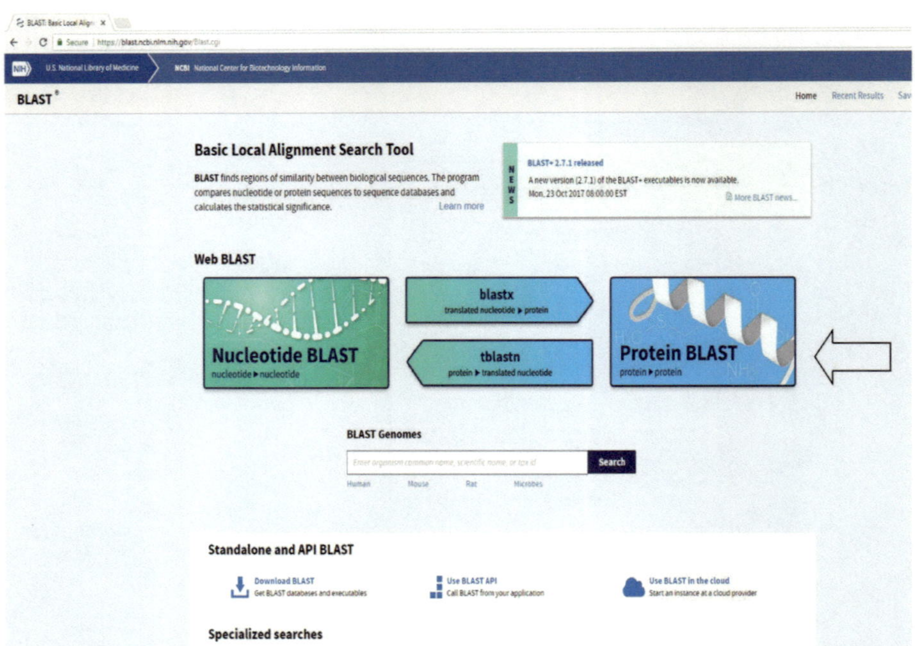

Figure 8. BLAST home page.

http://dx.doi.org/10.5772/intechopen.71011

The pathogen genome sequences that were compared with the human nerve proteins are as follows: HIV (Tax ID: 11,676), Polio (Tax ID: 138,950), Japanese Encephalitis (Tax ID:64,320), *M. leprae* (Tax ID: 1769), Human herpes virus 1 (Tax ID: 10,298), Human herpes virus 2 (Tax ID: 10,310), Rabies virus (Tax ID: 11,292), Zika virus (Tax ID: 64,320), Corona virus (Tax ID: 11,118), Varicella zoster virus (Tax ID: 10,335).

Select program PSI BLAST as the BLAST algorithm for a more position-sensitive search. It looks deeper into the database to best match to your query. Click on the BLAST button and wait for the results. Take screen shots of your result and also download the provided excel format (**Figure 9**).

The output of the BLAST identified the significant peptide sequence similarities between the human protein and its pathogenic counterpart **Figure 10**. These peptide sequence similarities are identified by amino acid positions, in which amino acids exist in single-letter codes. The BLAST provides us with the number of sequence similarities between the pathogenic genomic sequence and its host proteins. It also identifies viral counterpart peptides and the region of similarity on the host proteins.

Further interpretations of the results can be made by referring to the Uniprot database to obtain the biological and functional aspects of the host and the pathogen proteins (**Figures 11** and **12**).

1.2.5. Ascribing a biological role and application

The results show a number of sequence similarities existing between host proteins and various pathogen proteins. The maximum number of peptide sequence similarities were found between host protein caprin-2 which had 495 similarities with polio; neurogranin had 230

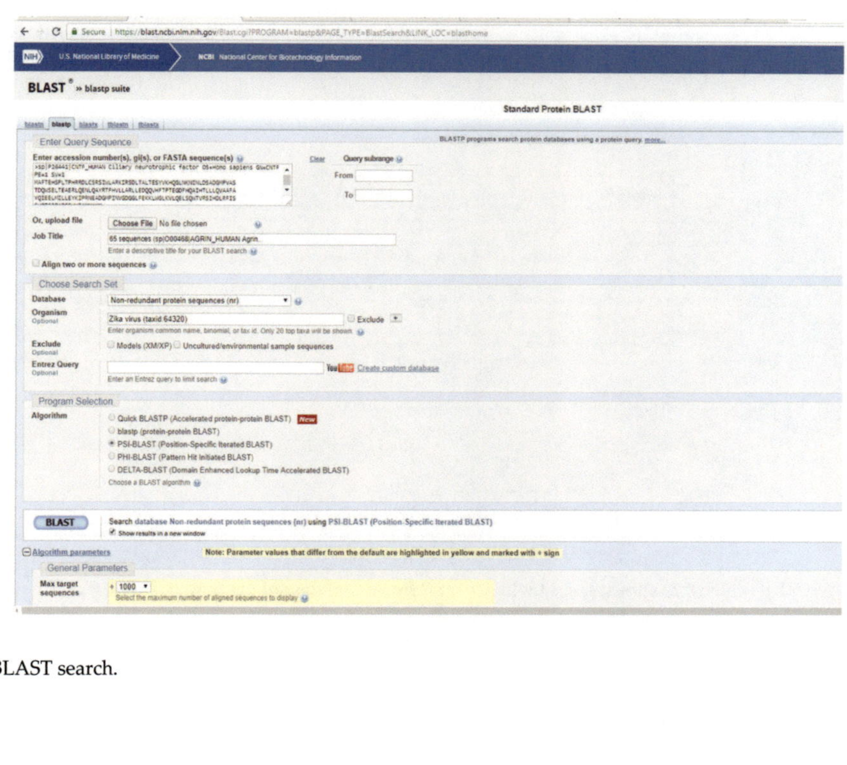

Figure 9. BLAST search.

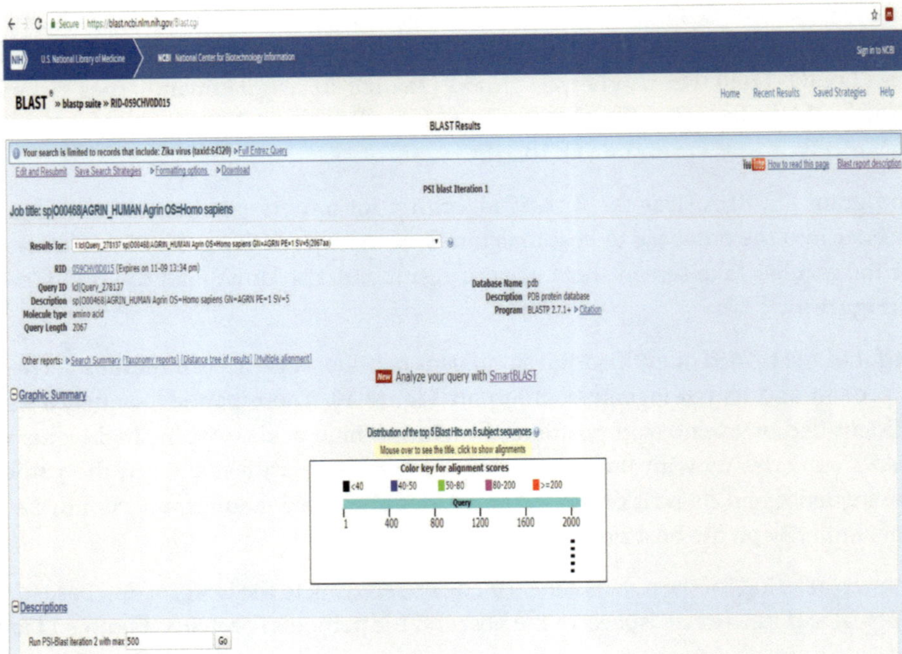

Figure 10. BLAST results of nerve proteins showing similarity to pathogen proteins.

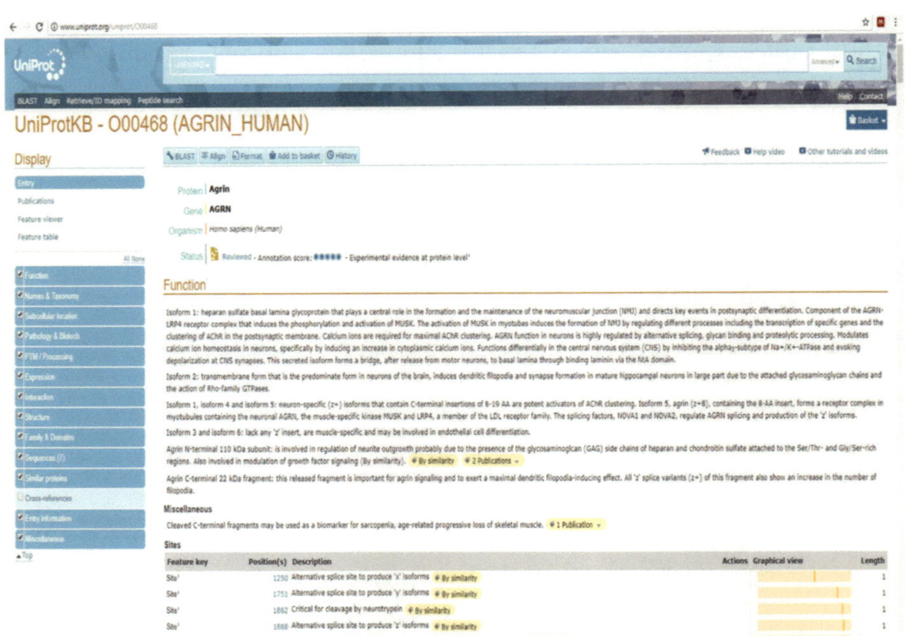

Figure 11. UniProtKB screenshot showing the biological and functional data of the human protein.

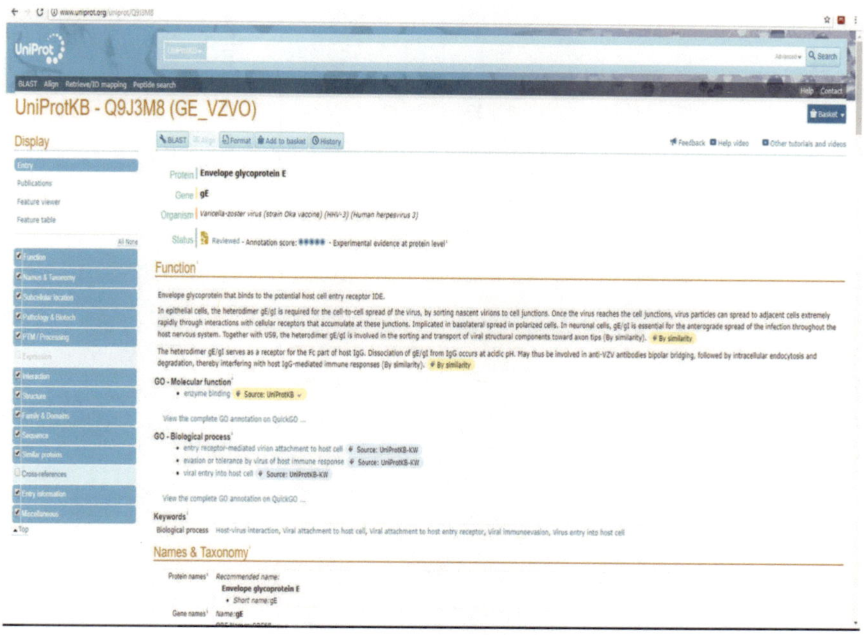

Figure 12. Uniprot screenshot showing the biological and functional data of the viral protein.

similarities with HHV2; secretogranin-3 had 221 similarities with Japanese encephalitis; agrin had 212 similarities with varicella; caprin-2 had 198 similarities with rabies virus; galanin peptides had 87 similarities with Zika virus; kinesin had 54 similarities with HIV; neurofilament heavy polypeptide had 46 similarities with corona virus; neurogranin had 39 similarities with HHV1; and 2′,3′-cyclic-nucleotide 3′-phosphodiesterase had 21 similarities with *M. leprae*.

This method identifies significant virulent factors which have sequence similarities to human nerve tissue proteins. The nerve proteins that exhibited sequence similarities with four or more pathogenic virulent factors are displayed in **Table 1**. All 63 proteins are found to have sequence similarities with *M. leprae* proteins.

Agrin is a heparin sulphate basal lamina glycoprotein with a molecular mass of 217,232 Da. It plays a central role in the formation and maintenance of the neuromuscular junction. It is known to direct events in postsynaptic differentiation. Agrin also induces the phosphorylation and activation of muscle-specific kinase (MUSK), the clustering of Acetyl choline esterase receptor (AChR) in the postsynaptic membrane, regulates calcium ion homeostasis in neurons, and is involved in regulation of neuritis outgrowth [22, 23].

1.2.6. HHV3 peptide similarity to human protein agrin

Agrin UniProtKB-O00468 (AGRIN_HUMAN) (AA position 1269–1326) (**Figure 13**) has a similarity to membrane glycoprotein C (Sequence ID: AEW88711.1 AA Position 43–122) of the varicella zoster virus UniProtKB-Q9J3M8 (GE_VZVO) which by its similarity has the

S. No	Query No.	Proteins	HIV	Polio	JE	HHV 1	HHV 2	*M. leprae*	Corona	Zika	Rabies	Vericella
1	O00468	Agrin	0	0	4	0	0	6	1	0	1	212
2	P17677	Neuromodulin	1	1	0	1	3	6	28	1	0	75
3	Q9BW19	Kinesin	54	1	0	0	0	9	0	0	0	0
4	P10636	Tau protein	0	1	0	0	14	5	9	0	0	19
5	P25189	Myelin protein P0	2	0	0	1	22	7	1	0	0	0
6	P23515	Oligodendrocyte-myelin glycoprotein	0	2	0	1	0	9	0	0	1	23
7	P48681	Nestin	0	0	3	2	0	8	2	30	0	22
8	P04271	Protein S100-B	0	26	0	2	11	7	0	0	0	12
9	P17600	Synapsin-1	0	1	7	11	2	13	0	0	5	0
10	P02686	Myelin basic protein	0	0	0	0	2	9	4	3	0	5
11	Q16620	BDNF/NT-3 growth factors receptor	0	0	0	23	8	11	0	0	1	15
12	Q5VV43	Dyslexia-associated protein KIAA0319	0	0	0	37	21	5	5	0	2	1
13	P07196	Neurofilament light polypeptide	0	0	0	1	1	2	4	0	0	77
14	Q8WXD2	Secretogranin-3	3	5	221	0	10	8	0	0	9	0
15	Q00973	Beta-1,4 N-acetylgalactosaminyltransferase 1	1	29	0	1	2	8	0	0	0	0

Table 1. Sequence similarities of human nerve tissue proteins with human virulent factors. Multiple alignments obtained in a single BLAST search could result in identities of the amino acids or substitutions of the amino acids in the same peptide region.

http://dx.doi.org/10.5772/intechopen.71011

Alignments

membrane glycoprotein C [Human alphaherpesvirus 3]
Sequence ID: **AEW88711.1** Length: 520 Number of Matches: 2
Range 1: 43 to 122

Score	Expect	Method	Identities	Positives	Gaps	Frame
45.4 bits(106)	2e-05()	Composition-based stats.	29/80(36%)	37/80(46%)	6/80(7%)	

Features:

```
Query  1269  ATARATTASRLPSSAVTPRAPHPSHTSQPVAKTTAAPTTRRP-PTTAPSRVPGRRP-PAP  1326
             A A  + ASR P  AV P +          VA T  +  TR+P P  AP+    R+P PA
Sbjct  43    AVAPTSAASRKPDPAVAPTSAASRKPDPAVAPTXTSAATRKPDPAVAPTSAASRKPDPAA  102
```

```
Query  1327  Q----QPPKPCDSQPCFHGG  1342
                  QPP   ++  C HGG
Sbjct  103   NTQHSQPPFLYENIQCVHGG  122
```

Figure 13. BLAST output of membrane glycoprotein of HHV3 showing similarity to human protein agrin.

potential to bind to the tissue cell receptor. Experimental evidence in epithelial cells shows that the hetero demonization of viral receptors could spread the virus by sorting nascent virion to nerve tissue cell junctions. The virus particles can spread to adjacent cells through interactions with cellular receptors at these cell junctions. The virus at cell junctions spreads extremely rapidly into the tissues [24, 25]. Sequence mimics of agrin to the varicella membrane glycoprotein could have an effect on either viral entry into host cell, evasion or on tolerance of host immune response to the virus and virion attachment to the host cell. These similarities in peptide regions warrant further exploration to understand pathogenesis and to identify target peptides for antibody engineering [26].

1.2.7. Poliovirus and rabies virus peptide similarities to human protein caprin-2

Caprin-2UniProtKB-Q6IMN6 (CAPR2_HUMAN) is a protein of molecular mass 68,429 Da. The structure of caprin-2 was found to be similar to the polio and rabies viruses. Caprin-2 (AA position: 136–176) has a similarity to the polyprotein of polio virus UniProtKB–E0WCG5 (E0WCG5_9ENTO) (polyprotein sequence ID: ACZ05040.1 AA position: 1994–2070) (**Figures 14** and **15**). Caprin-2 (AA position: 13–54) also has a similarity to the phosphoprotein of rabies virus UniProtKB-Q80JL8 (Q80JL8_9RHAB) (phosphoprotein sequence ID: AAO60615.1 AA position 76–110) (**Figure 15**). Caprin-2 has a significant role in influencing phosphorylation of the Wnt-signaling pathways (PubMed:18,762,581) [27]. Caprin-2 also facilitates LRP6 phosphorylation by CDK14/CCNY during G2/M stage of the cell cycle, which may potentiate cells for transport or translation of mRNAs, modulate the expression of neuronal proteins involved in synaptic plasticity [28], while simultaneously influencing cell cycle signaling and regulation of viral transcription and replication [29, 30].

Alignments

polyprotein [Human poliovirus 1]

Sequence ID: **ACZ05040.1** Length: 2209 Number of Matches: 1

Range 1: 1994 to 2070

Score	Expect	Method	Identities	Positives	Gaps	Frame
30.4 bits(67)	1.7()	Compositional matrix adjust.	22/77(29%)	32/77(41%)	19/77(24%)	

Features:

```
Query  136   IEKKKLKLE--------DYKDRLKSGEHLNPDQLEAVEK-----------YEEVLHNLEF  176
              E  KL LE        DY D L    HL  +++  V+            +  +++NL
Sbjct  1994  FEALKLVLEKIGFGDRVDYIDYLNHSHHLYKNKIYCVKGGMPSGCSGTSIFNSMINNLII  2053

Query  177   AKELQKTFSGLSLDLLK  193
                 L KT+ G+ LD LK
Sbjct  2054  RTLLLKTYKGIDLDHLK  2070
```

Figure 14. BLAST output of polyprotein of poliovirus showing similarity to human protein caprin-2.

1.2.8. *Mycobacterium leprae peptide similarity to 2′, 3′-cyclic-nucleotide 3′-phosphodiesterase*

2′, 3′-cyclic-nucleotide 3′-phosphodiesterase UniProtKB-P09543 (CN37_HUMAN) is a protein of molecular mass 47,579 Da. 2′, 3′-cyclic-nucleotide 3′-phosphodiesterase (sequence ID: WP_010908292.1 AA position 191–261) has a similarity to thiamin pyrophosphokinase of *M. leprae* UniProtKB A0A197SEI9 (A0A197SEI9_MYCLR) (AA position: 170–2166) (**Figure 16**) 2′, 3′-cyclic-nucleotide 3′-phosphodiesterase is involved in RNA metabolism of the myelinating cell, CN37 (2′, 3′-cyclic-nucleotide 3′-phosphodiesterase) is the one of the most abundant myelin protein in nervous system. The sequence similarities identified could impact cell signaling and also regulate energy metabolism [31].

Alignments

phosphoprotein, partial [Rabies lyssavirus]

Sequence ID: **AAO60615.1** Length: 116 Number of Matches: 1

Range 1: 76 to 110

Score	Expect	Method	Identities	Positives	Gaps	Frame
29.3 bits(64)	1.4()	Compositional matrix adjust.	14/42(33%)	25/42(59%)	7/42(16%)	

Features:

```
Query  13   ELTSVEKSLREWSRLSREVIAWLCPSSPNFILNFPPPPSASS  54
            ++ S E+ L+ WS+   E+I+++       ++NFP PP  SS
Sbjct  76   QMRSGERFLKIWSQTVEEIISYV-------MVNFPNPPGRSS  110
```

Figure 15. BLAST output of phosphoprotein of rabies virus showing similarity to human protein caprin-2.

thiamin pyrophosphokinase [Mycobacterium leprae]

Sequence ID: **WP_010908292.1** Length: 393 Number of Matches: 1

See 5 more title(s)
Range 1: 191 to 261

Score	Expect	Method	Identities	Positives	Gaps	Frame
28.5 bits(62)	0.70()	Compositional matrix adjust.	24/75(32%)	33/75(44%)	17/75(22%)	

Features:

```
Query  170  SADDLKKLKPGLEKDFLPLYFGWFLTKKSSETLRKAG-----------QVFLEEL--GNH  216
            +ADDLK LKP + K++ P+  G        ++LRKAG           Q+  E L  G H
Sbjct  191  AADDLKSLKPFI-KEYQPVLVG---VSGGADVLRKAGYRPQLIVGDPEQISTEALRCGAH  246

Query  217  KAFKKELRQFVPGDE  231
                 +     PG E
Sbjct  247  VVLPADADGHAPGLE  261
```

Figure 16. BLAST output of thiamin pyrophosphate of *Mycobacterium leprae* showing similarity to human protein 2′, 3′-cyclic-nucleotide 3′-phosphodiesterase.

1.2.9. Zika virus peptide similarity to human protein galanin

Galanin peptide UniProtKB-P22466 (GALA_HUMAN) is a protein of molecular mass 13,302 Da. Galanin (AA position 53–99 position) has a similarity to polyprotein envelope protein E of Zika virus UniProtKB-Q73880 (Q73880_9HIV1) sequence ID: ARB07952.1 (AA position: 729–765) (**Figure 17**). Galanin is involved in the smooth muscle contraction of the gastrointestinal and genitourinary tract, regulation of growth hormone release, modulation of insulin release, and might also be involved in the control of adrenal secretion [32]. The envelope protein E of the Zika virus is responsible for binding to host cell surface receptors and mediating fusion between viral and cellular membranes. It is synthesized in the endoplasmic

Alignments

polyprotein, partial [Zika virus]
Sequence ID: **ARB07952.1** Length: 1939 Number of Matches: 1
Range 1: 729 to 765

Score	Expect	Method	Identities	Positives	Gaps	Frame
24.3 bits(51)	2.2()	Compositional matrix adjust.	14/47(30%)	23/47(48%)	10/47(21%)	

Features:

```
Query  53   SFSDKNGLTSKRELRPEDDMKPGSFDRSIPENNIMRTIIEFLSFLHL  99
            SF  K+G     E+RP          R  PE+N++R+++   S  H+
Sbjct  729  SFRAKDGCWYGMEIRP----------RKEPESNLVRSVVTAGSTDHM  765
```

Figure 17. BLAST output of polyprotein of Zika virus showing similarity to human Galanin peptide.

reticulum with protein prM and forms a heterodimer. Galanin's similarity with the ZIKA polypeptide could subsequently affect neural regulation of muscle function and play a role in immune evasion pathogenesis and viral replication [33].

1.2.10. HIV 1 peptide similarity to human kinesin-like protein

Kinesin-like protein KIFC1 UniProtKB-Q9BW19 (KIFC1_HUMAN) is a protein of molecular mass 73,748 Da. Kinesin-like protein (AA position: 411–470) has a similarity to HIV virus envelope glycoprotein UniProtKB-D6QPK9 (D6QPK9_9HIV1) sequence ID:ADG63850.1 (AA position:270–387)(**Figure 18**). KIFC1 along with microtubules contributes to movement of endocytic vesicles. These similarities could affect viral attachment to the host cell, membrane fusion, and entry into the cell and the nucleus [34, 35].

1.2.11. Corona virus peptide similarity to human neurofilament heavy polypeptide

Neurofilament heavy polypeptide UniProtKB-P12036 (NFH_HUMAN) is a protein of molecular mass 112,479 Da. Neurofilament heavy polypeptide (AA position: 819–872) has a similarity to ORF1a UniProtKB-A0A0F6SKM6 (A0A0F6SKM6_9GAMC) of Corona virus sequence ID: AKF17723.1 (AA positions: 890 –1031) (**Figure 19**) neurofilament of the nerve tissue usually contain three intermediate filament proteins: L, M, and H (NFH-human) which is involved in the maintenance of neuronal caliber. NFH-H has an important function in axon maturation. These similarities could affect viral replication, protein processing, and could generate autoantibody production [36, 37].

1.2.12. HHV 1 and HHV 2 peptide similarity to human protein neurogranin

Neurogranin UniProtKB-Q92686 (NEUG_HUMAN) is a protein of molecular mass 7618 Da. The structure of neurogranin at identical regions has a similarity to envelope glycoprotein M of

Alignments

envelope glycoprotein, partial [Human immunodeficiency virus 1]

Sequence ID: **ADG63850.1** Length: 414 Number of Matches: 1
Range 1: 270 to 387

Score	Expect	Method	Identities	Positives	Gaps	Frame
36.2 bits(82)	0.90()	Compositional matrix adjust.	35/145(24%)	55/145(37%)	39/145(26%)	

Features:

```
Query  411  QTGSGKTFTMEGGPGGDPQLEGLIPRALRHLFSVAQELSGQGWTYSFVASYVEIYNETVR  470
            Q G+ KT  +    GGDP++       +RH F+   E         F  +  +++N T +
Sbjct  270  QFGNNKTIIFKQSSGGDPEI-------VRHSFNCGGEF--------FYCNTSQLFNSTWK  314

Query  471  DLLATGTRKGQGGE-------CEIRRAGPGSEELTVTNARYVP-----VSCEKEVDALLH  518
            +    GT  G  G        C I++     +E  V  A Y P     +SC   +  LL
Sbjct  315  N--NNGTWNGTAGSNNTITLPCRIKQIINMWQE--VGKAMYAPPISGNISCSSNITGLL-  369

Query  519  LARQNRAVARTAQNERSSRSHSVFQ  543
                   + R   N+ SS     F+
Sbjct  370  -------LTRDGGNDNSSNGTETFR  387
```

Figure 18. BLAST output of envelope glycoprotein of HIV 1 showing similarity to human kinesin-like protein.

http://dx.doi.org/10.5772/intechopen.71011

Alignments

ORF1a [Duck coronavirus]
Sequence ID: **AKF17723.1** Length: 3981 Number of Matches: 18
Range 1: 890 to 1031

Score	Expect	Method	Identities	Positives	Gaps	Frame
79.3 bits(194)	2e-14()	Composition-based stats.	58/155(37%)	78/155(50%)	26/155(16%)	

Features:

```
Query  819   EIPKKEEVKSPVKEEEKPQEVKVKEP------PKKAEEEKAPATPKTEEKKDSKKEEAPK  872
             E PK+E  K    EE+KP+E  V+ P      P+K EE+K   TP           E PK
Sbjct  890   ETPKEETQKPQKVEEQKPKETPVETPKEETQKPQKVEEQKPKETPV----------ETPK  939

Query  873   KEAPKP-KVEEK--KEPAVEKPKESKVEAKKEEAEDKKKVP--TPEKEA--PAKVEVKED  925
             +E  KP KVEE+  KE  VE PKE   + +K E +  K+ P  TP++E   P KV   E+
Sbjct  940   EEIQKPQKVEEQKPKETPVETPKEETQKPQKVEEQKPKETPVETPKEETQKPQKV---EE  996

Query  926   AKPKEKTEVAKKEPDDAKAKEPSKPAEKKEAAPEK  960
              KPKE     +  PD +   EP K + + +  P K
Sbjct  997   RKPKETLLNKQFLPDSSSDDEPRKKSFRFKLKPTK  1031
```

Figure 19. BLAST output of ORF1 of corona virus showing similarity to human neurofilament heavy polypeptide.

HHV1 and envelope glycoprotein M of HHV2 at partially overlapping positions. Neurogranin (AA position: 38–63) has a similarity to the envelope glycoprotein M of HHV1(UniProtKB-A0A181ZHE7 (A0A181ZHE7_HHV11) (sequence ID: SBO07578.1 AA position: 347–376) (**Figure 20**). Neurogranin (AA position: 38–64) also has a similarity to the envelope glycoprotein M of HHV2 (UniProtKB-A0A0Y0R357 (A0A0Y0R357_HHV2)) (sequence ID: AMB66044.1 AA position 389–416) (**Figure 21**). Neurogranin functions as a signaling messenger, a substrate for protein kinase C and has affinity to calmodulin in the absence of calcium. These similarities

Alignments

Envelope glycoprotein M [Herpes simplex virus (type 1 / strain 17)]
Sequence ID: **SBO07578.1** Length: 455 Number of Matches: 1
Range 1: 347 to 376

Score	Expect	Method	Identities	Positives	Gaps	Frame
27.7 bits(60)	0.11()	Composition-based stats.	13/30(43%)	16/30(53%)	4/30(13%)	

Features:

```
Query  38    RGHMARKKIKSGERG----RKGPGPGGPGG  63
             R H A K+++S  RG    R  P PG P G
Sbjct  347   RAHSALKRVRSSMRGSRDGRHRPAPGSPPG  376
```

Figure 20. BLAST output of envelope glycoprotein of HHV 1 showing similarity to human protein neurogranin.

of HHV1 & 2 with neurogranin could have an interaction with viral transport into the host cell Golgi network and subsequently to the host nucleus [38].

1.2.13. JE 2 peptide similarity to human protein secretogranin-3

Secretogranin-3 UniProtKB-Q8WXD2 (SCG3_HUMAN) is a protein of molecular mass 53,005 Da. Secretogranin-3 (AA position: 139–190) has a similarity to the polyprotein of Japanese encephalitis virus (UniProtKB-G3LHD8 (G3LHD8_9FLAV) (sequence ID: SBO07578.1 AA position: 2744 to (**Figure 22**). Secretogranin-3 is a member of the chromogranin/secretogranin

Alignments

envelope glycoprotein M [Human alphaherpesvirus 2]
Sequence ID: **AMB66044.1** Length: 491 Number of Matches: 1
Range 1: 389 to 416

Score	Expect	Method	Identities	Positives	Gaps	Frame
29.3 bits(64)	0.024()	Composition-based stats.	13/28(46%)	18/28(64%)	1/28(3%)	

Features:

```
Query  38   RGHMARKKIKSGERG-RKGPGPGGPGGA  64
            R H A ++++S  RG R+G  PG PG A
Sbjct  389  RAHSALRRVRSSMRGSRRGGPPGDPGYA  416
```

Figure 21. BLAST output of envelope glycoprotein of human alpha herpes virus 2 showing similarity to human protein neurogranin.

Alignments

polyprotein [Japanese encephalitis virus]
Sequence ID: **AEO72439.1** Length: 3432 Number of Matches: 1
Range 1: 2744 to 2833

Score	Expect	Method	Identities	Positives	Gaps	Frame
29.3 bits(64)	0.77()	Composition-based stats.	21/90(23%)	45/90(50%)	9/90(10%)	

Features:

```
Query  139   HQLDGTPLTAEDIVHKI---AARIYEENDRAVF-DKIVSKLLNLG----LITESQAHTLE  190
             H++ G    A ++VH +    +  +    DR V+       + +NLG     + + + H+ +
Sbjct  2744  HEMYGVSGAAGNVVHAVNMTSQVLLGRMDRTVWRGPKYEEDVNLGSGTRAVGKGEVHSNQ  2803

Query  191   DEVAEVLQKLISKEANNYEEDPNKP-TSWT  219
             +++ + +QKL  + A  + +DP  P  +WT
Sbjct  2804  EKIKKRIQKLKEEFATTWHKDPEHPYRTWT  2833
```

Figure 22. BLAST output of polyprotein of JE 2 showing similarity to human protein secretogranin-3.

family of neuroendocrine secretory proteins comprising a number of significant cellular functions. In an experimental mouse model, autoimmunity with secretogranin was associated with encephalitis [39]. These similarities identified in the host-pathogen could affect neuro endocrine secretory protein release and autoimmunity.

2. Creating a schematic model

The sequence similarities in agrin,caprin-2,2′,3′-cyclic-nucleotide 3′-phosphodiesterase, galanin peptide, kinesin-like protein, neurofilament heavy polypeptide, neurogranin and secretogranin-3 with its corresponding pathogenic peptide/s could have a number of cellular-level implications which include alternations in receptor binding, signaling/synaptic transmission, metabolic alteration, inflammation, resulting in autoimmunity and consequently neuropathy (**Figure 23**) [11, 40].

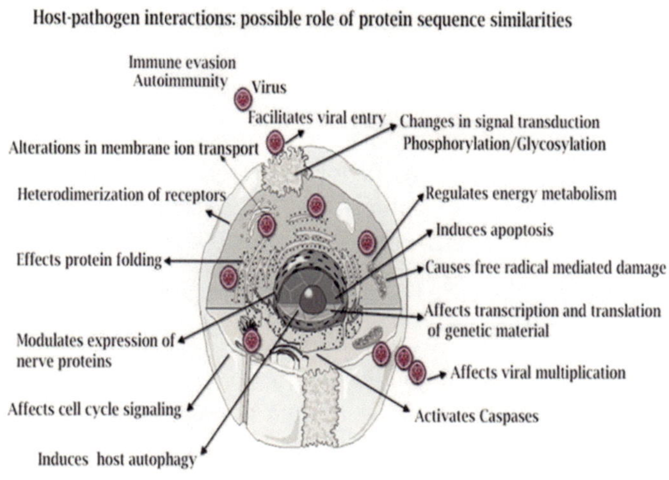

Figure 23. A model for the modes of host-pathogen interaction and possible intracellular regulation of metabolic activities.

3. Conclusion

In conclusion, it is important to conduct bioinformatic searches and design wet experiments with the objective of identifying a vast number of functionally significant peptides for further comparison and study. Bioinformatic search tools and various available databases are to be extensively explored to rapidly develop possible neuroprotective or pathogenic peptide sequences. These peptides can be further explored as targets to generate recombinant antibodies. This exercise can also be used to develop an efficacious and safe vaccine against pathogens that demonstrate no autoimmune cross-reactions. It can also contribute to design peptide/drug molecules to neutralize the effects of neurotoxins. Bioinformatics is the key to open the door of understanding medical and biological processes in the future.

Acknowledgements

We acknowledge short-term project works of Do Eon Lee of York University, 700 Keele St, Toronto, ON M3 J 1P3, Canada and Logeshwaran Vasudevan of Bharathidasan University, Palkalaiperur, Tiruchirappalli, Tamil Nadu 620024, and Dr Sharon Bushi of Morristown Med CtrIntnlMedcn, 100 Madison Ave, Morristown, NJ 07960 on the preliminary work of nerve protein pathogen similarity searches.

Author details

Lavanya Suneetha*, Prasanna Marsakatla, Rachel Supriya Suneetha and Sujai Suneetha

*Address all correspondence to: drlavanyasuneetha@gmail.com

Infectious Disease Research Laboratory, Nireekshana ACET, Hyderabad, India

References

[1] Pardy RD, Rajah MM, Condotta SA, Taylor NG, Sagan SM, Richer MJ. Analysis of the T cell response to Zika virus and identification of a novel CD8+ T cell epitope in immunocompetent mice. PLoS Pathogens. Feb 2017;**13**(2):e1006184

[2] Iversen T-G, Skotland T, Sandvig K. Endocytosis and intracellular transport of nanoparticles: Present knowledge and need for future studies. Nano Today. 2011;**6**(2):176-185

[3] Bullman S, Meyerson M, Kostic AD. Emerging concepts and Technologies for the discovery of microorganisms involved in human disease. Annual Review of Pathology: Mechanisms of Disease. Jan 2017;**12**(1):217-244

[4] Luscombe NM, Greenbaum D, Gerstein M. What is bioinformatics? A proposed definition and overview of the field. Methods of Information in Medicine. 2001;**40**(4):346-358

[5] Wilson MR, Zha L, Balskus EP. Natural product discovery from the human microbiome, Journal of Biological Chemistry. May 26 2017;**292**(21):8546-8552. DOI: 10.1074/jbc.R116.762906. Epub 2017 Apr 7

[6] McManus RM, Heneka MT. Role of neuroinflammation in neurodegeneration: New insights. Alzheimer's Research & Therapy. Mar 2017;**9**(1):14

[7] Martinez-Martin N. Technologies for proteome-wide discovery of extracellular host-pathogen interactions. Journal of Immunology Research. 2017;**2017**:1-18

[8] Stanfield BA, Luftig MA. Recent advances in understanding Epstein-Barr virus. F1000 Research. Mar 2017;**6**:386

[9] Briken V. Molecular mechanisms of host-pathogen interactions and their potential for the discovery of new drug targets. Current Drug Targets. Feb 2008;**9**(2):150-157

[10] Barel M, Charbit A. Role of glycosylation/deglycolysation processes in *Francisella tularensis* pathogenesis. Frontiers in Cellular and Infection Microbiology. Mar 2017;**7**:71

[11] Yu X, Decker KB, Barker K, Neunuebel MR, Saul J, Graves M, Westcott N, Hang H, LaBaer J, Qiu J, Machner MP. Host–pathogen interaction profiling using self-assembling human protein arrays. Journal of Proteome Research. Apr. 2015;**14**(4):1920-1936

[12] Gutlapalli VR, Sykam A, Nayarisseri A, Suneetha S, Suneetha LM. Insights from the predicted epitope similarity between mycobacterium tuberculosis virulent factors and its human homologs. Bioinformation. Dec 2015;**11**(12):517-524

[13] Suneetha LM, Singh SS, Vani M, Vardhini D, Scollard D, Archelos JJ, Srinivasulu M, Suneetha S. *Mycobacterium leprae* binds to a major human peripheral nerve glycoprotein myelin P zero (P0). Neurochemical Research. Sep 2003;**28**(9):1393-1399

[14] Su MA, Davini D, Cheng P, Giang K, Fan U, DeVoss JJ, Johannes KPA, Taylor L, Shum AK, Valenzise M, Meloni A, Bour-Jordan H, Anderson MS. Defective autoimmune regulator-dependent central tolerance to myelin protein zero is linked to autoimmune peripheral neuropathy. Journal of Immunology. May 2012;**188**(10):4906-4912

[15] Raju R, Devi SK, Mehervani C, Kumar AS, Meena AK, Reddy PP, Pranay P, Jain S, Archelos-Gracia JJ, Suneetha S, Suneetha LM. Antibodies to myelin P0 and ceramide perpetuate neuropathy in long standing treated leprosy patients. Neurochemical Research. May 2011;**36**(5):766-773

[16] Vardhini D, Suneetha S, Ahmed N, Joshi DSM, Karuna S, Magee X, Vijayalakshmi DSR, Sridhar V, Karunakar KV, Archelos JJ, Suneetha LM. Comparative proteomics of the *Mycobacterium leprae* binding protein myelin P0: Its implication in leprosy and other neurodegenerative diseases. Infection, Genetics and Evolution. Mar 2004;**4**(1):21-28

[17] Rigden DJ, Fer Andez-Sú Arez XM, Galperin MY. The 2016 database issue of nucleic acids research and an updated molecular biology database collection, Nucleic Acids Research, 2016;**44**

[18] Alpi E, Griss J, da Silva AWS, Bely B, Antunes R, Zellner H, Ríos D, O'Donovan C, Vizcaíno JA, Martin MJ. Analysis of the tryptic search space in UniProt databases. Proteomics, Jan 2015;**15**(1):48-57

[19] Boutet E, Lieberherr D, Tognolli M, Schneider M, Bansal P, Bridge AJ, Poux S, Bougueleret L, Xenarios I. UniProtKB/Swiss-Prot, the manually annotated section of the UniProt KnowledgeBase: How to use the entry view. Methods in molecular biology (Clifton, N.J.). 2016;**1374**:23-54

[20] Foulger RE, Osumi-Sutherland D, McIntosh BK, Hulo C, Masson P, Poux S, Le Mercier P, Lomax J. Representing virus-host interactions and other multi-organism processes in the gene ontology. BMC Microbiology. Jul. 2015;**15**:146

[21] Altschul SF, Madden TL, Schäffer AA, Zhang J, Zhang Z, Miller W, Lipman DJ. Gapped BLAST and PSI-BLAST: A new generation of protein database search programs. Nucleic Acids Research. Sep 1997;**25**(17):3389-3402

[22] Zhang W, Coldefy A-S, Hubbard SR, Burden SJ. Agrin binds to the N-terminal region of Lrp4 protein and stimulates association between Lrp4 and the first immunoglobulin-like domain in muscle-specific kinase (MuSK), The Journal of Biological Chemistry. Nov 2011;**286**(47):40624-40630

[23] Kröger S, Pfister H. Agrin in the nervous system: Synaptogenesis and beyond. Future Neurology. Jan 2009;**4**(1):67-86

[24] Alfsen A, Yu H, Magérus-Chatinet A, Schmitt A, Bomsel M. HIV-1-infected blood mononuclear cells form an integrin- and agrin-dependent viral synapse to induce efficient HIV-1 transcytosis across epithelial cell monolayer. Molecular Biology of the Cell. Sep 2005;**16**(9):4267-4279

[25] Kenyon TK, Cohen JI, Grose C. Phosphorylation by the varicella-zoster virus ORF47 protein serine kinase determines whether endocytosed viral gE traffics to the trans-Golgi network or recycles to the cell membrane. Journal of Virology. Nov 2002;**76**(21):10980-10993

[26] Zerboni L, Sen N, Oliver SL, Arvin AM. Molecular mechanisms of varicella zoster virus pathogenesis. Nature Reviews Microbiology. Mar 2014;**12**(3):197-210

[27] Ding Y, Xi Y, Chen T, Wang J, Tao D, Wu Z-L, Li Y, Li C, Zeng R, Li L. Caprin-2 enhances canonical Wnt signaling through regulating LRP5/6 phosphorylation. The Journal of Cell Biology. Sep 2008;**182**(5):865-872

[28] Wang X, Jia Y, Fei C, Song X, Li L. Activation/proliferation-associated protein 2 (Caprin-2) positively regulates CDK14/Cyclin Y-mediated lipoprotein receptor-related protein 5 and 6 (LRP5/6) constitutive phosphorylation., The Journal of Biological Chemistry. Dec 2016;**291**(51):26427-26434

[29] Ono EAD, Taniwaki SA, Brandão P. Short interfering RNAs targeting a vampire-bat related rabies virus phosphoprotein mRNA. Brazilian Journal of Microbiology. Jul - Sep 2017;**48**(3):566-569. DOI: 10.1016/j.bjm.2016.11.007. Epub 2017 Feb 5

[30] Kammouni W, Wood H, Jackson AC. Serine residues at positions 162 and 166 of the rabies virus phosphoprotein are critical for the induction of oxidative stress in rabies virus infection. Journal of Neurovirology. Jun 2017;**23**(3):358-368. DOI: 10.1007/s13365-016-0506-8. Epub 2016 Dec 19

[31] Teles RMB, Krutzik SR, Ochoa MT, Oliveira RB, Sarno EN, Modlin RL. Interleukin-4 regulates the expression of CD209 and subsequent uptake of *Mycobacterium leprae* by Schwann cells in human leprosy. Infection and Immunity. Nov 2010;**78**(11):4634-4643

[32] Bersani M, Johnsen AH, Højrup P, Dunning BE, Andreasen JJ, Holst JJ. Human galanin: Primary structure and identification of two molecular forms. FEBS Letters. Jun 1991;**283**(2): 189-194

[33] Routhu NK, Byrareddy SN. Host-virus interaction of ZIKA virus in modulating disease pathogenesis. Journal of Neuroimmune Pharmacology. Jun 2017;**12**(2):219-232. DOI: 10.1007/s11481-017-9736-7. Epub 2017 Mar 27